Morphogenesis and Human Flourishing

Social Morphogenesis

Series Editor:

MARGARET S. ARCHER
Centre for Social Ontology, University of Warwick, Coventry, UK

Aims and scope:

To focus upon 'social morphogenesis' as a general process of change is very different from examining its particular results over the last quarter of a century. This series ventures what the generative mechanisms are that produce such intense change and discusses how this differs from late modernity. Contributors examine if an intensification of morphogenesis (positive feedback that results in a change in social form) and a corresponding reduction in morphostasis (negative feedback that restores or reproduces the form of the social order) best captures the process involved.

The series consists of 5 volumes derived from the Centre for Social Ontology's annual workshops "From Modernity to Morphogenesis" at the University of Lausanne, headed by Margaret Archer.

More information about this series at http://www.springer.com/series/11959

Margaret S. Archer
Editor

Morphogenesis and Human Flourishing

Springer

Editor
Margaret S. Archer
Centre for Social Ontology
Department of Sociology
University of Warwick
Coventry, UK

This volume V follows the book "Social Morphogenesis", edited by Margaret S. Archer, which was the first book in the series published in 2013 http://wwww.springer.com/social+sciences/book/978-94-007-6127-8, the volume "Late Modernity", edited by Margaret S. Archer, published in 2014, the volume "Generative Mechanisms Transforming the Social Order", edited by Margaret S. Archer, published in 2015 and the volume "Morphogenesis and the Crisis of Normativity", edited by Margaret S. Archer, published in 2016.

ISSN 2198-1604 ISSN 2198-1612 (electronic)
Social Morphogenesis
ISBN 978-3-319-49468-5 ISBN 978-3-319-49469-2 (eBook)
DOI 10.1007/978-3-319-49469-2

Library of Congress Control Number: 2017934071

Printed on acid-free paper

This Springer imprint is published by Springer Nature
The registered company is Springer International Publishing AG
The registered company address is: Gewerbestrasse 11, 6330 Cham, Switzerland

Acknowledgement to the Independent Social Research Foundation

With grateful thanks from all contributors to our book series on 'Social Morphogenesis' for the funding and support that we have received from the ISRF for over 6 years.

Without this help, we could not have met in different European cities for the first week in January every year, enjoyed our exchanges immensely and managed to produce a book a year:

Archer, Margaret S. (Ed.), 2013, Vol 1, *Social Morphogenesis,* Dordrecht, Springer.

Archer, Margaret S. (Ed.), 2014, Vol 2, *Late Modernity: Trajectories Towards Morphogenic Society,* Dordrecht, Springer.

Archer, Margaret S., (Ed), 2015, Vol 3, *Generative Mechanisms Transforming the Social Order*, Dordrecht, Springer.

Archer, Margaret S., (Ed.), 2016, Vol. 4, *Morphogenesis and the Crisis of Normativity,* Dordrecht, Springer.

Archer, Margaret S., (Ed.), 2017, Vol. 5, *Morphogenesis and Human Flourishing,* Dordrecht, Springer.

Thank you from us all for supporting our independent research and the foundation of the Centre for Social Ontology.

Contents

Chapter 1
Introduction: Has a Morphogenic Society Arrived?

Margaret S. Archer

Preface

This is the last of five books in the series on 'Social Morphogenesis'. So far we have explored the intensification of morphogenetic processes on a global scale from the 1980s onwards, but have refrained from claiming that these announce transition towards a new social formation replacing late modernity – the world-wide Morphogenic Society. The time has come to remove this question mark, if not definitively. Since the social sciences can rarely be predictive, because of the intrinsic openness of the social order, the interplay of multiple generative mechanisms and the constant intervention of unforeseen contingencies, the most we have offered in the previous four volumes are evaluations of whether or not there are marked tendencies consistent with the eventual emergence of a Morphogenic Society. Nevertheless, it could coherently be maintained that there are a multiplicity of social orders, ones which could now qualify as being 'morphogenic' and thus display as much variation as the multiple forms of modernity have done to date.

For those readers who have not followed the five Volumes as they have appeared annually, it is reasonable for them to ask: 'So what is the difference between Morphogenesis and Morphogenetic Society?' The Morphogenetic/Morphostatic framework (M/M) was developed (Archer 2013a [1979], 1995) as an explanatory framework; a means for analytically breaking up the processes – that always occur over time – into tractable phases in order to explain their outcomes in relation to some change or continued stability of a social feature that is problematic to the researcher(s) in question. The M/M framework is not a theory; in itself it explains nothing, any more than does the Critical Realist ontology upon which it is based

M.S. Archer (✉)
Centre for Social Ontology, Department of Sociology, University of Warwick, Coventry, CV4 7AL, UK
e-mail: margaret.archer@warwick.ac.uk

M.S. Archer (ed.), *Morphogenesis and Human Flourishing*, Social Morphogenesis,
DOI 10.1007/978-3-319-49469-2_1

(Porpora 2013, Vol 1, p. 26). To recapitulate, what we have been examining over the last six years is indeed a theoretical question; namely, are we globally moving towards a social formation that could justifiably be termed a Morphogenic Society? First and foremost, this would mean a world in which *morphogenetic processes increasingly predominated over morphostatic ones in terms of their outcomes*. The new reader's likely response is a good one; 'How is one to say and on what basis?'

In earlier epochs, it would have been easier to point to the fact that transformatory mechanisms were exogenous rather than endogenous, that is reliant upon conquest, colonization or climatic disasters. With globalization, it is much more difficult because our one world nullifies the endogamous/exogenous distinction. What happens in one part is affected by what happens in other parts, even though it is undoubtedly the case that one may benefit at the expense of the other(s). Moreover, some may rightly wish to point out that morphogenesis has been with the social order forever. They would be correct because without it there would have been no change at all, apart from those exogenously induced or introduced Thus, to answer our new reader's hypothetical question, it is necessary to engage in some recapitulation about the theoretical propositions developed and assessed throughout the series. Only then will it be possible to appreciate how well the thesis stands up to scrutiny and where the present discussion of Eudaimonia stands in relation to the theory as a whole.

Summary Characteristics of Morphogenic Society

No Morphogenic social formation has yet been realized that accords with the Concrete Utopia and the conditions propitious to its emergence are stringent, though for the first time in history their realization is conceivable. For the sake of clarity it seems useful to re-emphasize the distinction between the process of morphogenesis and the defining characteristics of a Morphogenic social formation. Morphogenesis has always been with us, despite being a slow process historically because usually swamped by morphostatic mechanisms. Otherwise, there would be no trajectories of change to trace from early societies onwards and no need for the M/M approach. The M/M mode of analysis *is not a theory*, it merely proffers an explanatory framework or analytical toolkit intended to assist theorists to sort out the plethora of data that surrounds every problem about why there is change or its absence at any level of the social from the micro- to the macroscopic. Conversely, the potential advent of Morphogenic society, with its origins in the late twentieth century is a theory, but what it theorises is a possibility and not the inevitability of social 'progress'. To advance it draws upon the transcendental argument of Critical Realism (Bhaskar 1979) by asking what needs to be the case for global Morphogenic society to become instantiated for the first time. What follows is the sketchiest summary of the required characteristics, ones that have been spelt out in the four previous volumes. It goes without saying that the conditions upon which the realization of these characteristics depend may be found not to obtain – at least yet.

1. Morphogenetic processes increasingly predominate over morphostatic ones. In other words, positive feedback exceeds negative feedback, meaning that 'change' prevails over mechanisms restoring 'stasis' (Buckley 1967); it also often entails 'morphonecrosis', i.e. the extinction of certain social forms (Al-Amoudi and Latsis, Vol 3 2015) The term *morphogenesis bound* refers to circumstances in which it is restrained by morphostatic pressures, whereas *morphogenesis unbound* is free from such restraints.
2. A great leap forward takes place in late modernity; one based upon 'variety fosters greater variety', in ideas, techniques, skills, products and life-styles. As morphogenetic change gathers in momentum and penetration, there is a shift away from the Competitive situational logic typical of modernity, with its zero-sum production of winners and losers in almost every field. Instead, a new situational logic of Opportunity engages based upon the option of generating further novel variety through innovative syntheses.
3. This tendency intensifies dramatically when Structure and Culture[1] both become morphogenetic and enter into synergy with the other, rather than reinforcing one another's morphostatic consequences or the lag of one constituting a drag upon the other. Synergy grows because the pool of 'complementary compatibilities' is enlarged as novel items are added to the structural and cultural domains. As the 'variety' of new items increases, so does the probability of 'pairs' being complementary – although not in any fixed proportion – which commends their joint exploration and induces new changes.
4. When Morphogenesis becomes predominant, shared Normativity can no longer serve as a basis for social order. Laws, rules, norms and conventions become increasingly disparate and often divisively contested. Consequently, social integration plummets. In response to the normative crisis, resort is increasingly made to anormative forms of regulation, to reinforcing a 'Macro-Moral Disconnect', to confining religious beliefs to the private domain and to expelling morality from public life. Behavioural regulation prevails over the encouragement of cooperation or redistributive measures.
5. The 'new' is not automatically commensurate with the 'good'. Some forms of synergy are predominantly beneficent, such as the systematic use of pain-killers in palliative medicine; others are the reverse, for example, digital crime and the Dark Net. What needs to be the case for a Morphogenic social formation to promote human flourishing or Eudaimonia and promote the Common Good?

Baldly, the first four propositions constitute the backbone of the thesis and are open to empirical substantiation but also to both substantive and theoretical contestation. What follows is akin to a brief Executive Summary on each point in turn, including reservations and elaborations. It would be improbable to imagine, given twelve distinguished authors collaborating over six years that all of the following would be whole-heartedly endorsed by everyone, but no sociological enterprise makes a

[1]Structure and Culture are viewed by me as different entities with their own distinctive properties and powers and thus cannot be elided (Archer 1988) as they are by Porpora in his new book (2015).

contribution on the basis of complete unanimity. Summarizing our discussions on the first four theses serves as a broad *résumé* of the previous Volumes published in the Series and takes the form of answers given to hypothetical questions raised by new readers. This section identifies the main processes that we have learned are crucial in prolonging the struggle over transformation and are responsible for delaying transition to a new social formation, perhaps indefinitely.

The next section specifically considers Eudaimonia (in relation to proposition 5). Any future increase in the scope and intensity of morphogenetic change comes with no guarantee that it will augment the human well-being or flourishing of all. Thus, if and when it is asserted that a Morphogenic global society has the potential for increasing human thriving, we should treat this statement cautiously. Objective and confirmatory indices in the third-person do not suffice and neither does any hype attached to 'opportunity' and 'novelty'. For us and fellow members of humanity, our thriving turns upon first-person acknowledgement that our social circumstances are conducive to what we care about (or recognition that our changing social context has generated new concerns that matter to us). This necessarily entails working in terms of both objectivism and subjectivism because we are strong evaluators and the process of reflexivity by which we deliberate about our social context in relation to ourselves and vice versa is the root cause of the courses of action we adopt, i.e. it is the ultimate source of the social order being activity-dependent.

1. Morphogenetic processes increasingly predominate over morphostatic ones

   QUESTION: *How is this proposition substantiated?*

This is reasonable to ask, given that inveterate problems attach to any empiricist metrics of social change. Such metrics will necessarily be incomplete because the causes of change may have engaged without yet producing their outcomes (e.g. the distribution of diseases); social changes are incommensurables precluding their comparison or weighting (e.g. in Europe, more people came online in the last 30 years and less got married, but empirically we cannot say which was the bigger change); social change often involves displacement (from Radio listening to watching TV to PC streaming), but we cannot use a 'rate of displacement' to measure change because of the deliberate obsolescence of many new products.

The majority of theorists, originating from informatics/cybernetics who ventured to replace a metrics of social change by a societal increase in *variety* were objectivists, individualists, and dismissive of social relationality because the definition of *variety* rested upon atomism and aggregation that make for scientistic empiricism.[2]

Objectivism was marked in Ross Ashby's introduction of the term 'variety' itself from information theory where its quantity could always be enumerated. In his

[2]Nonetheless, it is worth a side glance at the post-Second World War development of cyberneticians because, to their credit, these were among the theorists who broke through the futile but prolonged divide among social scientists between materialism and idealism as to which was the motor of social change by simply brushing it aside. (these comments are found in more detail in Archer 2013b, Chap. 8.)

definition, variety is represented by how many distinct 'elements' were contained in a given set, that is the number of subsets with different 'identities' and the recognition that this was increasing over time, with the growth in 'differences' (Ashby 1956:124–5). Thus, variety was an objective, atomistic and aggregate concept in which the *social distribution of these 'elements'* played no part. This was of obvious concern to social theorists brought up on Durkheimian anxiety that the generation of 'differences' served to reduce social integration, unless restorative policy interventions were undertaken. The objectivist response that when or once a given new element of variety exceeded a distribution of 50%, then its further diffusion generated similarities (such as the spread of literacy or television), simply did not solve the 'problem of integration'. Crucially, this is because there is no guarantee that the two processes generating differences and their diffusion as similarities would keep up with one another overall.

The connection between the objective and measurable definition of variety, produced by increased positive feedback was developed by Maruyama into a formula for maximizing social change based upon the growth of heterogeneity amongst a population. In short, the more heterogeneous any population became in terms of the distribution of non-overlapping elements of variety, the greater the synergy and the creation of new information (2003 p. 618).

This preoccupation with the spread of *differences* and disregard for *similarities* between people clearly indicates the individualism of this approach because the acme of heterogeneity would be when every last person was differentiated from every other by their unique combination of 'elements'. What would bond them were no longer things they shared ('identities' as Ashby had put it) but the existence of those sufficiently different from them to whom they were attracted for the sole purpose of transacting in synergy with them. Not only was this a peon of praise to individualism but also a social policy to promote it. 'Heterogenistics', as Maruyama named it, would network marriages of symbiotic convenience for those who had failed to locate their own 'trading partners'. Not only does this approach nullify human relations, but it is clearly antipathetic to emergent relational goods, of which the earliest to be recognized sociologically was social integration. Relations are never considered as the generators of emergent 'relational goods', unobtainable in any other manner, such as trust, caring and reciprocity (Donati and Archer 2015).

In contradistinction, we have eschewed metrification throughout the Series and confined ourselves to qualitative assessments about whether there is more or less reproduction or transformation of the status quo (sectionally or societally) and likelihood of either diminishing or increasing. In other words, our analysis of social change is theory led in relation to our theoretical objective – but so we would argue is any other.

2. A great leap forward takes place in late modernity; one based upon 'variety fosters greater variety', in ideas, techniques, skills, products and life-styles.

   QUESTION: *Does this mean that everyone participates in this process and what happens to society if they do?*

Certain political scientists (Teune and Mlinar 1978), working on a theory of social development, explicitly introduced concepts dealing with the *distribution of variety* to produce *diversity* and its significance for *integration.* We can approach the hypothetical question above by asking if this approach comes closer to the conception of Morphogenic society, where both the possibilities of making and benefitting from new opportunities are open to all. Simultaneously, we ourselves can begin to query if this leap forward was towards the advent of a good society – characterized by both system and social integration – both of which are predicates of human flourishing.

The key points they make are their emphases on the 'distribution of variety' (producing diversity) and the difference between 'diversity' and 'differences'. *Undistributed* variety is where 'object properties' (home ownership or having a degree) are concentrated among one sub-set of some social entity – a city, country or the world – rather than being dispersed to some extent throughout them. Diversity (i.e. the extent of *distributed variety)* is thus the degree to which the sets of properties belonging to components of a set are not identical. Conversely, if differences alone differentiate between sets (let's say socio-economic groups) then two important distinctions follow for relations between sets: 'similarities and differences taken together are a structural condition for interdependence', whereas 'differences by themselves define cleavages or breaks in the structure of a social system' (Teune and Mlinar p. 35). This seems to have far-reaching consequences; Hofkirchner, heir of the Bertalanffy strand of systems thinking, has consistently emphasized throughout our volumes the importance of the former – 'Unity through Diversity' – for the emergence of the Good Society.

However, what becomes a matter of contention is when it is claimed that real relational properties between people that are not material in kind – ones crucially connected with their thriving – '*such as equality and hierarchy*, will change as a result of changes in the aggregative relational properties' (Teune and Mlinar, p. 54 my italics). In other words, it is the concentration of house ownership or the possession of a degree etc. that make for the upper class and not the other way around. Here Lazega in particular has repeatedly underlined in previous volumes how valued 'variety' can be 'hoarded', meaning access to it is controlled by those in a *prior position* to do so, meaning inequality and hegemony remain unchanged.

3. This tendency intensifies dramatically when Structure and Culture[3] each becomes morphogenetic and enters into synergy with the other

   QUESTION: *How does synergy come about and does everyone participate in it and benefit from it?*

Contrary to most commentators who identify a single 'factor' as the driver and then, as empiricists, seek to establish or persuade us that many other characteristics change because of their association with it, we work in terms of generative

[3] I have maintained that Structure and Culture are entities with distinctive properties and powers that must not be elided. Doug Porpora makes the same point in his new book (2015).

mechanisms that explain how it is that there are some such correlations at the level of events.[4] Basically, by refusing to elide Structure and Culture because of their distinctive and emergent properties and powers (the former being materially grounded and the latter ideationally grounded), it is possible to talk about 'contingent complementarities' developing between them. In other words, there are objective advantages in combining these new elements to produce further novel developments. Whether or not this does occur is, of course, dependent upon active agents who see this as being advantageous to their current vested interests. Thus, the concrete generative mechanisms that some of us advance are all conceptualized in terms of SAC, unlike ones based upon other social ontologies (e.g. that emanating from Analytical Sociology (Hedström and Swedberg 1998), which rejects Structure, Neo-Pragmatism (Neil Gross 2009) that reduces Agency to aggregates, or Mario Bunge (2004) who denies any independent role to Culture).

Our questioner may well persist and ask what those who detect potential benefits deriving from examining and exploiting a given 'contingent complementarity' actually do to reap them. Fundamentally, those in this position match the requirements of their current vested interests with the affordances of some relatively independent development and generate synergy by incorporating them (through recruiting some of their developers, purchasing their products and sometimes patents or establishing new research enterprises for their conjoint exploration and later exploitation). This was my own way of unpacking the Silicon Valley story (2014, 2015). Obviously, other generative mechanisms would be required to account for the origins of such symbiosis in different parts of the social order. However, 'working together', which is the root meaning of synergy, does not imply mutual respect or reciprocity between the parties concerned; instead, these are relations of instrumental convenience. Today, synergy works in such terms and thus means that some agents may distance themselves and pursue an entirely different and sometimes oppositional agenda (such as those digital pioneers who repudiated collaboration with multi-national capitalism in favour of free cultural diffusionism; Open Access and the Cultural Commons in various forms).

Nevertheless, considerable morphogenesis was the outcome in both cases; importantly the rapid growth of financialized capitalism and the unanticipated but even faster development of the social media. Did these advances imply a proportionate recession in morphostatic institutions, processes and practices? Certainly this is so if we think in overall SAC terms; of the demise of traditional social classes (S), of the displacement of routine and habitual action in response to the loss of 'contextual continuity' and its replacement by the Reflexive Imperative (A), or of the devaluation of traditional 'cultural capital' (C). But as Maccarini (2014) pertinently asked, 'Did nothing survive the fire?' Some things did, when associated with contrary vested interests, because this is not an automatic or mechanical relationship. Some groups typically fight on, and may enjoy resurgence (the aftermath of the

[4]Nevertheless, 'tendencies may be possessed and unexercised, exercised unrealized, and realized unperceived or undetected'.

'Arab Spring' or the release of xenophobia and racism, and defending national boarders in the face of mass migration). Some do become entirely self-defensive; forming what Maccarini (2015) termed 'enclaves'. And some survived, as Lawson (2016) showed for econometrics, through the convenience of their irrelevance to powerful capitalist interests, or could be built upon to capitalist advantage (2015) as in the fiction of the firm as a Legal Person.

In the above, it should be clear to our questioner that everyone in the global social world was affected by these morphogenetic surges and transformations but that far from everybody was a participant in these changes, let alone a beneficiary of them. To do or be so would imply that the groups in question (local, national or international) did have articulate and oppositional vested interests plus sufficient access to decision-making power to defend them.

4. When Morphogenesis becomes predominant shared Normativity can no longer serve as a basis for social order

   QUESTION: *Can't a new corpus of laws, rules and norms be developed that are compatible with Morphogenic society?*

In both early legal philosophy and sociology, *morphostasis* was held to be (or more accurately, presumed to be) the precondition of a harmonious relationship between legal validity and normative consensus. This was the case regardless of whether it was maintained that shared values underwrote social integration and stability or, rather, that social stability fostered normative consensus. Conversely and increasingly, morphogenesis (under whatever term it is known) was held to be problematic, if not positively hostile, to the establishment of a new normative corpus of laws, rules, norms or conventions given that it precludes stable and durable contexts to which they apply or in which they could develop. By the end of the last century, most legal normativists had conceded that the bindingness of legal provisions in the eyes of many addressees had become 'shaky' and less effective.

A principal reason for this growing 'shakiness' could be attributed directly to the intensification of morphogenesis itself because legal provisions simply could not keep pace with the variety of novel practices it introduced over the last three decades. Novel opportunities for crime created a novel problem for legislative regulation, namely 'how to keep up?' This inverted the traditional relationship between the legal order and the social order. Increasingly, the law lags behind innovative malfeasance and, since variety generates more variety in ways that are unpredictable, it outdistances the possibility of jurisprudence ever catching up. There are two legal alternatives. Either the law can try to 'run faster', but this greatly inflates the quantity of legislation and still remains a retrospective tidying up operation. It has been attempted and abandoned in Britain[5]. Whilst the volume

[5]For example, between 1983 and 2009 the British Parliament approved over one hundred criminal justice bills and over 4000 new criminal offences were created. In response to that trend, the Ministry of Justice established a procedure to limit the designation of new crimes (Cabinet Office 2013).

of Government primary legislation diminished between 1979 and 2009, conversely the quantity of Statutory Instruments augmented (House of Lords 2011). The latter is the alternative to futile legislative frenzy. It consists in an increasing cascade of regulations, passing downwards through a plethora of Agencies, culminating in increased bureaucratic rather than legal regulation.

This growth in anormative regulatory provisions (dependent upon fines and prohibitions and entailing neither personal shame nor social sanction) encouraged an individual cost/benefit approach; namely was a breach (such as a parking ticket) worth it to the subject? (Archer 2016a, b). Growing reliance on bureaucratic regulation was an acknowledgement that the assumptions of the old 'Command and Control' model as the preserve of the state, using legal rules backed by criminal sanctions, no longer held good. In Julia Black's words, this model had been '"centered" in that it assumes the state to have the capacity to command and control, to be the only commander and controller, and to be potentially effective in commanding and controlling. It is assumed to be unilateral in its approach (governments telling, others doing), based on simple cause-effect relations, and envisaging a linear progression from policy formation through to implementation.' (Black 2001: 106).

Simultaneously, two other processes tightly linked to morphogenesis fundamentally undermined 'shared normativity' as a basis for a return to the former mode of legal regulation. One was the 'escalation in cultural abundance' (Carrigan 2016) stemming from the diversification of digital outlets that further decreased socio-cultural integration and fostered 'fragile social movements', cut off the previous process by which old-style movements had maintained steady pressure for legal changes in the interests of large sections of the population (enfranchisement, civil rights, unionization etc.). Another was the increase in migration, resulting in the dis-embedding and re-embedding of peoples with the same consequences for novel forms of cultural syncretism as displayed by earlier religious Diasporas (Gorski 2016).

If these three processes *inter alia* prevented any return to the earlier top-down 'command and control' form of jurisprudence, can our reader's question be answered by a bottom-up alternative? Moreover, could this change its preoccupation with social regulation and co-ordination to focus, instead, upon encouraging novel forms of sociality and the new 'relational goods' generated by them through cooperation? Donati (2016) changes the perspective from deontic normativity (stable and shared), constituting the infrastructure upon which legal systems depended, to consider the processes of nomos-building within morphogenesis, which raises the level of social integration as agents recognize the benefits of the relational goods they produce and can share in only as participants (such as the conviviality shared in a public garden residents have created together).

However, rather than such initiatives cumulatively contributing to a new legal framework, what prevents the higher authorities from taking advantage of these voluntary contributions and reducing their own, as seemed to be the case in Britain when the Food Banks spread as humanitarian provisions were reduced to become part of austerity measures?[6] Since that instance is hardly conclusive, the paradox of 'relational evils' remains. Can we simply deny that neighbourhood gangs are lacking in sociality, that belonging is involuntary and none of their outcomes are desirable without over-indulging our own moral values?

I am only indicating that this bottom-up alternative ineluctably leads us to considering Eudaimonia (individual and collective) and the good life in (morphogenic) society. Unless we can answer this without either advocating or indulging in moral relativism we would be endorsing the complete separation of facts and values that Critical Realism has always resisted. Until we have done that, I am afraid that our hypothetical reader has to wait for an answer to his question.

Morphogenesis and Eudaimonia

Why should any social theorist hold that the increased intensity of morphogenetic change in society would or could be the source of growing well-being for its (global) members? To answer this question we have first to backtrack to what our group of collaborators have come to understand and endorse over our six years of discussions about the concept of a Morphogenic society and the likelihood of its advent. How it is conceptualized is closely related to whether or not it is viewed as closely linked to furthering human flourishing. Two meanings have been developed in the course of this book series.

1. The **full blown Morphogenic Society** would be one in which the production, exploration and exploitation of 'contingent compatibilities' constitutes novel **opportunities** (jobs, roles, *modi vivendi*) whose take-up follows a **situational logic of opportunity** (the new being found more attractively advantageous than the old) and meets with little **opposition** because no vested interests have yet been consolidated on this novel terrain. Consequently, those exploring it are not constrained by a pre-structured context, either materially or culturally. In turn, what they make of it is not necessarily locked in conflict with what others seek to do, thus potentially allowing for **win-win outcomes**. Minimalistically, these would be conflict-free and maximally they would generate **relational goods**, emergent from their **positive social relationality**.

This interpretation of the Morphogenic Society is a Concrete Utopia (Bloch 1959–1986). Within Critical Realism, such Utopias 'pinpoint the real, but non-actualized, possibilities inherent in a situation, thus inspiring grounded hope to inform emancipatory praxis' (Hartwig 2007). That is a fair description of what I was doing when initially floating the idea of Morphogenic Society (Archer 2007, 2012). Such Utopias are not predictions but attempts to illustrate a divergent form of social structuring – to show that there is an alternative to the tribulations of Late Modernity

[6] However, in Italy, their legal status was reinforced by the Good Samaritan Law.

and adduce some realistic exemplars of how it is already at work in certain domains. This was also the route taken by Donati and Archer in *The Relational Subject*, 2015, along with reviewing some of the obstacles to its realization. Indeed, Donati's contributions to this series of books have fleshed out the relationship between Morphogenesis and Relationality, especially in developing the concept of 'relational steering' (2013) and the pivotal role of reflexivity in the morphogenesis of normativity. In this volume, he defends the thesis that 'the good life coincides with the creation of relational goods' (Chap. 7, [p1]). It does so by creating new life opportunities within the social relations that orient the conduct of our lives towards sociability. However, he is only too aware of the resistance and resilience of previous (*lib/lab*) social forms makes generalized sociability (un)realistically utopian and thus much of the time takes Morphogenetic Society in its second meaning below.

2. **Unbound morphogenesis** is the meaning favoured by the majority of our contributors (leaving two agnostics). This interprets Morphogenic society as one where morphogenetic processes intensify until they predominate over morphostatic ones, becoming less and less constrained by them and hence will proceed to generate increasing variety. It follows that social action becomes less governed by routinization, by habitus or habits and that it lies in the hands of individuals and groups to seize their own means of flourishing or implicitly to accept that they will not thrive, or at least as well as they might.

Most of the contributors see good reason to regard the relationship between intense Morphogenesis and Eudaimonia as being far from a direct one. It is puzzling (see Maccarini Chap. 5) because the lack of association derives from two different causal mechanisms: the new dilemmas of choice now confronting all agents and actors, stemming from morphogenesis itself, and the stubborn endurance of institutions and vested interests from the past whose influence suffuses the present.

Yet why would it be thought at all that intensified Morphogenesis could foster Eudaimonia rather than the two lacking any determinate relationship? Their connection hangs on Critical Realism's portrayal of humankind (individually and collectively) as the bearers of 'capacities' and 'liabilities', both of whose potentials can be extended or exacerbated through their relations with natural reality and its three orders: the natural, the practical (our heritage of material culture) and the social (Archer 2000). Here we are concerned with the social order and the potential for Morphogenesis unbound to enable the development or fuller use of people's 'capacities'. As I briefly argue in Chap. 6, this hinges on the new opportunities that are opened up (new experiences, novel jobs, newly recognized skills etc.), which elasticated subjects' existing 'capacities' and acknowledge some forms of ability that previously gained no recognition and may not have been recognized even by their possessors. In other words, ascribed characteristics will diminish in importance and achieved ones increase as the notion of achievement itself diversifies. Thus, if more people can do more of what they do best – for remuneration, for pleasure, or for pro-social ends – this provides a stepping stone towards the 'good life' in society and the enhancement of their flourishing.

However, this is not only a matter of what people do best but also about what they care about most. In other words, social subjects as 'strong evaluators' invest themselves in their *concerns* and derive their identities from their specific constellation of such concerns. Hence, I am in full agreement with Andrew Sayer that 'our own flourishing comes to be dependent upon the flourishing of our commitments… There is thus no clear distinction between our own flourishing and that of our commitments; they are fused' (2011, p. 125). It is a feature of every normal human being to inspect and to evaluate reflexively the social context in which they find themselves involuntarily at birth in terms of whether or not that natal context enables or frustrates the realization of what they come to care about and to what degree.[7]

Things always matter to people, although the importance of what they care about (Frankfurt 1988) need not be noble or commendable, such as the availability of drugs. Agential subjectivity is crucially important, but it is not an infallible guide to Eudaimonia; subjects' reflexive definitions of the good life are epistemic, whereas their flourishing (or lack of it) has an objective ontological status; consider the ill-health of habitual drug-users who can come to recognize the discrepancy between their own epistemology and ontology (and voluntarily enter rehab). Nevertheless, it remains the case that their self-defined concerns are what guides and prompts their actions and produces different courses of action amongst those inhabiting much the same social context. Another way of putting this is that subjects do indeed have first-person authority about what motivates their concerns and subsequent life-choices, but to any third-person this may not be deemed to constitute the good life for them or anyone else.

Therefore, our concerns do not establish a direct link between Morphogenesis and Eudaimonia. That was Dahrendorf's mistake (1994), namely the assumption that the good life consists in the possibility of increasing access to as many opportunities as possible for everybody. Such a view makes two fallacious assumptions. It takes it for granted that all people want everything as it becomes available, which is untrue because many do not, rejecting popular entertainment, celebrity 'culture', foreign food, meat, recreational drugs etc. Furthermore, it presumes the existence of a welfare safety net if the nature of their concerns proves damaging to them (Donati, Chap. 7). None of our contributors fall into these traps. On the contrary, they accentuate three reasons why Morphogenesis and Eudaimonia are not necessarily in close association.

[7]This is my own definition: 'reflexivity is the regular exercise of the mental ability, shared by all normal people, to consider themselves in relation to their (social) contexts and vice versa' (Archer 2007, p. 4).

Why Morphogenesis Does Not Entail Eudaimonia

First, many experience too much choice and lack the reflexivity necessary to exceed their first-order inclinations and to develop second-order concerns, which entails prioritizing some, subordinating others and excluding further contenders that initially appeared desirable. Instead, consumerism, commodification and the digital surfeit now on offer condemns some to the status of digitalized 'wantons', in Frankfurt's terms (1988), namely people who cannot discipline their first-order desires into a volitional hierarchy of what really matters to them. Instead, they become victims of 'digital distraction' that Carrigan (Chap. 8) understands as an induced crisis in which today's presentism yields an immediate expressive response that defeats the shaping of their lives tomorrow and successive tomorrows by enveloping them in a 'data smog'.

What these 'distracted people' share is the problem of 'cultural abundance' and their inability to exercise any means of 'bounding variety', or for that matter recognizing that much of it is not new variety at all but a 'proliferation of spam'. Indeed, this discursive explosion is additive rather than substitutive (there is no 'quotient of replacement', as argued earlier.) In their disorientation, they tend to turn away from the algorithmic 'guidance' of the commercial search engines ('having bought X, you will likely enjoy Y'), only to turn towards others on social media, whose traffic now outstrips that of the former, but whose users are wantons like themselves, particularly amongst the young who know insufficient about both themselves and the world. Since like initially turns to socio-economic like, this serves only to intensify their expressive reactions rather than to extend their knowledgeability or to diminish uneven access to it throughout society. This lack of commitment amongst large tracts of the population is thus broadly associated with the next reason why some if not all contributors see no direct connection between Morphogenesis and Eudaimonia.

Second, and as is always the case with relationally contested morphogenesis, those whose dominance is challenged do not cede their positions or their assets because their basic vested interests remain largely unchanged. At most, they alter in form but not in nature. One consequence is that in defence of their interests, new variety is most quickly appropriated by those with the resources to do so. As Gorski (Chap. 2) insists from a neo-Aristotelian approach to Eudaimonia, human flourishing is substantive rather than formal; access to resources and an infrastructure is required to develop skills and to engage in new activities. Yet as all sociologists know, these are both very unevenly distributed within and between the various nation states and even regions of the world. In other words, T^1 in the basic morphogenetic cycle never finds the parties involved lining up, as it were at the starting gate, equally endowed in terms of resources. (This is why analysis can only pretend to be entirely synchronic if it incorporates the enduring historical 'winnings' of some groups, acquired diachronically along with their ideological convictions, including that they have an acquired right to perpetuate their privileged access to the infrastructure). If, in shorthand, we simply call this 'power', the uneven access to resources and powerful ideas can readily be linked with which groups have preferential chances of attaining Eudaimonia.

In last year's volume, devoted to Normativity, Ismael Al-Amoudi (2016) produced an economical and creative diagram explaining why, in brief, when Administrative authorities introduced a new regulation at T^1, those possessing more power at that time can transform their practices to circumvent it much faster than those with less power (starting at the same T^1). The more powerful continue to do so (keeping ahead of the rest of the field) even when the regulatory authority tries to tighten the instruments in force to prevent this outcome. I believe this can be used more generally as an extension to the M/M approach to explain why those who are better-off in terms of resources, repute and organizational representation also do better than those less powerful when morphogenesis is underway, even if they were not its progenitors and even when there is little affinity between their interests and the aims of those initiating the change in question (as in old-style two party democracies).

The fact that they remain closer to the winners than the losers in terms of outcomes implies that the situational logic of Competition retains its hold, precisely because they are acting fast and successfully, hence avoiding becoming losers. Simultaneously, this also has the implication that there are gradations in power and influence (perhaps dissimilar in different sectors of society), usually meaning that there is a disparate category below them who bear the brunt of both those responsible for initiating morphogenetic changes and of those best placed at any T^1 to protect their own interests adaptively to them. Such differences in outcomes would tend strongly to correspond with the distinction between Corporate and Primary Agents (Archer 1995) (Fig. 1.1).

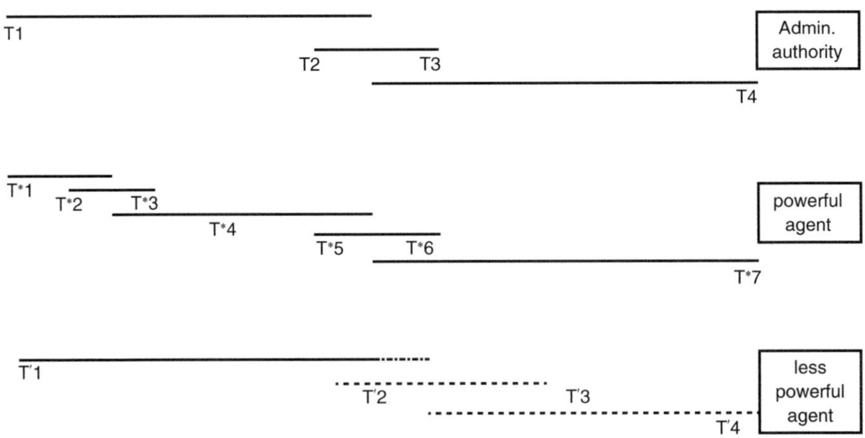

Fig. 1.1 Power differences and who benefits most from morphogenesis (Source: Al-Amoudi 2016: p. 129)

Gross differences in the structured distributions of resources, repute and representation serve to entrench the 'winners' and the 'losers', reflecting the dynamics depicted in the above diagram. As a recursive outcome, meaning that winnings and losses accumulate over time, this also results in social divisions becoming deeper and structural barriers to the achievement of universal participation in morphogenetic decision-making becoming steeper. This is exactly what has been witnessed in the developed world during the current millennium, where few strong countervailing mechanisms have intervened to mitigate this consequence. Instead, multi-national and increasingly financialized capitalism have generated the paradox whereby substantial growth in global aggregate wealth has been accompanied by an increase in worldwide inequality, despite the decrease in absolute poverty. Clearly, this situation is paralleled in International Relations; in the Morgenthau school of thinking, the possibility of a 'good international society' is not even acknowledged (Wight, Chap. 12).

However, misunderstandings can arise when the structural process, for example, of morphogenesis is elided with the role of power in determining which group gains or benefits most from any given morphogenetic cycle. (This is a kind of re-run of the old conflationary structure and agency debate, which the M/M approach was intended to resolve). Thus in volume III, Lawson (2015) introduced the strange status of the capitalist company as 'a legal person', despite it being non-conscious and non-intentional, but conferring material advantages upon the firm's executive in terms of restricting their legal liabilities, which encouraged them to defend this status – successfully.

Taking this up in the present volume, Morgan and Sun (Chap. 9) begin by noting that the dominant tendency in late modernity is to locate the corporation as falling primarily within processes of morphogenesis. That seems to me correct; the digitalized and financialized form of capitalist enterprises today has undergone considerable transformation from the early days of the multi-national firm, let alone the earlier days of capitalism's inception. In short, capitalist enterprise has itself been profoundly morphogenetic. The fact that it indeed remains competitive, adheres to the wage form etc. and its new corporations have retained their peculiar legal status are all testimonies to its enduring power and capacity to defend entrepreneurial vested interests through transformations such as entering into (or better, buying into) digitalization (see Archer 2014a, b, Chap. 5) or tax avoidance through the strategic location of where taxes are paid. It does not, I think, justify the conclusion that 'the primary form of the elaborations seems to involve change in order to stay, in many respects, the same'. Much less does it lead to the conclusion that 'morphogenesis is also a type of morphostasis' under a different description of the process, namely elaboration to resist transformation understood as resistance to shifts in power. Such shifts are undoubtedly a synchronic motive during competitive conflict in which the capitalist corporation largely continues to win out, but these successful manoeuvres should not be represented as morphostasis. Staying ahead in the power play is not to stay the same, in fact, precisely the opposite. Instead, one can maintain that the capitalist corporation has been a prime exemplar of morphogenesis: dispensing with producing anything (except profit), shifting from the real to the virtual economy and currently busy dispensing with workers in favour of robotics. Only the Nominalist would invoke 'sameness' when the referent has changed so drastically.

Morgan and Sun are not Nominalists, nor do they accept that the enduring legal status of the corporation means it is effectively 'out of control' as Lawson maintained. For example, its tax avoidance depends upon another power-play between states to attract businesses, but could be seriously reduced by the introduction of 'unitary taxation' that the EU plans to adopt. Of course, this will entail another round of competitive conflict between state and market. Nevertheless, whichever proves the more powerful party this time around, it is a very different challenge to modern capitalism to design a modern economy that does not require labour but remains dependent upon wage earners in their role as consumers. Whilst this must prompt further morphogenesis, relations with nation states over taxation will likely generate compromise, concession and creativity in this trial of strength, but the outcome is unlikely to be morphostatic – things will not revert to the way they were before, which ever party wins in this new confrontation.

Third, however difficult it may be for readers to deny the intensification of various manifestations of morphogenesis in their own life times and the simultaneous demise of morphostasis, although they may evaluate this emergence of Morphogenic Society very differently, it seems likely that many would agree with us about the lack of a direct connection with Eudaimonia. Their reasons may sometimes be the same; namely the absence of equality (and growth in inequality) that prevents many deriving any benefit from the social changes taking place. Some also add that the beneficiaries are only such at the expense of the poor and this is undoubtedly the case for the poorest suffering from Climate Change (Dunlap and Brulle 2015). Thus, to derive a benefit or to suffer harm from morphogenesis cannot be construed in cash terms alone or exclusively materially (including the rolling back of welfare provisions), but may entail institutional elaborations that confine access to a privileged group, whist creating a large category of the excluded (such as the shift towards private pension schemes) or the redrawing of cultural boundaries (from which Western women have largely benefitted).

Equality, Participation and Eudaimonia

It is this that leads Andrew Sayer to conclude that a necessary condition of dignity for all 'therefore implies far-reaching equality, not just in what people get in resources, but in terms of what they are allowed and expected to *do*. It requires contributive, as well as distributive justice,' (2011, p. 214). It is also this that leads Gorski (Chap. 2) to endorse Critical Realism's departure from the Aristotelian elitist Eudaimonia that excluded women and slaves from consideration. Note that what is advocated by Sayer above is 'far-reaching equality', not absolute equality, because a *just* society is neither *just* nor *good* if unequals are treated equally. Such was the case in Lepelltier's plan for enforced egalitarianism in public instruction advocated during the *Convention*, the most militant Jacobinist phase of the three revolutionary Assemblies; education for all would cease after Primary schooling and before any more advanced instruction enabled the higher intellectual abilities of some allowed them to outdistance others (Vaughan and Archer 1971, p, 121ff). Not only did this mean denying their capacities the freedom to develop, but it simultaneously prevented the use of their abilities from contributing to the common good. In short, the *good* society cannot be legislated or regulated into being.

In advocating 'far-reaching equality', whilst defending the right of all to develop their capacities both for their own good and for their contribution to the good society requires an appropriate conceptualization of Eudaimonia for the person and for the social context that can be deemed 'good', the two being necessarily linked.

As Zamagni – another theorist who seeks 'far-reaching equality' alone – maintains in the economic context, what will not do are: 'Our familiar theories of contracts, of industrial organization, of prices, and more, have no need to bother with the category of the person: an informed, rational individual is sufficient... we have come to the point where even the most 'abstract' of economists cannot but admit that if we want to attack the almost totally new problems of our society – such as the endemic aggravation of inequality, the scandal of human hunger, the emergence of new social pathologies, the rise of clashes in identity in addition to the traditional clash of interests, the paradoxes of happiness, unsustainable development, and so on – research can no longer confine itself to a sort of anthropological limbo. One must take a position on the matter' (Zamagni 2008, p. 468). The position cannot be one endorsing the 'monistic' individual (operating in a social environment, affecting it but unaffected by it) and, above all, someone whose 'relations' with others make no difference to their trajectory through the world or consequences for it. Goodness requires relationality because it is not an aggregate property but a quintessentially generative one.

Hence, to Donati[8], 'the good is a common good because *only together* can it be recognized and acted upon (generated and regenerated) as such, by all those who have a *concern* about it. At the same time, it must be produced and enjoyed by all those who have a stake in it. For this reason, *the good resides within the relations that connect the subjects*' (2008, p. 661). Or, more briefly; 'Only if we see the common good as a relational good, can we understand its inner connection with the human person' (ibid p. 662) in the social order.

However, it seems to me and to Porpora (Chap. 3) that we must tread carefully with Critical Realism's ethical universalism in which the free flourishing of each is held to be the relational condition of universality, which spells the free flourishing of all. This often repeated formulation from Marx should cause us to pause, in particular over the use of the word 'all'. Is 'flourishing' not similar to 'equality' as discussed above; something we would wish to see becoming society-wide but

[8]Donati's Relational conception, one quite distinct from Emirbayer's Manifesto for relational*ism, whose denial of emergence*, confines relations to an infinite series of transactions between people.

accept cannot be truly universal (outside Concrete Utopia). Therefore we have good reason for not advocating that it be more than 'far-reaching'?

As concerned 'equality', the reason was that its enforcement would deprive *both* talented individuals and society of the fruits of their fully developed capacities. The reason is different here. It is disclosed in the quotation from Donati above; relational goods require *participation* in their generation and *concern* for their realization. Even if one adds 'stakeholders' to participants, as he does, this does not add up to the universalism of 'all'. Why not? This is because some will opt for the furtherance of relational evils that they deem preferable for themselves. We can challenge their reasoning ('false consciousness' or 'mystification' if preferred); we can agree with Maccarini (Chap. 5) that human subjects require institutional help to nurture their flourishing; and none of us disagrees that the extension of thriving is largely a social matter – something we promote 'together'. Nevertheless, full-blooded universalism flounders on those furthering relational evils, and not only on the psychopathology of the indiscriminate gun-man or the greed of the rational actor and their equivalents in any age. These can be contained and immobilized (imprisonment, institutionalized medication or the most compassionate of care) but the best of medico-legal outcomes for them pronounces some to be 'no longer a threat to the community', it does not assure that they are capable of becoming part of the 'we' that together generate relational goods.[9] In brief, moral universalism has to cede realistically to 'far-reaching participation'.

Ultimately, the *good society* is one which promotes the Common Good (Donati 2008). What makes it 'good' is that a large majority contribute to generating it (thus entailing a high level of *social integration* because without most participating by contributing there would be a substantial category of the 'excluded' – of non-beneficiaries who cannot even be 'free riders' because to experience relational goods entails being in-relationship)[10]. What also makes it 'good' is that the relational goods produced in one sector do not conflict with those generated in any other, thus entailing a high level of *system integration* without which the goods in question would clash, damaging both – as when the conditions for sustaining a high quality of family life conflict with those for maintaining equivalent work relations[11].

These are demanding conditions because although a potentially 'good' society *is by definition morphogenetic because relational goods are (new) emergent properties*, it may well lose its claim to 'goodness' owing to the countervailing relational evils it is equally capable of generating, which can be just as morphogenetic (novel varieties of harm introduced relationally). Were the latter to predominate, both social and system integration would decline in consequence; the population in

[9]They are not deprived of the human right to 'good care', which would be provided in a good society.

[10]This does not preclude them from benefitting from certain subsidiary features such as peaceful neighbourhoods or work relations, providing they do nothing to disrupt them.

[11]Note that this cannot be reduced to the individualistic terms in which the so-called 'work-life' balance is supposedly worked out by each employee in an organization.

question (now global) would be re-divided into (temporary) winners and losers and the situational logic of opportunity would be indefinitely postponed as adversarial groups clung to the defence of their vested interests – thus prolonging zero-sum competition and tenaciously defending competitive advantages. Thus, intense morphogenesis alone, even when matched by parallel retreats in morphostasis provides no warrant for announcing the advent of the *good* Morphogenic society. Reluctantly, that is where it seems we (the global we) are stuck at present.

In dwelling upon relations and relationality above a preliminary linkage has been made between 'far-reaching equality' between persons and 'far-reaching' participation of persons', and their relationships that promote both social solidarity and the social order that fosters Eudaimonia. Before pursuing it further, let us contrast this with the objectivist (metrified), individualistic and purely distributive approach to equality of the heirs to the cybernetic heritage. Consider a diagram that Teune and Mlinar present for the purposes of illustrating their key concepts of the *Developmental Logic of Social Systems* (1978). This illustrates a situation where there is substantial 'distribution of variety', where 'diversity' is also more than counterbalanced by 'similarities'. Thus, the figure represents *ceteris paribus* the conditions for relatively stable social development, in the aggregate, objective and individualistic terms used. Note that although sub-sets could be made up of individual persons, even where they are not (e.g. cities), these are defined as an aggregate of them (Fig. 1.2).

First, let us suppose, for illustrative purposes, that this was a static snapshot of a city's properties and their distributions at some historic T^1. Empirically, the quantity of objective properties and their variety, pre-selected by the investigators for their research purposes, could have been found to be completely different in both number

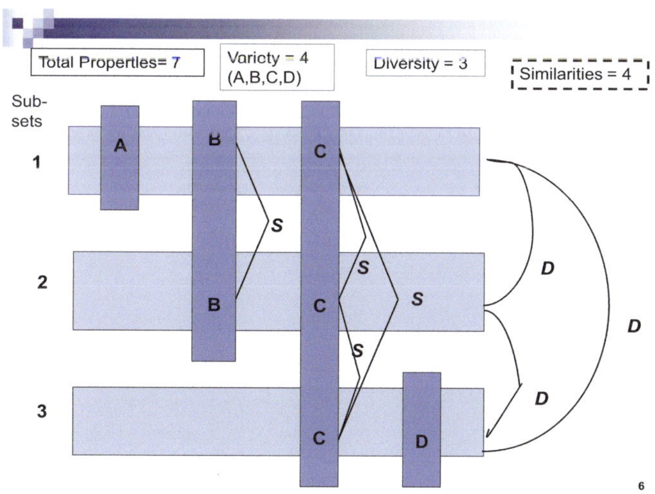

Fig. 1.2 Variety, Diversity and Similarities amongst sib-sets (Source: Teune and Mlinar, *The Developmental Logic of Social Systems*, Figure1, p. 3)

and distribution. However, if a variety of only three properties was recorded – 'those owning land', 'those who are householders' and 'those bearing a title' – there would have been two sub-sets alone, corresponding to the 'nobility and the rest', with no similarities or diversity between them. At the opposite extreme, an egalitarian city would be constituted by a single set in which the same three properties were possessed by all, hence every member shared 'similarities' but this population had no diversity (as measured). In that case it would in fact be a Morphostatic Society.

However, these authors are as interested as we are in how matters change over time and hope to have advanced a 'developmental logic' in the course of their book. It is cleverly articulated, using few further concepts than those contained in the above figure and advances formulations such as 'The Law of Diminishing Diversity' and 'The Law of Attractiveness of Variety (Teune and Mlinar 1978, p. 60–61). Thus, the latter states 'that the components will tend to interact more with those components with nearly equal, or greater variety and less with those with less variety' (p. 61). Since I have introduced this work strictly for purposes of comparison and not of critique, the point is to note that what does not appear in this particular example is *who* is attracted to *whom* and *why* and *who else* joins them, or what *reasons prompt* this quest for the variety in question. As a theory it is entirely unpeopled, completely objective and exclusively in the third-person. This means, that it abrogates the terms of the acronym I coined in the Introduction to our first volume (Archer 2013a, b) for all M/M analysis, emphasizing that any explanation must come in a SAC (meaning it incorporates Structure, Culture and Agency). Agency is the missing element here (reduced to 'components'), as is any distinction between Structure and Culture; all of these are dissolved into an unstratified ontology reduced to properties and their bearers. In short, this may make for a quiet city, but the question of Eudaimonia is not allowed to arise within it.

Networking Eudaimonia: The Processes of Participation

A stratified social ontology (as in Critical Realism and neo-structuralism) is required in which different properties and powers pertain to different strata (conventionally, the micro-, meso- and macro-levels) and exert a causal influence upon the processes governing participation and therefore upon who can express their concerns within each stratum. Without robust social linkages between the 'levels', participation is blocked, meaning potential participants are confined to exercising their agency lower down. Social theory has frequently replicated this situation, and necessarily in its conflationary versions, whether these represent downwards, upwards or central conflation (Archer 1988, 1995). These I have critiqued at length elsewhere. However, for our present discussion, their specific deficiency concerns 'the missing middle', in both theory and practice where participation is concerned. The lack of a meso-level, constituted by organizations, institutions and associations is the biggest blockage to participation or barrier to our understanding of its effects.

Two concrete examples serve as illustration. On the one hand, nothing looks more participatory than political 'populism', but numerous Latin American examples show that it can easily be hijacked by monocratic regimes, frequently dependent upon support of the military. In the absence of a robust meso-level, these bottom-up demands – in line with a quest for Eudaimonia – may experience complete blockage. The scenarios can be extremely complex, but what the protesters lack is any participatory route that leads from street protest to the Presidential Place. On the other hand, in the West, the case of representative democracy is one where the populace is now confronted with centrist governments and declining party organizations forming weaker and weaker conduits for 'bottom-up' participation. This fosters top-down decision-making and anormative bureaucratic control, the formation of new 'ultra' parties and policies preying on the lowest common denominator of public prejudices.[12] Both are very different instances of the 'missing middle'.

Giddens' central conflationism (1979) that maintained structures had only a 'virtual' ontology until 'instantiated' by agents, clamped structure and agency together in a conceptual vice, by disallowing any stratum operative between them. With the middle ground cleared of structures (organizational or associational), diagrams such as the one re-produced below became common (Fig. 1.3).

Structuration theory is indefinite and indeterminate about *who* is responsible for social change, *how*, *why* and *what they do* in relational opposition to others in order to attain transformation. What then flourishes is 'actor-based modelling' using large data-sets and powerful software. Why? Because, in Epstein's words: 'Agent-based

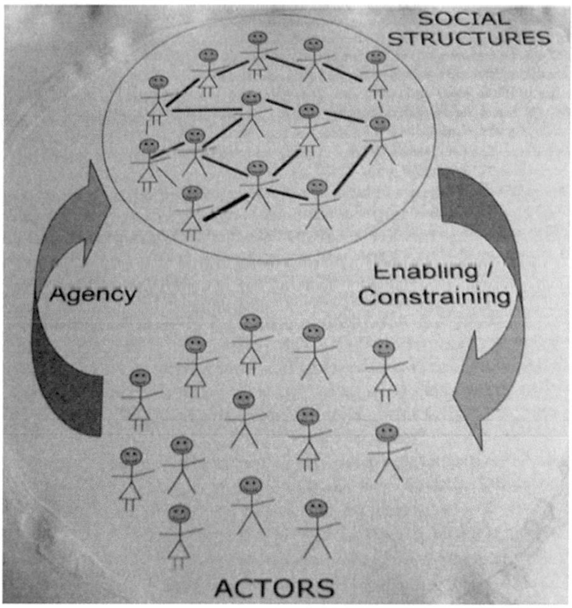

Fig. 1.3 The Absence of the Meso-level (Source: Christian Fuchs, *Internet and Society: Social Theory in the Information Age*, 2008: 52)

[12]The 2016 Brexit Referendum illustrated everything about the 'missing middle', from the decision to call it, the blatant lies of all parties during it, to the sheer political ignorance of those voting for it.

models allow us to study the micro-to-macro mapping' (1999), without reference to any form of social organization lying between them.

Emmanuel Lazega has done sterling service by consistently demonstrating through various case studies how crucial meso-level organizations are for mediating both top-down and bottom-up decision-making by facilitating or blocking participation. What he illustrates in the overtly hierarchical structure of a French Diocese (Chap. 10) is how the variety of priestly orientations towards expressing their vocation at the Parish level then crystallize into networks with like-minded parishioners, thus shaping very different forms of grass roots collegiality . The Bishop (meso-level) makes a trade-off between the animosities potentially threatening their relations against increasing their participation, by co-opting some from each orientation onto the diocesan bureaucratic committees, on pain of cutting himself off from a large part of the faithful. Through the cooptation of these diverse impulses for change, which then have to work in co-operation, new variety enters the diocesan system from below. Equally, as these networks do more than co-exist, but rather thrash out cooperative solutions, negotiated together, the way is open for some of these initiatives to be passed upwards and to modify future 'top-down' policies of the higher ecclesiastical authorities by a similar process. Through such a networked increase in participation, 'bottom-up' and 'top-down' influences 'can be said to drive each other's evolution in a morphogenetic sense. If the structure of the network changes but the diocese survives, then the diocese as a system is morphogenetic' (Lazega, Chap. 10).

Wight hints at how a parallel analysis of new networks penetrating the macro-level, such as UN agencies and INGOs more generally, advance both participation and equality, inducing morphogenetic changes in the legislative policies of nation states (Chap. 12). This was born out in August 2015 during the UN process of designating new Sustainable Development Goals (accentuating targets that would introduce more equity for the most globally disadvantaged) and the Paris Agreement in December 2015 on the reduction of carbon emissions that was dependent upon the participation and co-operation of member states as it will be for its efficacy.

Conclusion

Thus, it can be seen that over the five volumes in the series, the contributors have reached the following three broad conclusions[13] about our original question: are we globally moving towards a social formation that could justifiably be termed a Morphogenic Society? (Perhaps it would be fairer to represent these as the majority view).

[13]As Editor, I am acutely aware of having failed to do justice to the nuanced views and positions taken by individual friends and collaborators, especially in this final and summary volume, for which I apologise.

1. Firstly, we have come to a necessary working definition of a Morphogenic Society as a world in which morphogenetic processes increasingly predominate over morphostatic ones and is reflected by their outcomes.

Broadly we are agreed that these are the lineaments towards which today's global social formation has already moved in contradistinction to Late Modernity. This agreement includes acceptance that 'morphonecrosis' has been characteristic of certain prior social forms that previously underwrote morphostasis (Al-Amoudi and Latsis 2015). However, some also wish to signal that morphostatic forms and processes can be (at least temporarily protracted) by and within defensive 'enclaves' and 'vortices', protecting them from the intrusion of morphogenetically induced change (Maccarini 2015). Nevertheless, the majority accept the predominance of morphogenesis and anticipate that the emergence of new 'contingent complementarities', particularly between Structure and Culture, will continue to spawn ever novel forms of variety that may have differential impacts and different tempos in various parts of the world, but that their knock-on effects will indeed be global in scope.

2. Our first collective reservation is that without 'far-reaching' increases in both equality and participation, however Morphogenic it may be, it will be a divided society characterized by 'winner' and 'losers'. Equality and participation are linked; those with least resources in terms of remuneration and repute will also find their representation increasingly confined to restricted channels such as voting in general elections. Correspondingly, change will be predominantly 'top-down', to the detriment of participants from lower socio-cultural levels. This also works the opposite way around; participants with least equality will be obstructed in attempts of introduce 'bottom-up' initiatives. Forms of elaboration emanating from the top-down need to be counterbalanced by those instigated from the 'bottom-up'. Otherwise, sectional interests will replicate or augment their initial advantages/disadvantages as in Fig. 1.1, which effectively shows 'the rich getting richer and the poor, poorer' in a variety of currencies. Our problem is that without a level playing field at T^1, then interactional dynamics during $T^2 - T^3$ will mean outcomes at T^4 are likely to be even less fair for subsequent interaction. This major problem is not simply confined to the historic (diachronically acquired) vested interests being perpetuated from past to present, but also that new objective interests (synchronically pursued) are acquired on that basis and transmitted onwards from the present to the future.
3. The root question raised by this volume can be put conditionally. Even were a new social formation that qualified as 'Morphogenic' on the two criteria above held to have emerged from late modernity, does it tend to enhance generalized human flourishing or the reverse? It is probably our reservations about the changes taking place in relation to the Eudaimonia clause that accounts for our lack of enthusiasm in proclaiming a new age. Because the characterization of any social change is both theory and value laden, any form of morphogenic society can be welcomed or abhorred. Since every such change is activity-dependent, then its evaluation will be decisive for the support or opposition that it attracts

whilst in *statu nascendi.* Unless the Morphogenic Society does promote general Eudaimonia then none of the present collaborators would deem it 'good'. This is obviously not the case for many adhering to mainstream economics, Rational Choice Theory or Neo-Pragmatism, for example, or for any whose prime concern is limited to the advancement of their own interest group alone.

To link the 'good society' to 'general human thriving' is to impose a demanding criterion upon a Morphogenic social formation for it to gain our approbation. Other exemplars of intense morphogenesis that have already been realized would not meet this demand. Few would deny that the transformation of multi-national capitalist production into financialized, digital capitalism was powerfully morphogenetic, though it is not the end of capitalism. Nevertheless, the fact that it continues to exploit, to increase inequalities, to engender many varieties of ill-being cannot be attributed to the endurance of previous morphostatic factors. Indeed, some of the factors responsible for contemporary inequality are themselves morphogenetic, most notably Climate Change[14].

The Eudaimonic criterion is not demanding simply because it unites intense morphogenetic change with the fostering of global human well-being, but because it deals with two very different ontologies. A society or a social formation has an *objective mode of existence;* despite the fact that some of its most important features are non-observables – in particular, aspects of their generative mechanisms. Nonetheless, what can be discovered or ventured about them takes place in the third-person, that is, they are voiced by the investigator(s). Conversely, beyond that which is biologically grounded about human flourishing, has a *subjective mode of existence;* it is dependent upon and fused with our concerns and reflexivity and thus exists in the first-person, though no less real for that. Demanding as it may be, before it is considered good, a Morphogenic society should not only generate new opportunities but ones whose existence constitutes novel sources of fulfilment for more subjects (societally or sectorally). On the other hand, those defending 'business as usual' rest their arguments upon 'there is no alternative' and TINA is anything but value free; it condones the widening gulf of economic inequalities and in political participation and institutionalizes exclusion rather than inclusion. In effect, TINA assumes 'there is no alternative' to the frustration of their concerns for many if not most of those involved. This is not freedom from values in the least. Neither is ours, which are the reverse of theirs. But Critical Realism does not endorse the separation of facts from values nor allow the persistent denial of frustrated Eudaimonia for the many to be dismissed as inevitable collateral damage.

The point is whether or not the incontrovertible mess in which we find the current world as the Anthropocene heads towards finitude can be attributed to either the intensification of morphogenesis or the demise of morphostasis? In Volume II we maintained that the decline of previous (not necessarily traditional)

[14]The poorest three billion who contribute least to global warming do so because their poverty condemns them to traditional morphostatic practices for cooking and heating; what they suffer from are the carbon emissions of the rest and their novel appliances.

mechanisms underwriting social stability was not accountable for the current wars, xenophobia, terrorism, the migration of despair, hunger, torture, inter-generational hostility, political break-up and break down and many more 'pathologies'. Our reasoning was that morphogenetic changes could furnish their own modes of stabilization by means of the relational goods that they generated, providing these were generously distributed throughout the world. Certainly they can have this effect, but equally surely their current iniquitously unequal distribution intensifies relational contestation rather than the beneficent relationality of cooperation.

Should morphogenesis itself then bear the blame? Undoubtedly, change *per se* is disruptive to some and induces distraction and disorientation amongst others. However, there is a reason why we left discussion of Eudaimonia until this last volume and attach such importance to it. The initial speculative sketch of Morphogenic Society foresaw the mechanism of 'variety stimulating more variety' as generating historically unprecedented 'win-win' situations where benefits accrued to those seizing new opportunities, unopposed by the vested interests of other parties because this was *terra incognita.* Retrospectively, this was ingenuous; on the stock exchange, dealings in 'futures' pre-dated digitalization, in Research and Development Departments much is invested in attempting to stake a claim to the future, space research is already planning planetary vacations, and in horse-racing breeding a winner was a consistent historic attempt to commandeer the future. That future is not virgin territory; it is staked out with flags signifying new objective interests with which 'newcomers' will necessarily conflict. Whilst ever we remain a relationally contested social order, the zero-sum replication of winners and losers will continue. This cannot be minimized as a transitional phenomenon. Thus we are announcing without fanfare the advent of Morphogenetic Society – one that falls short of meeting the Eudaimonia criterion.

However, the future is made not found; in so far as flourishing is 'first person' it involves a subjective component. Optimism qualitatively influences what it is that we commit to and thus how reflexivity spreads forwards to foster relational goods. Morphogenesis and Eudaimonia are not locked in intrinsic enmity; in fact, much less so than were Morphostasis and human flourishing in earlier social formations. The real enemies today are 'politics without commitment' and 'economics without vision'. Our task is to help and to show that in practice the building up of civil society and a civic economy on the basis of reciprocity recommends itself to all through the generation of relational goods for all.

References

Al-Amoudi, I. (2016). In letter and in spirit: Social morphogenesis and the interpretation of codified social rules. In Archer (Ed.), *Morphogenesis and the crisis of normativity* (Vol. 4). Dordrecht: Springer.

Al-Amoudi, I., & Latsis, J. (2015). Death contested: Morphonecrosis and conflicts of interpretation. In Archer (Ed.), *Generative mechanisms transforming the social order*. Dordrecht: Springer.

Archer, M. S. (1988). *Culture and agency: The place of culture in social theory*. Cambridge: Cambridge University Press.
Archer, M. S. (1995). *Realist social theory: The morphogenetic approach*. Cambridge: Cambridge University Press.
Archer, M. S. (2000). *Being human: The problem of agency*. Cambridge: Cambridge University Press.
Archer, M. S. (2007). *Making our way through the world*. Cambridge: Cambridge University Press.
Archer, M. S. (2012). *The reflexive imperative in late modernity*. Cambridge: Cambridge University Press.
Archer, M. S. (2013a [1979]). *Social origins of educational systems*. Abingdon: Routledge.
Archer, M. S. (Ed.). (2013b). *Social morphogenesis* (Vol. 1). Dordrecht: Springer.
Archer, M. S. (Ed.). (2014a). *Late modernity: Trajectories towards morphogenic society* (Vol. 2). Dordrecht: Springer.
Archer, M. S. (2014b). The generative mechanisms re-configuring late modernity. In Archer (Ed.), *Late modernity* (Vol. 2). New York: Springer.
Archer, M. S. (Ed.). (2016a). *Morphogenesis and the crisis of normativity*, Vol.4, Dordrecht: Springer.
Archer, M. S. (2016b). Anormative social regulation: The attempt to cope with social morphogenesis. In Archer (Ed.), *Morphogenesis and the crisis of normativity*, Vol. 4, Dordrecht: Springer.
Ashby, R. (1956). *In introduction to cybernetics*. New York: Wiley.
Bhaskar, R. (1979). *The possibility of naturalism*. Harvester: Brighton.
Black, J. (2001). Decentering regulation: Understanding the role of regulation and self-regulation in a post-regulatory world. *Current Legal Problems, 54*(1), 103–146.
Bloch, E. (1959–1986). *The principle of hope* (3 vols), Oxford: Blackwell.
Buckley, W. (1967). *Sociology and modern systems theory*. Englewood Cliffs: Prentice-Hall.
Bunge, M. (2004). How does it work: The search for explanatory mechanisms? *Philosophy of the Social Sciences, 34*(2), 182–210.
Cabinet Office Paper. (2013). www.gov.uk/government/publicationd/when laws become too complex (downloaded 21.11.2014).
Carrigan, M. (2016). The fragile movements of late modernity. In Archer (Ed.), *Morphogenesis and the crisis of normativity* (Vol. 4). Cham: Springer.
Dahrendorf, R. (1994). The changing quality of citizenship. In B. van Steenberger (Ed.), *The condition of citizenship* (pp. 10–19) London: Sage.
Donati, P. (2008). Discovering the relational character of the common good. In M. S. Archer & P. Donati (Eds.), *Pursuing the common good: How solidarity and subsidiarity can work together*. Vatican City: Vatican City Press.
Donati, P. (2013). Morphogenesis and social networks: Relational steering not mechanical feedboack. In M. S. Archer (Ed.), *Social morphogenesis* (Vol. 1). Dordrecht: Springer.
Donati, P. (2016). The relational understanding of the origin and morphogenetic change of social morality. In M. S. Archer (Ed.), *Morphogenesis and the crisis of normativity* (Vol. 4). Cham: Springer.
Donati, P., & Archer, M. S. (2015). *The relational subject*. Cambridge: Cambridge University Press.
Dunlap, R. E., & Brulle, R. J. (2015). *Climate change and society: Sociological perspectives*. Oxford University Press: Oxford.
Frankfurt, H. G. (1988). *The importance of what we care about: Philosophical essays*. Cambridge University Press.
Fuchs, C. (2008). *Internet and society: Social theory in the information age*. Abingdon: Routledge.
Giddens, A. (1979). *Central problems of sociological theory*. London: MacMillan.
Gorski, P. S. (2016). Reflexive secularity: Thoughts on the reflexive imperative in a secular age. In M. S. Archer (Ed.), *Morphogenesis and the crisis of normativity* (Vol. 4). Cham: Springer.
Gross, N. (2009). A pragmatist theory of social mechanisms. *American Sociological Review, 74*, 358–379.

Hartwig, M. (Ed.). (2007). *Dictionary of critical realism*. Abingdon: Routledge.
Hedström, P., & Swedberg, R. (Eds.). (1998). *Social mechanisms: An analytical approach to social theory*. Cambridge: Cambridge University Press.
House of Lords. (2011). House of lords, Library Note, LLN 2011/028.
Lawson, T. (2015). The modern corporation: The site of a mechanism (of global social change) that is out-of-control. In M. S. Archer (Ed.), *Generative mechanisms* (Vol. 3). Cham: Springer.
Lawson, T. (2016). Collective practices and norms. In M. S. Archer (Ed.), *Morphogenesis and the crisis of normativity* (Vol. 4). Cham: Springer.
Maccarini, A. (2014). The emergent social qualities of a 'morphogenic' society, cultures, structures, and forms of reflexivity. In M. S. Archer (Ed.), 2, *Late modernity.*
Maccarini, A. (2015). Turbulence and relational conjunctures: The emergence of morphogenic environments. In M. S. Archer, (Ed.), 3, *Generative mechanisms.*
Maruyama, M. (2003). Causal loops, interaction and creativity. *Int Rev Soc, 13*(3), 607–628.
Porpora, D. V. (2013). Morphogenesis and social change. In M. S. Archer (Ed.), *Social morphogenesis*. Dordrecht: Springer.
Porpora, D. V. (2015). *Reconstructing sociology: The critical realist approach*. Cambridge: Cambridge University Press.
Sayer, A. (2011). *Why things matter to people, social science, values and ethical life*. Cambridge: Cambridge University Press.
Teune, H., & Mlinar, Z. (1978). *The developmental logic of social systems*. Beverly Hills/London: Sage.
Vaughan, M., & Archer, M. S. (1971). *Social conflict and educational change in England and France, 17-89-1848*. Cambridge: Cambridge University Press.
Zamagni, S. (2008). Reciprocity, civil economy, common good. In M. S. Archer & P. Donati (Eds.), *Pursuing the common good: How solidarity and subsidiarity can work together*. Vatican City: Vatican City Press.

Chapter 2
Human Flourishing and Human Morphogenesis: A Critical Realist Interpretation and Critique

Philip Gorski

Critical Realists sometimes claim that social science has an axiological concern with "human flourishing." Indeed, in practice, social science does often seek to explain the social origins of human ill-being, exploitation and oppression. And behind this concern there usually is a tacit concern with human well-being, development and emancipation.

But what exactly do we mean by terms like "well-being", "development" and "emancipation"? Critical Realists have only recently begun to spell out an answer. In doing so, they have drawn heavily on Aristotle and the neo-Aristotelian tradition. Understandably so: after all, the phrase "human flourishing" first entered into Anglophone discourse as a translation of the Ancient Greek *eudaimonia.*

The goal of this essay is to elaborate a theory of human flourishing that is broadly compatible with the meta-theory of Critical Realism, if not exclusively derived from it. This theory builds on five concepts that are constitutive of critical realism and distinguish it from rival meta-theories: ontological stratification, emergent powers, actualism, absence and spirituality. I will argue that Critical Realism has strong affinities with a vision of human flourishing that is: (1) pluralistic rather than monistic; (2) substantive rather than formal; (3) developmental rather than experiential; (4) egalitarian rather than elitist; and (5) transcendental rather than immanent.

Aristotle's ethics provides a good starting point for developing a pluralistic, substantive and developmental view of flourishing. But contemporary neo-Aristotelianism can – and sometimes does – take a tacitly elitist and radically immanentist view of flourishing that is at odds with Critical Realism. These tendencies are particularly evident in contemporary philosophies of transhumanism

P. Gorski (✉)
Department of Sociology, Yale University, 493 College Street, New Haven, CT 06520, USA
e-mail: philip.gorski@yale.edu

M.S. Archer (ed.), *Morphogenesis and Human Flourishing*, Social Morphogenesis,
DOI 10.1007/978-3-319-49469-2_2

and posthumanism. Critical Realists can counter these tendencies by drawing on other threads of the neo-Aristotelian tradition, including Hegel and Marx but also Nussbaum and Sen.

In the conclusion, I reflect on the implications of transhumanism for critical realist metaethics and the morphogenic society.

Human Flourishing I: Aristotelian Foundations

The term "human flourishing" is just one of the possible translations of the ancient Greek term "*eudaimonia.*" "Well-being" and "happiness" are sometimes used as well. The difficulty with the latter terms lies in their modern-day connotations. "Well-being" evokes a *passive physical state,* while "happiness" suggests *positive emotional experiences.* Aristotle himself was emphatic that *eudaimonia* is more than just well-being and pleasure.

The etymology of the term also points beyond any purely hedonistic or utilitarian reading. *Eu* means "good" and *daemon* means "spirit", so to be "eu-daemon" literally means to be "of good spirit." Eudaimonia is not just physical or psychological in the modern senses of those terms. It is something more. These are some of the reasons why many neo-Aristotelians believe that "human flourishing" is the best rendering of eudaimonia.

On its own, the word "flourishing" highlights the ways in which all life forms are similar to one another (Foot 2001; Kraut 2007). After all, human beings are not the only beings that can "flourish." One can just as easily apply the term to non-human animals or even to non-sentient life forms such as plants. It makes perfect sense to speak of a flourishing herd of dairy cows or a flourishing field of sunflowers. Flourishing is not specific to humans then; it pertains to all manner of living beings. So, another advantage of the flourishing concept is that it captures the naturalistic cast of Aristotle's philosophy.

Adding the word "human" highlights the ways in which the flourishing of human beings differs from that of other living creatures. While humans, cows and flowers can all flourish in their own ways they do not flourish in precisely the same ways. For example, a dairy cow that was constantly confined to a small wooden box could not easily flourish, even if it were exposed to sunlight and regularly fed. Biological research confirms this (Moberg 2000). But a sunflower could certainly thrive under such conditions. Similarly, a human being who was deprived of all conversation with its kind could not easily flourish, even if it were cared for in other ways. Imagine the effects if your friends, family, and colleagues subjected you to a "silent treatment" for an extended period. So, flourishing means different things for different kinds of living beings.

Does this mean that flourishing is a one-size-fits-all proposition for all those of the same kind? Do all members of the same kind flourish in just the same way? Plato seems to have thought so. His Academy defined *eudaimonia* as: "The good composed of all goods; an ability which suffices for living well; perfection in respect of virtue; resources sufficient for a living creature" (Plato 1997, p. 1676). The unity of the good stipulated in this definition does seem more logical than practical, insofar as it requires both "virtue" and "resources." Still, Plato is clear that the highest way of life is the life of the philosopher and that other forms of life are to be judged by the degree to which they approach that ideal. Non-philosophers may flourish to some degree, but not to the same degree as the philosopher. In short, Plato's vision of the human good was ultimately monistic.

Aristotle himself seems considerably more ambivalent (Aristotle 2000; Kraut 1989; Lear 1988). Like Plato, he firmly rejects a hedonistic account of *eudaimonia* and holds up the philosopher's vocation as a model of the good life. However, Aristotle also suggests that the life of politics may be equally good. Nor does he subordinate politics to philosophy as Plato does with the figure of the philosopher-king. He thereby opens the door to a pluralistic understanding of human flourishing, in which human beings can flourish in different ways and to the same degree. To be sure, it is a limited pluralism that identifies speech and reason as the distinctive powers of human beings and politics and philosophy as the highest activities. But it is a pluralistic vision nonetheless.

It should be clear by now why Aristotle would reject the modern-day folk theory that equates human happiness with positive emotion: because emotion is not one of the higher capacities that sets humans apart from animals. A dog or a cat can also experience positive emotion, as any pet owner well knows. But why would Aristotle reject the view of *eudaimonia* as "well-being"? Because flourishing is not a passive state of being; it involves *activity*, and in the case of human beings, *rational* activity. It is important to stress that this activity need not be physical; on Aristotle's definition, philosophizing would also count as a form of activity and, indeed, as a way of life (Hadot 1995). Nor is rationality necessarily philosophical; building a house would also count as a form of rationality. Indeed, for Aristotle, it is a paradigmatic model of rationality, insofar as it involves a skillful use of means towards certain ends.

Human flourishing also has social preconditions. On the Aristotelian view, the good life is only possible in a particular kind of human community, namely, a free state such as the Athenian Republic (Aristotle 1982, 1996). But free in what sense? Once again, it is important to distinguish Aristotle's position from the common wisdom of modern-day liberals. In the liberal tradition that begins with Hobbes and Locke, freedom is re-defined as non-interference: a person is free so long as she is not being physically coerced or actively hindered in formulating and executing her choices (Pettit 1997; Skinner 1998). But what if these choices are bad ones? Contemporary liberalism *à la* John Rawls simply refuses this question. It insists that a liberal polity must be neutral with respect to all questions about the human good (Rawls 2005). Political liberals presume that we cannot know anything about what is good for a particular person, much less for human beings more generally. The most that a liberal state can and should do is secure certain legal immunities for, and institutional relations between persons. Whether a person has the resources and infrastructure they need to make good decisions or execute personal plans is a matter of justice, not freedom. This is why Rawls and other "political liberals" follow Kant in arguing that the right is prior to the good.

"Freedom means being left alone and doing what you like": this is probably more or less how most citizens of Western liberal democracies would now define the term. But this is not how contemporary neo-Aristotelians understand freedom. Like Aristotle himself, they understand human freedom as skillful or rational activity (Nussbaum 2011; Sen 1999). From this perspective, individual rights might be seen as a helpful protection for individual freedom. But just as important would be access to the resources and infrastructure needed to develop skills and engage in activities. The fact that one is formally free to learn the piano or play football does not mean that one has the opportunity or skill to do so. That requires access to an instrument and lessons or a field and a coach. Aristotelians advance a substantive definition of freedom.

A liberal understanding of freedom often goes together with a utilitarian understanding of well-being. This understanding is experiential and aggregative. In the classical utilitarianism of the Benthamite school, individual utility is a simple of sum of pleasures minus pains (Bentham 2000). Pleasure and pain are understood in terms of bodily experience, be it physical or emotional. In the neo-classical utilitarianism of contemporary economics, individual utility is a function of individual preferences. Preferences are understood in terms of subjective desires, which are treated as irrational matters of taste (Becker 1996). In both cases, the sequencing of a person's experiences or the shape of a person's life are irrelevant to calculating their overall well-being. By this calculus, a person who spent their entire life hooked up to a pleasure machine that stimulated positive emotions or simulated desire fulfillment would be said to have lived a good life.[1] Similarly, a financier who achieved all the wealth and acclaim he aspired to, only be to exposed as a fraud and a liar upon retirement, would also be said to have lived well. Would Bernie Madoff and his family agree? It seems doubtful.

Such conclusions are at odds with common sense and also with a neo-Aristotelian account of flourishing. The neo-Aristotelian understanding of well-being is developmental, rather than experiential. From this perspective, flourishing arises out of activity. Psychological research supports this claim (Csikszentmihalyi 1996; Seligman 2012). From this perspective, a lifetime of passive pleasure spent hooked up to a machine would not be accounted a happy one. Similarly, the happy life has a coherent shape. It is not just a sum; it has a form. This is why Aristotle famously quipped that one could not know whether a person had led a happy life until after they were dead. In part, this was because the final judgment about a person' happiness is made by one's peers. But it is also because that judgment is based on the narrative arc of that life (Bruner 1987; Ricoeur 1991). Just as the final chapter of a novel can turn comedy into tragedy, so the final years of a person's life can transform an apparent success into a manifest failure. Of course the plot of a life

[1] This premise is explored in at least two science fiction movies: "The Matrix" and "Vanilla Sky."

has to do with the shape of its sub-plots. A person who becomes highly skilled at a particular activity – high finance, for example – but remains stunted in a more vital area – practical reasoning, say – may ultimately fail at life.

Human Flourishing II: Critical Realist Foundations and Elaborations

Critical realists come in many varieties: scientific and theological, Marxist and Thomist and so on. However, most strands of Critical Realism share an Aristotelian lineage. Thus, it should not be surprising that the Aristotelian view of human flourishing is easily translated into the language of Critical Realism. At the same time, Critical Realism also makes it possible to reconstruct certain elements of the Aristotelian view that are rightly regarded as politically or scientifically problematic, such as its inegalitarian implications and its biological foundations. In this section, I argue that Critical Realism leads to a view of human flourishing that is pluralistic, substantive, and developmental but also egalitarian and altruistic.

In a recent book on human personhood, sociologist Christian Smith uses the Critical Realist account of emergence to argue that human beings have as many as thirty distinctive capacities (Smith 2010). At the ground level of the human animal are two "existence capacities": "conscious awareness" and "subconscious being." These give rise to "primary experience capacities" such as "mental representation" and "volition" which in turn give rise to "secondary experience capacities" such as "intersubjective understanding" and "interest formation." From these there emerge "creating capacities" such as "language use" and "identity formation." The highest order capacities include "love", "aesthetic enjoyment" and "moral judgment." One can quibble with Smith's schema. One could argue that the list is too long, as some of his critics have.[2]

One might therefore prefer Martha Nussbaum's more parsimonious list of ten basic capacities instead (Nussbaum 2006). Or one could argue that some of these capacities are not specific to human beings. There is good reason to believe that other intelligent mammals such as dolphins are capable of language use and even practical reasoning (MacIntyre 1999). However, if we accept the premise that human beings are characterized by a high degree of (internal) ontological stratification, it then follows that they will also have an irreducible plurality of capacities many of which build on and emerge out of others. Nor would one need to evoke Aristotle's metaphysical biology to sustain this claim. Modern science provides plenty of evidence for it. There is little doubt that certain kinds of brain damage lead to certain

[2]In a subsequent book, Smith argues that human beings have six basic needs related to: "body", "knowledge", "integrity", "agency", "morality" and "sociality." However, these are inductively derived from existing research on human well-being and are not systematically grounded in his account of human personhood. See (Smith 2015).

kinds of incapacitation (e.g., an inability to make decisions) (Sacks 1998); that certain kinds of psychological ailments lead to other kinds of incapacitation (e.g., the psychopath's inability to feel empathy) (Baron-Cohen 2012); and that certain kinds of social deprivation lead to still other sorts of incapacitation (e.g., an inability to reason abstractly). In sum, an ontologically stratified view of human personhood points towards a view of human capacities, and thus of human flourishing, that is both pluralistic and hierarchical.

Critical Realism also has strong affinities with a developmental account of flourishing. In the "basic critical realism" of Roy Bhaskar, for example, a clear distinction is drawn between the "real", the "actual" and the "empirical" (Bhaskar 1997, 1998). The level of the real includes all structures or mechanisms, regardless of whether they are active or inactive, observable or non-observable. A key implication of Basic Critical Realism is that human persons and human societies will have underlying structures that are real, but not (yet) actual, because they have not yet been triggered.[3] A further implication is that human flourishing will not always be directly observable. In Bhaskar's dialectical critical realism, this insight is expressed somewhat differently, in the claim that the real is not exhausted by the present, by that which exists here or now; it includes absence as well (Bhaskar 1993, 1994, 2000). In other words, human persons and societies may have certain latent potentials whose development has been suppressed and whose absence manifests in ill-being. A more sociological version of this argument may be found in the M/M explanatory framework of Margaret Archer and more specifically in her theory of "Personal Emergent Powers" (Archer 2000, 2003). Archer argues that the capacity for intellectual reflexivity is developmentally dependent upon the capacity for "internal conversation" which is in turn dependent upon the capacity for abstract speech and so on. Further, Archer insists that individual action must be understood in relation to life plans, which are typically expressed in narrative form (Archer 2010). Of course, such plans and projections can go well or ill and may lead to faltering as well as flourishing. The crucial point, however, is this: a flourishing life is neither experienced nor lived as a disconnected series of discrete experiences. It has a shape or form that is itself (partly) the product of reflexivity and the internal conversation.

Given the influence of Aristotle, Hegel and Marx on Critical Realism, it is no surprise that Critical Realism would prove highly resistant to a purely formal definition of human freedom. The political thrust of Critical Realism has always been Social Democratic and/or Communitarian. On this view, human freedom has material as well as legal preconditions. Plainly put, most forms of human activity require access to some level of material resources. These resources might take the form of money. But they might also consist in infrastructure or artifacts required for certain activities, such as a musical instrument or a football pitch. Absent this access, and the underlying capacities (e.g., athletic or musical) cannot be activated.

[3]Note that this is quite similar to Martha Nussbaum's distinction between (real) "capacities" and (actualized) "functions" (Nussbaum 2011).

Of course, human freedom also has social preconditions that go beyond the strictly material. Because human beings are born helpless and remain vulnerable to illness and injury throughout their lives, it is vital that others be ready to care for them. Further, because human beings are inherently social, and cannot flourish without developing enduring and positive relationships with other people, it is vital that they live in stable communities. Needless to say, this is not always and everywhere the case. Indeed, in a morphogenetic society, the cultural preconditions of human flourishing may be seriously endangered, not because of a lack of material resources but due to the destabilization of human families and communities resulting from rapid and intensive social change and population movements.

One of the less appealing features of Aristotle's ethics, at least for citizens of modern liberal democracies, is its patently inegalitarian character (Aristotle 1982). Aristotle regards "barbarians" (i.e., non-Greeks) as unfit for life in the polis because their powers of speech are inadequate (i.e., they do not speak Greek). Women are likewise barred from citizenship because they are supposedly lacking in reason. Slaves he regards as slaves "by nature." They must be governed by others because they are unable to govern themselves. At the pinnacle of this pyramid is the free, Greek man. He, alone, is able to participate in public life, manage a private household and rule over other, lesser men and over women and children.

As a form of ethical naturalism, which bases its ethical postulates on naturalistic foundations, Critical Realism has an easy answer to this problem: the factual premises of Aristotle's ethics have been scientifically disproven. We now know that women are the intellectual equals of men; that the intellectual "backwardness" of slaves is due to a lack of education; and that human languages are functionally equivalent in most respects. (That children need supervision by their parents and other adults seems equally clear, though a few would dispute this.)

This argument is sufficient to rebut claims about natural inequality based on sex, ethnicity and class; but Aristotle's ethics can also be read in a more "meritocratic" fashion that authorizes a natural aristocracy based on biological endowments. On this argument, first formulated by Nietzsche and then elaborated by modern libertarians, some individuals are superior to others by nature (Nietzsche 2008; Rand and Branden 1965). (Today, we would be more apt to say that they are "genetically" superior.) These individuals have a wider range and higher level of human powers. It is a law of nature that they should rule over and even prey upon others. Their relationship to the masses of humanity is like that of wolves to sheep. Ultimately, they are destined to overcome their humanity altogether, to become "supermen" or, in modern parlance, "transhumans."

There is no shortage of counter-arguments. There is the theological argument that humans beings are fundamentally equal because they are made in the image of God (Waldron 2002). There is also the Kantian argument that human beings qua rational agents are inherently deserving of equal respect (Kant and Gregor 1998). Martha Nussbaum has now given the Kantian argument an Aristotelian twist. She contends that human persons are deserving of equal respect because they all possess a basic level of human capacities.

Nussbaum's argument may be sufficient to ground the claim that all healthy and fully-abled people should be treated as equals. But what of those who lack or lose key capacities due to disablement, injury or illness? Are they also deserving of equal respect? Alasdair MacIntyre supplies an answer (MacIntyre 1999). All human beings are also dependent and vulnerable *by nature*. More than any other animal offspring, human infants are born helpless and in need of care if they are to survive and thrive. Human adults remain physically vulnerable; they all experience incidents of injury and illness, particularly as they grow older. To do well, then, humans must be able to give and receive care from others. Thus, one of the cardinal virtues of human beings is what MacIntyre calls "acknowledged dependence."

Of course, many people are unable to recognize this state of dependence or unwilling to acknowledge it. As Durkheim recognized long ago, the problem is especially acute in modern societies with their highly elaborated divisions of labor (Durkheim 1933, 1958). The problem is that relations of social dependency do not necessarily lead to feelings of moral obligation. Modern societies do have several mechanisms for addressing this problem. The first is nationalism, which expands traditional notions of fictive kinship to the national community. The problem with this solution, of course, is that feelings of national solidarity are often sustained through the demonization of national "others" and through the idolization of national leaders. Xenophobic and patriarchal nationalisms of this sort are irreconcilable with a civic and democratic polity. The second is markets, which use self-interest as a means of coordinating action amongst anonymous parties. The problem with this solution, as we've learned again and again, is that free markets are not, in fact, "self-regulating"; they require state regulation as well. As Polanyi long ago saw, the idea of the self-regulating market is a self-undermining one (Polanyi 2001). Barring that, they will not operate efficiently, to say nothing of fairly. Durkheim himself proposed various remedies for this problem. One was to organize "national festivals", ritual commemorations of founding ideals (Durkheim 2001). Another was to organize citizens into corporate bodies based on occupational categories. The late work of Roy Bhaskar suggests a third means: spiritual experiences of self-transcendence (Bhaskar 2002). Indeed, for Bhaskar self-transcendence and acknowledged dependence were the defining features of spiritual experience.[4] Of course, those who undergo such experiences may understand them in religious or secular terms as well. In an increasingly morphogenetic society, characterized by high degrees of geographical mobility and labor market "flexibility", the old solutions of national and occupational solidarity, spiritual experiences of this sort may become an increasingly vital source of moral motivation and civic solidarity.

[4]For a similar view from a pragmatist standpoint, see also (Joas 2000).

Human Morphogenesis: The Transhumanist Challenge

Critical Realists have long been sensitive to the various ways in which social morphogenesis may impede human flourishing. Inspired by Marxian critiques of capitalism, early Critical Realism emphasized the alienation and ill-being that resulted from neoliberal reforms and the "market society." In the present juncture, Critical Realists remain concerned with the disruptions and dysfunctions caused by the globalization of neo-liberalism and market fundamentalism. The most obvious and consequential result of these developments has been the massive growth of economic inequality between and within nations over the last three to four decades. Billions of people are deprived of the basic resources and infrastructure they need to develop and flourish (Collier 2008). What is more, the globalization of the market has also weakened or severed many people's ties to kin and place, rendering them more physically and psychologically vulnerable than ever before. Meanwhile, capitalist exploitation of the natural environment has sparked a process of climate change that will lead to resource conflicts and population movements of unprecedented scale (Klare 2001)– indeed, it is already doing so.

However, with a few exceptions (Vandenberghe 2004, 2014), Critical Realists have paid little attention to another implication of the morphogenetic turn: the prospect of human morphogenesis. The decoding of the human genome and technical advances in genetics open up the possibility – perhaps the probability – that human beings will soon be able to clone their bodies, customize their offspring, upgrade their "wetware", replace worn-out body parts and, in general, to alter and/or enhance their bodily capacities. Similarly, the encoding of human cognition and the development of artificial intelligence holds out the promise of "hardware" upgrades to human "wetware" and perhaps even the emergence of self-reproducing and continually evolving forms of machine "life." Indeed, all of this is already happening, if not (yet) at the level envisioned by the prophets of transhumanism. Would-be parents use selective abortion and/or genetic testing to choose the sex of their offspring. Smart phones function as memory-enhancing prosthetic devices. Voice recognition software learns its users' vocal patterns. And so on. Tranhumanists may be overselling the scientific possibilities but they are not hawking science fiction.

Just who are the transhumanists (Elliott 2003; Hughes 2012)? Their intellectual leaders most often hale from the fields of science and engineering. As a result, they tend to be optimistic technophiles. Their political leaders usually lean towards libertarian views. Consequently, they are highly resistant to regulations and restrictions on the new technologies. Institutionally, they are most often housed in independent research institutes and think tanks, bankrolled by corporate managers and wealthy entrepreneurs. (Though a few have now managed to set up shop at respected universities as well). Conspicuous by their absence are humanists and social scientists, traditional conservatives or social democrats, and representatives from the helping professions and services.

How should Critical Realists respond to the transhumanist project? Intellectually, they should join other humanistic and social scientific intellectuals in pressing back against the naïve optimism of the transhumanist prophets. Perhaps because of their training in natural and applied science, most transhumanists seem blind to the potentially inegalitarian and dystopian implications of human morphogenesis. They seem quite unaware of how the conjuncture of genetic and technical enhancement with massive inequalities in wealth could lead to new forms of enslavement rather than new levels of emancipation. If the wealthy are able to afford the new enhancements, and perhaps even monopolize them, the result will be a deepening and even a re-naturalization of social class, rather than some sort of universal emancipation from biological constraints. In feudalism and other historic systems of aristocratic domination, the ruling classes often represented themselves as members of a higher race. And they may well have appeared as such to their subjects. Ready access to protein and time for vigorous exercise meant that aristocrats were often much taller and stronger than ordinary people. Likewise, (now) rudimentary "enhancements" such as cosmetic adornments, plastic surgery and colorful clothing will have reinforced this impression. A transhumanist future holds the prospect of a re-biologization and radical technologization of class inequality. It is not at all difficult to imagine a cognitively, physically, aesthetically and emotionally enhanced ruling class that maintains a massive underclass of servants and laborers in perpetual thralldom.

If the neo-Nietzschean prophets seem blithely unaware of what might happen when human enhancement meets up with capitalist markets, they appear equally obtuse about the potential conjunction between transhumanism and militarism. The enhancements they typically imagine are precisely the enhancements that an intellectual would fantasize about: heightened capacities for complex thinking, aesthetic experience, moral empathy and sexual pleasure. But why should human enhancements go in this particular direction? Why imagine the transhuman as a super-geek? What about heightened capacities for physical violence, spatial orientation, emotional deception and muscular development? This is how a 'defense' intellectual might envision a transhuman, namely, as a super-soldier instead of a super-geek. Indeed, defense agencies in Western countries are already planning for this future right now (McIntosh 2010).

The transhumanist community also seems unaware of the basic principles of social demography. Transhumanists wax delirious about the prospect of increased longevity, of lifespans measured in centuries instead of decades. But the massive declines in mortality rates that they envision would have equally massive effects on population structure. If current population levels are already pressing against a new set of Malthusian restraints set by natural resources, how much greater the pressure if the normal human lifespan were doubled or tripled. Of course, population size could be stabilized via radically lower birth rates. However, this would mean that many people would have to renounce reproduction altogether. Now, some citizens of affluent societies are already doing so voluntarily. Still, would a society in which the getting and raising of children was a privilege reserved for a minority be a thriving one? Nor is this the only reason to be somewhat skeptical about the overall effects of extended longevity on human flourishing. While many transhumanists espouse an Aristotelian cum Nietzschen view of human flourishing, their arguments about life extension are often based on a utilitarian calculus: longer life equals more experiences, and more experiences equal more utility. Obviously, things are not this simple as this. On the Aristotelian account, at least, the goodness of a life has as much to do with its shape as its length. There is no reason to believe that a longer life will always be a better life.

Morphogenesis and Metaethics

Over the course of 5 years and five books, participants in this project have discussed and debated Margaret Archer's "morphogenic society" question. Are morphogenetic mechanisms of social change effectively swamping morphostatic mechanisms of social reproduction? Certainly, the morphogenetic thesis resonates with subjective perceptions of social churn. Many of us feel as if all that is solid has already melted into air, and that the air itself no longer blows in any predictable direction.

There can be little doubt that the speculation about a coming morphogenic society corresponds to something in our lived experience, where by "our" I understand all of humanity and not just "we" Westerners. Global migrations, new technologies, "flexible" work, welfare retrenchment – morophogenesis is not just a figment of our imaginations. Still, at least two questions remain. (1) Is the present conjuncture just a brief interlude that will eventually give rise to a new era of stability? (2) Are the upheavals of our age really more severe than those of past ages, such as the early twentieth century or the early modern era? Both questions will take time to answer.

Certainly, one thing that is qualitatively new about our era is the prospect of *human* morphogenesis. Of course, human beings have been intentionally altering the macro- and surface-level properties of their bodies for millennia (e.g., by means of physical training and cosmetic decoration). And they have unintentionally altered the inner functioning and composition of their bodies as well through dietary changes (e.g., milk and glutens) and medical interventions (e.g., antibiotics). What is new today is the real prospect of intentional transformations at the genetic and neuro-electrical levels.

Should human morphogenesis become a social reality, social theory itself will undergo a radical morphogenesis. Again, we must not overstate the magnitude of the shift. Human beings as we know them have long been "cultural" and "social constructs." Individual identity has always and ever been cultural. Culture provides the material out of which we construct our identities. Outside a form of life, our lives would be formless. Inventorying and explaining cultural variations of this sort has long been a staple of social research. We now know that we are also "social constructs" in a truly biological sense. The burgeoning field of social epigenetics has begun documenting the influence of social conditions on our genetic make up. Evidently, genetic scripts have switches that can be turned on and off, with the position of the switch itself being a potentially heritable trait. We are all Lamarckians again.

Since its birth in the mid-nineteenth century, the social sciences have tacitly treated human beings as a kind of ontological bedrock on which social theories are constructed. To be sure, they have differed as to how soft and malleable a type of rock human nature is, with cultural anthropologists treating it like chalk and psychologists making it out as granite. But all the social sciences have taken "human actors" as an ontological given.

They will no longer be able to do in an age of human morphogenesis, at least not the degree they have they done until now. What if personal genetics is rendered a slave to fashion, alterable at the drop of a credit card? What if a human cloning becomes another form of "total makeover"? Hitherto hyperbolic language about "human self-fashioning" and the "construction of the body" may be rendered insufficient to describe the changes.

Of course, the challenges that would follow on the realization of radical morphogenesis of the human species would go well beyond social theory. They would extend to human ethics as well.

There has been a great deal of debate amongst professional philosophers in recent years about the relative merits of various ethical systems. The systems in question are three in number: (1) "deontological ethics" such as Immanuel Kant's which focus on moral duties; (2) "utilitarian ethics" such as Jeremy Bentham's which focus on the greatest good for the greatest number; and (3) "virtue ethics" in the Aristotelian tradition which focus on personal character. This debate has given rise to a new field: "meta-ethics."

One of the central questions that has vexed meta-ethicists is whether any or all of these systems are fully sufficient or whether they need to be combined in some fashion. For example, it has been argued that deontological ethics are too rationalistic to motivate right action for all but a handful of individuals and too absolutist to generate appropriate conduct in many situations. Who but a high-minded philosopher could really feel the full moral force of the categorical imperative for example? And aren't there situations where that force is better resisted – when it might be appropriate to shade the truth or even lie when it is the lesser of two evils? It has likewise been argued that utilitarian ethics is based on a faulty anthropology. Isn't moderation often a better recipe for fulfillment than maximization, for instance? And doesn't avoiding pain sometimes prevent growth? These are the sorts of questions that proponents of virtue ethics have often directed at their meta-ethical rivals.

The intellectual affinity of transhumanist ideologues for human flourishing raises troubling questions about the intellectual sufficiency of virtue ethics more generally. If the human good consists in the development of human powers, why not embrace technological means for expanding or enhancing those powers? If human freedom consists in the skillful exercise of human powers, then on what grounds could one prohibit such enhancements? Providing a strong response to these questions may require that we go beyond a focus on human flourishing per se.

Some forms of biological manipulation are objectionable on grounds of human dignity and human rights. For example, one could argue that cloning oneself violates the rights of the clone. Insofar as the clone is expected to replicate or extend the personhood of the cloner, the clone is not being treated as a separate person that is an end unto her- or himself. The same could be said about putative enhancements to minor children affected by their parents or other authorities. The child does not yet have the moral or intellectual capacity to make this decision himself and should not be deprived of a say in the matter.

But what about biological modifications that are voluntarily chosen by a mature adult? In this case, a counter-argument based on dignity or rights is not readily available. Instead, one might appeal to social ethics and political values. One might argue that certain forms of human inequality are so disruptive to the social order that they can be legitimately prohibited. For example, one might outlaw certain forms of physical enhancement on more or less the same grounds that most developed countries prohibit private citizens from carrying or even owning certain kinds of weapons: the harms that would follow from their misuse – and the near inevitability of such misuse – is simply too great to tolerate. Similarly, one might argue that other forms of human enhancement are so threatening to the political order that a community is justified in restricting them as well. A heightened capacity for dissimulation or a lowered level of empathy might well fit this description. It would make representative government even more subject to manipulation.

The concept of human flourishing has been attractive to critical realists, because it grounds a naturalistic and non-relativistic form of ethics. But the prospects that human nature itself may soon be subject to fundamental alteration suggests that a *critical* realism may need to borrow resources from non-naturalistic systems of ethics. It may need to draw on "critique" in the Kantian sense of an unconditional commitment to the dignity of the human person.

References

Archer, M. (2000). *Being human: The problem of agency*. New York: Cambridge University Press.

Archer, M. (2003). *Structure, agency and the internal conversation*. Cambridge, MA/New York: Cambridge University Press.

Archer, M. (2010). Routine, reflexivity, and realism*. *Sociological Theory, 28*(3), 272–303.

Aristotle. (1982). *The politics* (T. J. Saunders & T. A. Sinclair, Eds.). London: Penguin.

Aristotle. (1996). *The politics and the constitution of Athens* (S. Everson, Ed.). Cambridge, MA: Cambridge University Press.

Aristotle. (2000). *Nichomachean ethics* (R. Crisp, Trans.). New York: Cambridge University Press.

Baron-Cohen, S. (2012). *The science of evil: On empathy and the origins of cruelty*. New York: Basic books.

Becker, G. S. (1996). *Accounting for tastes*. Cambridge, MA: Harvard University Press.

Bentham, J. (2000). *An introduction to the principles of morals and legislation* Retrieved from http://site.ebrary.com/lib/yale/Doc?id=2001956

Bhaskar, R. (1993). *Dialectic: The pulse of freedom*. London/New York: Verso.

Bhaskar, R. (1994). *Plato etc.: The problems of philosophy and their resolution*. London/New York: Verso.
Bhaskar, R. (1997). *A realist theory of science*. London/New York: Verso.
Bhaskar, R. (1998). *The possibility of naturalism: A philosophical critique of the contemporary human sciences*. London: Routledge.
Bhaskar, R. (2000). *From east to west: Odyssey of a soul*. London/New York: Routledge.
Bhaskar, R. (2002). *Meta-reality: The philosophy of meta-reality*. New Delhi/Thousand Oaks: Sage Publications.
Bruner, J. (1987). Life as narrative. *Social Research, 54,* 11–32.
Collier, P. (2008). *The bottom billion: Why the poorest countries are failing and what can be done about it*. Oxford: Oxford University Press.
Csikszentmihalyi, M. (1996). *Flow and the psychology of discovery and invention*. New York: Harper Collins.
Durkheim, E. (1933). *The division of labor in society*. New York/London: Free Press/Collier Macmillan.
Durkheim, E. (1958). *Professional ethics and civic morals*. Glencoe: Free Press.
Durkheim, E. (2001). *The elementary forms of religious life*, trans. Carol Closman, abridged with an intro. and notes by Mark S. Cladis. Oxford/New York: Oxford University Press.
Elliott, C. (2003). Humanity 2.0. *Wilson Quarterly, 27*(4), 13–20.
Foot, P. (2001). *Natural goodness*. Oxford: Oxford University Press.
Hadot, P. (1995). *Philosophy as a way of life: Spiritual exercises from Socrates to Foucault*. Malden: Blackwell.
Hughes, J. J. (2012). The politics of transhumanism and the techno-millennial imagination 1626–2030. *Zygon, 47*(4), 757–776. doi:10.1111/j.1467-9744.2012.01289.x.
Joas, H. (2000). *The genesis of values*. Cambridge, MA: Polity Press.
Kant, I., & Gregor, M. J. (1998). *Groundwork of the metaphysics of morals*. Cambridge, MA/New York: Cambridge University Press.
Klare, M. (2001). *Resource wars: The new landscape of global conflict*. New York: Macmillan.
Kraut, R. (1989). *Aristotle on the human good*. Princeton: Princeton University Press.
Kraut, R. (2007). *What is good and why: The ethics of well-being*. Cambridge, MA: Harvard University Press.
Lear, J. (1988). *Aristotle: The desire to understand*. New York: Cambridge University Press.
MacIntyre, A. C. (1999). *Dependent rational animals: Why human beings need the virtues*. Chicago: Open Court.
McIntosh, D. (2010). The transhuman security dilemma. *Journal of Evolution and Technology, 21*(2), 32–48.
Moberg, G. (2000). Biological response to stress: Implications for animal welfare. In *The biology of animal stress: Basic principles and implications for animal welfare* (pp. 1–21). Wallingford: CABI Publication.
Nietzsche, F. (2008). *Thus spoke Zarathustra* (R. Pippin, Ed., A. D. Caro, Trans.) New York: Cambridge University Press.
Nussbaum, M. C. (2006). *Frontiers of justice: Disability, nationality, species membership*. Cambridge, MA: The Belknap Press, Harvard University Press.
Nussbaum, M. C. (2011). *Creating capabilities: The human development approach*. Cambridge, MA: Harvard University Press.
Pettit, P. (1997). *Republicanism: A theory of freedom and government*. New York: Oxford University Press.
Plato. (1997). *Complete works* (J. M. Cooper & D. Hutchinson, Eds.). Indianapolis: Hackett.
Polanyi, K. (2001). *The great transformation: The political and economic origins of our time* (2nd Beacon Paperback, Ed.). Boston: Beacon Press.
Rand, A., & Branden, N. (1965). *The virtue of selfishness*. New York: New American Library.
Rawls, J. (2005). *Political liberalism* (Expanded, Ed.). New York: Columbia University Press.
Ricoeur, P. (1991). Life in quest of narrative. In *On Paul Ricoeur: Narrative and interpretation* (pp. 20–33). London: Routledge.

Sacks, O. (1998). *The man who mistook his wife for a hat: And other clinical tales*. New York: Simon and Schuster.
Seligman, M. E. P. (2012). *Flourish: A visionary new understanding of happiness and well-being*. New York: Simon and Schuster.
Sen, A. K. (1999). *Development as freedom*. Oxford: Oxford University Press.
Skinner, Q. (1998). *Liberty before liberalism*. Cambridge, MA/New York: Cambridge University Press.
Smith, C. (2010). *What is a person?: Rethinking humanity, social life, and the moral good from the person up*. Chicago: University of Chicago Press.
Smith, C. (2015). *To flourish or destruct*. Chicago/London: University of Chicago Press.
Vandenberghe, F. (2004). Posthumanism, or the cultural logic of global neo-capitalism. *Complexitiés du posthumanisme: Pour une critique de la bio-économiquepolitique, 24–25*, 55–132.
Vandenberghe, F. (2014). *What's critical about critical realism?* London: Routledge.
Waldron, J. (2002). *God, Locke, and equality: Christian foundations in Locke's political thought*. New York: Cambridge University Press.

Chapter 3
Some Reservations About Flourishing

Douglas V. Porpora

When Tony Lawson emails me, he often asks whether I am flourishing. I usually respond, Not particularly. Actually, in contrast with Tony himself, I am not altogether comfortable with the word flourishing. In this paper, I work through my reasons why. In the end, I still do come down in support of the general move toward flourishing as an agenda for social science research but with qualification. I hope what I have to say will at least deepen understanding of flourishing even for those who remain untouched by my particular ambivalence.[1]

I expressed my ambivalence to Phil Gorski when our workshop ended last year, settling on flourishing as the topic for our current volume. Phil looked at me quizzically and showed me on the Internet Chris Smith's (2015) then new book *To Flourish or Self-Destruct*. Yes, I said, I already knew of the book and strongly support it. I just have reservations about flourishing as a designation.

Among critical realists, I seem alone in this regard. Besides Christian Smith, others too are writing about flourishing. Andrew Sayer (2011) speaks of flourishing in *Why Things Matter to People*. The concept is central to Roy Bhaskar's (2012) approach to meta-reality, and in that capacity has been adopted by Alan Norrie

---

[1]My thinking has definitely changed as a result of feedback I received at the workshop and from comments from Ruth Groff, Alan Norrie, and Christian Smith. As changes in thought will be reflected in a subsequent paper I am preparing for a subsequent Templeton workshop in flourishing, I am leaving this paper in the more provocative form in which it was originally presented. I will, however, indicate some initial responses to comments in footnotes. I will continue to be reflecting on them.

D.V. Porpora (✉)
Department of Anthropology, Drexel University, 3141 Chestnut Street, Philadelphia, PA, 19104, USA
e-mail: porporad@drexel.edu

M.S. Archer (ed.), *Morphogenesis and Human Flourishing*, Social Morphogenesis,
DOI 10.1007/978-3-319-49469-2_3

(2012). Phil Gorski (2013) himself has likewise written a defense of flourishing as a topic in social science.

Partly, in speaking of flourishing, all of the above initiatives are attempts to introduce values and morality into social science, which on a positivist and even Weberian line is enjoined to be value-free. With regard to the attempt to overturn value-neutral discourse, I am unequivocally in support of my comrades. I, too, think that morals and values ought to play a greater role in the social sciences.

It is just the word flourishing that discomforts me. It is not that I want people not to flourish. I certainly do not want people to languish or self-destruct.

So is my issue just semantic? Do I just not like that word as if I might also have some idiosyncratic aversion to the word "but"? I am not bothered just by the word, which as words go, is quite fine. I have no problem with talk of whether the tomatoes are flourishing this year. It is not as if flourishing were a trigger, prompting me automatically as in an old Vaudeville skit into an obsessive rant like, "Slowly, I turned . . ."

What discomforts me is talk of flourishing as an ultimate human end or ultimate concern – either personally or collectively. Personally, it does not identify what I consider my ultimate concern and therefore does not ultimately resonate with me.

I am actually even less comfortable with Aristotle's eudaimonia, which is what flourishing, like happiness, is meant to translate. At Maggie Archer's invitation as President of the *Pontifical Academy of the Social Sciences*, I recently presented a paper at the Vatican on how to reduce the normative demand for human trafficking. During questioning, economist Stefano Zamagni asked me why I had not spoken at all about happiness. I replied that as a Catholic, I don't care about happiness. Our happiness should not be our ultimate concern.

I was partly joking, and people laughed. But I was not entirely joking. Although I hardly speak on behalf of all Catholics, I do not think our ultimate concern should be our own happiness, not even an enlightened version of our own happiness, nor even our own, enlightened collective happiness.

Therein, for me, lies the rub, I think. Where I am coming from, we – not even the collective we – are our own end. For me, flourishing or happiness or eudaimonia with their Aristotelian roots in virtue ethics seem too much like enlightened self-interest.

Proponents of enlightened self-interest might pack into that concept all good things so that at the end of the day, there is nothing for me to oppose. I am afraid, however, I am so averse to egoism as to resist even an enlightened egoism that ends up being little different from altruism. I do not think our ultimate goal should be the cultivation of our own virtue. I think, rather that the cultivation of virtue comes not from aiming at it but through the pursuit of a higher good. That idea too perhaps may be ultimately Aristotelian.

What might such higher good be? When I teach *The Protestant Ethic*, I criticize how the Calvinists pursued the meaning of life as the glorification of God. I then go on to comment even more critically that we moderns have lost all meaning of life. When my students then ask me if I think life has meaning, I reply affirmatively.

When they next ask me what I think is the meaning of life, my students are both amused and very taken aback to hear me say the glorification of God.

This time, as amusing as I know my answer sounds, I am not joking at all. It is what I believe. Of course, by glorifying God I mean serving certain ideals, which can be served equally by those who do not believe in God. In any case, the flourishers will suggest, maybe that is just how I flourish: by serving those ideals. Maybe, but my point is that I am not trying to flourish. It is not my goal. My goal is to serve those ideals, and I resist that goal's being reduced to or translated into my own flourishing. If the pursuit of my goal leads to my own flourishing, great, but flourishing is not my aim.[2]

So here is another way to understand where I am going in this paper, which I had to write even to understand myself. I think it all to the good that flourishing has been placed on our agenda. It has thereby raised the stakes of discussion in social science discourse by introducing a moral element.

But it is not just a moral element that has been introduced. With talk of human flourishing, placed on the agenda as well is the idea of a human vocation. Yet once we have placed the human vocation on the agenda, the question becomes whether flourishing is the best name for it. And, for better or worse, the rivals include labels that are more specifically religious. It is this question I want to explore in this paper, and in the process, as we conclude our collection of Springer books, to comment as well on whether with morphogenic society, we are heading even for human flourishing if not for anything stronger. Let me begin, however with how flourishing has been introduced to recover a moral dimension within social science.

Flourishing and the Case Against Value Neutrality in the Social Sciences

Even apart from flourishing, critical realists have challenged both the fact/value distinction that goes back to Hume and the ideal of a value-neutral social science built upon it. Value-neutrality in social science has been upheld not just by the positivists but also by those much less associated with it, like Weber or even Russell Keat and John Urry (1975) who are otherwise opposed to positivism.

[2]Christian Smith (personal communication) is likewise eager to resist a reduction of flourishing to enlightened self-interest but suggests that that reduction can be avoided. If, he suggests, following Irenaeus that "the glory of God is the human fully alive," then we can avoid that collapse. I need to ponder that suggestion. Alan Norrie (personal communication) raises a different point, that no one individual can truly consider himself or herself to have had life go well if it does not go well for all. In fact, he suggests, there may be something ethically wrong in considering one's life gone well in such circumstances. If so, it seems to me, then there is some meta-normative constraint placed on flourishing, which is higher or deeper, although I understand those who favor talk of flourishing would say that collective flourishing is built into what they mean by individual flourishing. In fact, Norrie puts the point especially well. He says social justice precisely is about universal flourishing.

Keat and Urry's formulation of the position seems on the surface to be eminently reasonable: that explanatory claims are logically independent of political or moral judgments. One reply to this position is that political and moral judgments are at least not logically independent of explanatory claims. Value-claims are rather as Phil Gorski (2013, p. 543) nicely puts it, "fact-laden." It is a point also made by Charles Taylor (1967) and by Andrew Sayer (2011, p. 216–217). Sexist or racist values, for example, implicitly depend on certain ontological assumptions or factual claims and can therefore be undermined by sociological research that challenges those ontological or factual assessments.

Of course, the counter-argument is that the consideration above just calls into question the converse of Keat and Urry's claim and not the claim itself. The strongest argument, I think, against the claim itself, again voiced by a number of us (Gorski 2013, p. 547; Smith 2015; Porpora 2015), is that there are ineluctable thick descriptors or moral facts for which the moral and the factual cannot be disentangled. It is, for example, an entirely empirical matter whether any particular case is an instance of rape, murder, or genocide, but each of these designations is, nevertheless, strongly evaluative morally.

The moral element, moreover, cannot be stripped from these designations without serious injury to them. If not, then as both Roy Bhaskar (1994, p. 110) and Andrew Collier (2004) have further argued, objectivity cannot be equated with neutrality. On the contrary, if, by objectivity we mean that description most true to the object of description, then in such cases as rape, murder, and genocide, the most objective description may well be the most value-laden. In such cases then, a posture of value neutrality will be positively injurious to epistemic objectivity.

Although I think the above reasoning is the strongest line against value-neutrality in the social sciences, flourishing also finds its way into the debate. It begins with Bhaskar's notion of explanatory critique (see, for example, Bhaskar 1989). Bhaskar points out that if our research shows some social fact to be harmful to human flourishing, then we naturally will be disposed to oppose it, such opposition constituting a value judgment. As that value judgment is an intrinsic part of what lends our finding its import, Bhaskar maintains that again with explanatory critique, social science research is not merely descriptive but also evaluative and in some cases even morally evaluative.

In *Why Things Matter to People*, Sayer makes a similar argument. His argument in this connection proceeds by unpacking what is meant by "critical" in what is called Critical Social Science (CSS).

> Given the passion for attaching the prefix 'critical' to any kind of study, it might seem that at the minimum it could merely indicate a critical attitude to other, earlier approaches to social science. But then it has always been the job of any academic to be critical of existing ideas, and not only radicals but conservatives have always done this, so the adjective is redundant. However, if it goes further to the critical evaluation of concepts and accounts that are influential in society itself, and not merely in academic discourse, showing that some are false or at least that they ignore something significant, then this suggests something more distinctive, namely critique as oriented toward *the reduction of illusion* in society itself. (Sayer 2011, p. 220–221)

So the first thing Sayer is saying here is that the most robust understanding of critique in what is called CSS implies a critique of illusion in society. He next unpacks what is presupposed by critique in that sense.

> This kind of critique implies a minimalist normative standpoint, insofar as it assumes it is better to believe what is true or more true than what is false or less true, or better for beliefs and practices to be consistent than inconsistent or contradictory, and for them not to produce unwanted consequences, at least not harmful ones. (Sayer 2011, p. 221)

There are, Sayer is saying, minimal normative stances built into this understanding of critique. He argues, furthermore, that "critique cannot avoid such standpoints, though it may hide or fail to notice them; we need to make them explicit" (Sayer 2011, p. 219).

It is Sayer's next sentence, however, that brings the point home. To make explicit the normative standpoint in such critique, he says, "requires a consideration of ethics and *eudaimonia*" (Sayer 2011, p. 219). In relation to our discussion, it is an interesting phrasing. To the extent that eudaimonia indexes virtue ethics, which is itself a subset of ethics, Sayer's addition of eudaimonia seems redundant. Unless of course Sayer is trying to emphasize eudaimonia as the specific ethical perspective required. Required is not just an ethical perspective in general, Sayer may be suggesting, but that one in particular.

I think in fact Sayer is suggesting a particular need for eudaimonic ethics. Gorski (2013) likewise moves from the need to incorporate a non-relativist ethical dimension in sociology to a defense specifically of ethical naturalism based in eudaimonia. Smith (2014) as well moves straightforwardly in this direction as does Bhaskar (2008).

The question is why this particular ethical direction. Why will not deontological or utilitarian or some other approach to ethics do? Why this need for eudaimonia particularly? I think the reasons are diverse. To begin, let us continue with Sayer, whose reasoning is very explicit.

> In practice, the targets of the critiques developed by substantive CSS are not merely false ideas and their supports and consequences, or lack of freedom, but injustices and avoidable suffering . . . What would 'domination', 'oppression', 'abuse', 'racism' and 'sexism' – all familiar terms in social science discourse – mean, if they had nothing to do with suffering? Yet this connection between critique and suffering (and by implication, flourishing) is inadequately addressed in CSS's self-understandings, that we have addressed so far, for they do not indicate such grounds for critique. (Sayer 2011, p. 228–229)

Sayer is making several points here. First, CSS does not just critique any old false beliefs but false beliefs that matter in some way. Second, the way in which those beliefs matter is in their contribution to injustice and avoidable suffering.

It is, however, again Sayer's final point that brings the issue home. Of course, it shows up only elliptically in the parenthesis. That final point is that conceptually, concern for suffering implies concern for flourishing. Although unstated, the reason would seem to be that one suffers insofar as one fails to flourish.

Sayer thinks in fact that the whole of human rights discourse is to be grounded in the concept of flourishing. He says, "The human rights discourse can be defended in principle insofar as it adequately identifies the minimal, basic prerequisites of human flourishing" (Sayer 2011, p. 231). In the end, Sayer maintains, because humans are "vulnerable beings capable of flourishing and suffering," "some conception of flourishing is unavoidable" (Sayer 2011, p. 239).

Bhaskar (2008) arrives at universal flourishing via a parallel argument in his *Dialectic: The Pulse of Freedom*. Admittedly, the specific moves and ultimate ontology are different, from both of which I think Sayer would demur.

> Insofar as an ill is unwanted, unneeded and remedial, the spatio-temporal-causal-absenting or real transformative negation of the ill presupposes universalizability to absenting agency in all dialectically similar circumstances. This presupposes in turn the absenting of all similar constraints. And by the inexorable logic of dialectical universalizability, insofar as all constraints are similar in virtue of 'their being constraints', i.e. qua constraints, this presupposes the absenting of all constraints as such ... And this presupposes in its wake a society oriented to the free development and flourishing of each and all, and of each as a condition for all, that is to say, universal autonomy as flourishing ... So the goal of universal human autonomy is implicit in every moral judgment. (Bhaskar 2008, p. 663)

What I find similar to Sayer in Bhaskar's argument above is the underlying logic. Although Bhaskar is speaking in much more elevated language than Sayer, Bhaskar's basic point seems the same: If an ill is an ill, then it is unwanted – and not just unwanted by any one individual for idiosyncratic reasons but universally unwanted by what lawyers would call a reasonable person. That universality of the unwanted-ness embodied by the reasonable person implies a stance toward the ill that is not just prudential but actually normative or moral. And insofar as what makes the ill an ill is its inhibition of human flourishing, we arrive at Sayer's own conclusion above that "some conception of flourishing is unavoidable."

Admittedly, Bhaskar is less careful here than Sayer. Thus, Sayer (2011, p. 226) is right to complain that Bhaskar speaks of absenting all constraints and not just those specifically that inhibit flourishing. I would also object – and imagine Chris Smith (2014) would as well – to characterizing human autonomy as a universal goal "implicit in every moral judgment." It is not simply that, like Smith, I think human autonomy has its moral limits – and that as Haidt (2013) would tell us, there are also other moral values to be served. It is also for me precisely the connotation of an ethic of self-fulfillment that puts me off flourishing talk.

I will come back to that last point, but for now let me say along those lines that, like Sayer, Bhaskar accords flourishing a central moral place. In fact, for Bhaskar, flourishing becomes vocational. Mervyn Hartwig nicely captures this element of Bhaskar's thought.

> Dialectic builds on an ethics based upon ontology, the nature of dialectic as the absenting of absence, dialectics of truth, desire, and freedom, and explanatory critique. These lead to a moral theory, that moves 'from primal scream to universal flourishing' (D: 180), in which 'concrete singularity {the free flourishing of each} is the relational condition of concrete universality {the free flourishing of all}. (Hartwig 2007, p. 136)

I remain a bit put off here by a dialectics of "freedom" and especially "desire," although I am quite okay with truth and explanatory critique. The central point of the passage, though, echoing Marx, is that the "free flourishing of each" depends ontologically on the "free flourishing of all." In the next section, I will contest this claim. I am not sure it is true. In any case, however, the passage founds on this claim an entire human vocation toward universal flourishing. With that vocation, we are fully within an ethics of eudaimonia.

Christian Smith arrives at virtue ethics via a more straight-forward route, beginning with basic, existential questions.

> What does it mean for a human person to live a good life? Can people find direction outside of their immediate desires for genuinely reliable guidance on how to live a good life? Does life have any real purpose anyway? (Smith 2015, p. 201)

I consider these exactly the right questions to ask and am excited finally to have a fellow sociologist asking them. I like it that Smith is directing us morally away from our immediate desires, although I would adamantly prefer to move away from desire altogether. I especially like Smith's directing us to ultimate purpose. Moral purpose – as opposed to mere moral procedure – reflects my own preoccupation in moral philosophy. With the question of ultimate purpose, we are again dealing with what I have been calling a human vocation, something we humans are jointly meant to realize (see Porpora 2001, 2004).

Whether that locution – something we humans are meant to realize – has any meaning is also, I think, an important question that Smith places on the table. I personally do think there is something we humans are meant to accomplish together. My question is whether flourishing – even our collective flourishing – is the best name for that collective task.

Smith, on the contrary, does suggest human flourishing as our final end. It is thus to Aristotle's eudaimonia that Smith specifically takes us: "A good way to convey the character of this final end or purpose in life is to name it *flourishing*, also sometimes called here 'thriving' or 'a good life well lived'" (Smith 2015, p. 202). "Eudaimonia," Smith tells us, "refers not to a moment in time but to an entire life well lived" (Smith 2015, p. 203).

I have no problem with the phrase "a good life well lived." Depending on how that is unpacked, I would say it could get at what I, too, consider the meaning of life. My reservations relate to how Aristotle actually does unpack it. As Smith (2015, p. 203) tells us, "the purpose of human life in this sense also involves not only living well but to some extent having life go well, expressing right conduct and prosperity."

I resist having prosperity and having life go well packed into the purpose of life. Socrates was neither prosperous, and nor in the end did his life go well. He was after all sentenced to death. Still, I think, we would want to say he flourished. Thus, as the Stoics would say – and they were partly inspired by the example of Socrates, one's happiness is entirely an internal affair and not a function of what happens outside oneself.[3]

[3]Chris Smith responds (again personal communication) that he would continue to refer to a life having gone well by the idea of flourishing "as long as we remember that different lives have different callings, vocations, paths, roads, etc. that define well for them." For some, he suggest, that may involve sacrifice. I agree that there is something to this idea, that even by sacrificing,

But it is not only the element of prosperity that I resist. I also resist the more basic rationale through which Aristotle arrives at flourishing as the meaning of life. Again, Smith directs us.

> How can anyone know or have good reason to believe that flourishing is the proper telos of human life? That, Aristotle observed, is *self-evident*. Ask people why they do whatever they do (given constraints) and *ultimately* one will hear one version of the answer, "Because I want a life that is happy, flourishing, enjoying well-being." (Smith 2015, p. 203)

Smith goes on to say carefully that Aristotle is assuming the people asked above are normal. Perhaps therein lies the problem: I have come to realize that in a number of respects, I am not normal. Certainly, I want to be happy and to enjoy well-being. But I do not consider those the ultimate ends of my life. On the contrary, I try at least to serve something higher.

I am somewhat more comfortable with Phil Gorski's (2013) take on what he calls ethical naturalism, which he likewise grounds in Aristotle's eudaimonia. What makes me more comfortable is in the first place, Gorski's acknowledgement that ethical naturalism cannot account for the whole of ethics, that at most it speaks only to "the good" and not to "the right."

In a footnote, Gorski (2013, p. 549) explains that ethical naturalism is naturalistic in being non-theistic. I think that an important admission. I suspect that generally flourishing is being commended in large part precisely because it is grounded in a naturalistic, i.e., non-theistic ethic. It is not that its promoters are all atheists. In fact, we know otherwise. Gorski's footnote is even careful to point out that his naturalism is "not necessarily a-theistic" but "compatible with certain forms of theism as well." Even that last qualification is careful. Ethical naturalism is certainly compatible with certain forms of theism. I just don't know if it is compatible with mine.

The main point, however, is that if ethical naturalism is being promoted in part because of its independence from theism, I think it is because ethical naturalism is judged on that ground more palatable to social scientists, who certainly want no truck with theism. That strategy makes eminent sense. The question is whether we who answer to a higher authority can, qua social scientists, be satisfied with this more neutral ground.

I am also somewhat comforted by Gorski's attempt to distance ethical naturalism from the "utilitarian ring" he acknowledges it bears. He accordingly denies that eudaimonia is equivalent to "an aggregation of emotional states or experiences." For Aristotle, Gorski (2013, p. 550) says, happiness rather concerns the "overall shape of one's life."

I like the ring of that last locution. Why then am I only somewhat comfortable with it? In part again because of the way Aristotle unpacks the "overall shape of one's life." Gorski (2013, p. 550) says that happiness for Aristotle is "satisfaction

---

we may affirm our better selves. The question for me concerns motivation. Are we sacrificing ultimately to affirm our better selves or to further the cause for which we are sacrificing? Can't it be both? Yes, but I would like to say there is only one supreme cause I feel called to serve.

that one has 'lived well', that one has lived a life of 'virtue', not only in one's own eyes but in those of one's peers as well."

I do not challenge the take on Aristotle presented by Gorski and Smith. I think they are right. Rather, I challenge Aristotle and side here more with Plato. Ruth Groff actually pointed out to me last summer that on "the good," I am more "a Plato than an Aristotle guy." As Plato argued in the *Republic*, a virtuous life and a reputation for it do not always coincide and may often in fact conflict. As I believe with Plato that the former takes precedence over the latter, I am uncomfortable with the Aristotelian conflation of the two.

More basically, however, I remain uncomfortable with the moral target in virtue ethics being our own virtue. Gorski speaks in Aristotelian terms of ethics as involving moral aim. My discomfort concerns what we are aiming at. East and West are agreed that to save one's soul, one must ultimately abandon it. Even in the happiness literature Gorski cites, it is acknowledged that one is less likely to achieve one's own happiness by aiming specifically at it (see Frankl 2006; Sidgwick 1981). Paradoxically, one achieves happiness rather by aiming at certain ideals. What are those ideals? Are they not virtues? Is the difference between virtue ethics and an ethic of idealism only semantic? Maybe, but let us not go there directly.[4]

So What's My Issue?

I have several issues. Let me begin with Sayer. I concede to Sayer that we sociologists are often critical of various aspects of society; that we – certainly, I include myself – often focus our work on such critiques; and that at bottom we are critical of what causes suffering.

But then Sayer goes on to suggest that to the extent that we are interested in suffering, we must likewise be interested in flourishing as suffering implies a failure to flourish. Maybe, but I am not so sure. Consider the admonition below to the people of Israel from the prophet Isaiah, which definitely does move me. In the passage, as a prophet, Isaiah is purporting to speak on behalf of God.

> 'Why have we fasted,' *they say*, 'and You have not seen? *Why* have we afflicted our souls, and You take no notice?'
>
> In fact, in the day of your fast you find pleasure, And exploit all your laborers. Indeed you fast for strife and debate, And to strike with the fist of wickedness. You will not fast as *you do* this day, To make your voice heard on high.
>
> Is it such a fast that I have chosen, A day for a man to afflict his soul? *Is it* to bow down his head like a bulrush, And to spread out sackcloth and ashes? Would you call this a fast, an acceptable day to the Lord?

[4]For a sociological confirmation of this point, see Christian Smith's (2014) *The paradox of generosity: Giving we receive, grasping we lose*.

> "*Is* this not the fast that I have chosen: To loose the bonds of wickedness, To undo the heavy burdens, To let the oppressed go free, And that you break every yoke?
>
> *Is it* not to share your bread with the hungry, And that you bring to your house the poor who are cast out; When you see the naked, that you cover him, And not hide yourself from your own flesh? (Isaiah 58: 5–7)

I, for one, am greatly stirred by these lines. They are a call to social justice. As such, I do not think they are aptly summarized as "Look guys, I, the lord, want you all to flourish, and currently not all of you are doing so."

Better might be, "I, the lord, have created a world in which you all might flourish, and you have forsaken that end." I like that summary better if only because the word forsaken suggests an obligatory moral edge beyond collective prudence. Still, I do not think the summary completely apt. That for which the prophet is demanding redress is so far removed from flourishing as to place that condition beyond relevance. To feed the hungry and clothe the naked is hardly to secure their happiness. More urgent here is their basic survival.

That as a society Israel was neglecting the basic survival of its people was, from the prophet's perspective, not just unfortunate but a scandal, a moral outrage. Why so? Because, from the prophet's perspective, the poor exert a moral claim on us. Millennia before the enlightenment, we have here in the Bible an articulation of basic human rights.

Sayer, we saw, wants to ground human rights in flourishing. Brian Turner (1993) previously sought likewise to ground human rights in human vulnerability. Such moves cannot work on their own. The reason is that as Ayn Rand was known to argue, the need of others does not by itself constitute an ethical demand on us. After all, like us, plants and animals are vulnerable with definite prerequisites for flourishing. Prerequisites that we routinely ignore or sabotage. We sabotage them, for example, to put food on our plates and clothes on our backs. So something's need alone does not constitute any kind of moral demand on us. Flourishing alone does not get us there.

What is needed is a thicker moral ontology (see Joas 2013; Taylor 1994). As Smith (2010, 2015) himself argues, we need an ontology of the person that makes clear why persons as such do constitute a moral claim on us. Provision of such a fuller ontology is a way of going from *is* to *ought*.

Although as an atheist, Ayn Rand was unmoved by it, the Biblical tradition does supply such an ontology. It was, as encapsulated by Thomas Jefferson in the *American Declaration of Independence*, that we humans are the special creation of God, created in God's own image. That putative ontological status confers a sanctity on all human persons, and it is on that sanctity in turn – and not just on our requirements for flourishing – that Jefferson founded our human rights.

Remove that ontology and fail fully to replace it as has been done by our entire secular, liberal, cosmopolitan culture, and human rights are left without moral grounding. It is a groundlessness from which the secular denizens of that culture have just agreed to turn their heads (see Ignatieff 2003).[5]

Bhaskar (2012) has not turned his head. His meta-reality answers to the need by providing just the sort of moral ontology required. Bhaskar makes that provision precisely via his elevated, mythic language that Sayer expressly eschews. Sayer eschews such language because it is the language of us religious, and Sayer expressly does not include himself among our number.

The religion Bhaskar invokes is of course not theistic, not Biblical, not even Western. Although, it too, is rooted in flourishing, this time the ultimate source is not Aristotle but the *Bhagavad Gita*. According to the *Gita*, the dualisms of the world, especially the duality that separates each from all others, is illusion, the kind of illusion that Sayer says is the job of CSS to critique. If, per the Hinduistic perspective of Bhaskar's meta-reality, we see through the illusion of our own separate identities, we will be drawn to the unconditional love that realizes that our own full flourishing depends on the full flourishing of all. The free flourishing of all thus becomes our human vocation.

Although I was originally somewhat averse to this talk of meta-reality, I have, largely owing to Alan Norrie's (e.g., 2015) sensitive treatment of it, come to appreciate it much more. I think there is much to commend about it. It answers, as I have said, a philosophical need that secular liberalism fails to fill. And I fully support unconditional love. Even the case Bhaskar makes from love to universal flourishing makes sense to me.

Still, meta-reality does not work for me. That is because I hear a different drummer and march to a different tune. As a Christian, my sensibility is ultimately Jewish rather than Hindu, by which I mean, *Kabbala* aside, I resonate more with an ineluctable I-Thou relationality than with a cosmic union of identities. When the Good Samaritan encounters the hapless victim on the road, I do not think it is the Samaritan's own flourishing he is principally thinking about. It seems to me rather the call of the other in all his otherness to which the Samaritan responds and not to himself.[6]

But let us return to Isaiah. If I have not been satisfied with other renditions of Isaiah's words in terms of flourishing, nor do I favor the summary that would follow from Bhaskar's meta-reality: "Look, guys, especially you rich in your castles warm, you cannot flourish fully as long as among you there are suffering widows and orphans; for your own sakes, see to their needs."

---

[5]Smith (2009) makes the same point.

[6]Alan Norrie points out to me here that my talk of the other in all his or her otherness sounds a lot like Levinas. While I certainly end up in much the same place as Levinas in the importance I place on the I-Thou relationship, I do not arrive there via the same heavy metaphysics. I do agree minimally with Levinas and, more recently with Donati and Archer (2015) that we are relational beings from the start and so find it natural to respond to the thou-ness of others, however much we are very capable are of turning 'them' into 'its'. Of course we can also respond to a thou with antagonism as In Hegel's *Phenomenology of the Spirit*.

The problem for me with this Bhaskaresque summary is that it converts the speech act Isaiah performs from moral summons to prudential counsel. In so doing, the Bhaskaresque summary makes attendance to the needs of the poor one's own interest, one's enlightened self-interest to be sure, but one's own interest nevertheless.

One problem with that conversion is that as prudential counsel I do not quite buy the admonition – either socially or personally. Socially, I can imagine saying a society is flourishing even if not everyone in that society is. Take ancient Greece, for example. Say Athens of the fourth century B.C.E. Would we not say that during that time it flourished? I would. It experienced a colossal cultural explosion to which in so many ways we are still indebted. Yet it was built on slavery.

Nor as prudential counsel do the prophet's words work on me personally. I confess that in this life I may just not have attained what Eastern thought considers to be full enlightenment (see you in the next life, brother), but were I one of the rich, I could imagine myself saying, "As I am a satisficer rather than a maximizer, I'm flourishing quite enough, thank you, without worrying about the widows and orphans. Let them look out for themselves."

But if the prophet's words do not work at all on me as prudential counsel, they do work on me very powerfully as moral critique and moral summons.

What's the difference? The difference is marked by Smith in a short footnote. In the footnote, Smith (2015, p. 325) distinguishes eudaimonic ethics from the ethics of Kant, who in turn sharply distinguishes morality from self-interest.

Once we mention Kant, it all becomes clear. On questions of morality, my sensibilities align strongly with his. Well, I thought so. Both Ruth Groff and Chris Smith tell me I am not a Kantian as it is not his secularized categorical imperative that drives me nor duty as such. But I do hold with Kant that morality drives us beyond self-interest to a higher call. Maybe it is enough to cite Hillel ("if I am only for myself, what am I?"). In any case, although I do not think that morality and self-interest necessarily conflict, they do so frequently enough. And when they do conflict, self-sacrifice is the offering we make to our higher moral calling, a measure in fact of our devotion to it. This, at least, is what I believe.[7]

In the same footnote, Smith cites Kant saying what I said earlier: That we achieve full contentment or our proper telos or flourishing by pursuing not them but rather higher ideals. I think Plato would agree. If so, then to invoke a distinction from anthropology, it might still remain correct *etically* – i.e., from the outside – to describe flourishing as our human telos without its being correct *emically*, i.e., from the inside. Emically, in pursuing ultimately something beyond our own self-perfection, I stand with Kant and against, say, Foucault (1988), whose *The Care of the Self* ought to confound his followers who for decades maintained there was no self to care for – or at least no unitary self, which also makes me wonder about

[7] Here, at least Alan Norrie seems to agree with me. Among the number of interesting things Norrie says on this point is the bite of deontology in Kant that Aristotle seems to lack. In this regard, he goes on to talk of the importance of collective responsibility that he finds in the work of Jaspers (again see Norrie 2015).

Foucault's (1988, p. 65) use of "one" in such formulations as "One had best keep in mind that the chief objective one should set for oneself is to be sought within oneself, in the relation of oneself to oneself." What in standard Foucauldian terms is this essentialist "one" – and "oneself" – of which Foucault speaks? We must ask Judith Butler.

Sorry. I confess that the Foucauldians if not Foucault himself do set me off on a rant. Let me return to the point. Leave aside the wonder of Foucault's suddenly speaking of unitary selves or of selves that potentially at least can be unified. I would also dispute Foucault's history. I do not think that either Socrates or the Stoics were concerned ultimately with self-cultivation.

To be sure, they were concerned with self-cultivation. I am not denying that that they were. I am denying that self-cultivation was their *ultimate* concern. I am denying that Socrates and the Stoics were engaged in self-cultivation for its own sake. Rather they sought to cultivate themselves and their own virtue to put themselves right with God and the world.

Socrates and the Stoics were expressly not atheists. They worshipped what is variously called order, reason, *logos* – and even God – and sought to make of themselves an homage to that higher good. To achieve this result the Stoics particularly worked on themselves to narrow or minimize their own desires, to be happy with less, all the better to serve. Thus, as Epictetus says, quoting Euripides, "Lead me, O Zeus, and thou O Destiny, the way that I am bid by you to go: To follow, I am ready."

So it is similarly for me. My own self-cultivation is not for its own sake but in *imatatio dei*, in imitation of God's own inspiring example. What is it about God I seek (certainly unsuccessfully) to emulate? God's self-forgetting, even self-sacrificing love. Is that holy quality ultimately in God's own enlightened self-interest?

So What Words Are Better?

Again I am not so much suggesting that there are words better than flourishing as words with which I, for one, given the kind of theist I am, better resonate.

What are those words? What do I think is the human vocation? When I contemplate the vastness of the universe and consider further that this vastness might have been required to insure the appearance even just once of intelligent life, it seems to me we have been entrusted with a great vocation. We are the universe conscious of itself. That station is an exalted one and as such a calling.

To what are we called? To whatever it is, I do not think it can be just individual, nor even just the sum of individual realizations. The human vocation, whatever it is, must be social, something we are meant to accomplish together.

What might be that social accomplishment? Certainly, I am moved by the Biblical ideal of social justice, a designation introduced into modern discourse by the Jesuit priest, Luigi Tapparelli. Perhaps, however, social justice is too narrow a designation. As a Christian, I do feel called to help build the reign of God that Jesus announced, but the Jewish *Tikkun Olam* also works for me. The Hebrew expression, Tikkun Olam means repair of the world. That repair is definitely an encompassing goal.

I said earlier that I thought the purpose of life is to glorify God. How do we do that? In Hegelian terms, I would say the collective purpose of our lives is to reflect back to the Absolute Spirit the Absolute Spirit's own perfection.

What is the Absolute Spirit's own perfection? The reign of God, the repaired world: The reign of love and justice and unconditional welcome into community. I thus also would go along here some way with Feuerbach: enough to say that even if there is no divine person, there are at least qualities I consider divine, namely love and justice, and mercy. So our personal goal is to live by them and our collective goal to realize those attributes fully in our institutions.[8]

Okay, great, it may now be said, I am for love and justice and all other good things. But are love and justice and suchlike not virtues and would a world built on them not constitute universal flourishing? I think I must answer both questions affirmatively. Love, and justice, and suchlike are virtues and a world built on them would constitute human flourishing. Yes, I agree.

So have I then put us through this long journey for nothing? Just to conclude at the end that I am no longer uncomfortable with flourishing? Not entirely. Let me recapitulate the positions at which I think I have arrived by writing this paper. Do I think flourishing is enough to ground human rights? No. Do I want to flourish? Yes, certainly, but it is not my top priority. Do I think we should be cultivating our virtues? Yes, but not as an end in itself. We only know, moreover, which virtues to cultivate from the larger good or ideals we serve. So in some sense, the larger ideals – and our emotional call to them – come first. That was Plato's position, and ultimately, I think, Aristotle's too. It was Aristotle's unmoved mover, the perfect goodness of which draws us emotionally that is to be the ultimate object of our devotion. We are to become like that which we love, and the virtues honoring that love develop accordingly.

I also asked earlier whether social scientists who answer to a higher authority can be satisfied with universal flourishing as a more neutral moral goal for the social sciences. I myself can be satisfied: universal human flourishing is certainly close enough for me to the ultimate goal toward which I think we and all humanity should be working. I would only add that for me, universal flourishing does not satisfactorily in itself designate the full significance of that goal. To me, universal human flourishing is important because it represents the *good society*, reflecting the divine qualities we are meant to institutionalize. For me, without that or some

[8]These are all relational concepts. So in terms newly set out by Pierpaolo Donati and Margaret Archer (2015), it may be said that our human vocation is to achieve certain relational goods.

such elevated, cosmic significance, universal human flourishing alone sounds like collective prudence without any edge of moral binding-ness.[9]

In *What Is a Person*, Christian Smith urges on us the perspective of *Personalism*. Since as a matter of record (Porpora 2015) I have already signed onto that program, let me put the point of the previous paragraph in Personalist terms. In *Person and the Common Good*, Jacques Maritain (1973), one of the founders of Personalism, insists, as I have, that we are not our own end. Even the common good, for Maritain, cannot be equated with earthly flourishing. It signifies something more. So, for me similarly, if I, too, fight for universal human flourishing, it is because universal flourishing signifies something more, and it is at that more that I ultimately aim.

Is Our Current Trajectory Toward Flourishing?

So I said I would end with commentary on the course of our books in relation to flourishing and the human good. Although, again perhaps peculiarly I disclaim the self-description, I am what others would call a person of faith. I do have faith at least that, God with us, we will in the end achieve the good society we were placed here to achieve.

In the short and medium terms, however, the signs toward that end are definitely mixed. We are now deeply locked in the struggle Benjamin Barber (1995) termed Jihad vs. McWorld, neither pole of which being that which we want. A recent piece in the *New York Times* reported that even if we changed our ways completely now, a definite rise in global temperature will last for millennia, the end likely resulting in an aggravated ice age. Humankind is thus in for a rocky ride. And all of the adverse mechanisms we in our previous books described as part of intensified morphogenesis are still with us.

So our situation is fraught. We are nowhere near the good society or universal human flourishing, certainly nothing I would term the reign of God. Hegel thought history consummated with the Prussian state and Francis Fukuyama (2006) with contemporary America. On the contrary, clearly, we have a long way to go. Yet, there are some promising signs, such as, for example, fragile as it is, developing worldwide consensus on such matters as human rights, global warming, and even terrorism.

The question comes down to the question of moral progress. Are we making it? Are we as a world moving in a progressively moral direction? It is a question that social science has largely repudiated, although Stephen Pinker (2012) has taken a

[9] Again, Alan Norrie seems to agree with me "that universal flourishing is valid insofar as it signifies something more," which he agrees is something like universal love overall and authenticity here and now. I'll take that.

stab at putting it back on the agenda. Perhaps attention to flourishing will place it more squarely on the agenda. I hope so. Now that I have arrived at a qualified comfort with flourishing, human progress toward that end does indeed interest me as a topic.

References

Barber, B. (1995). *Jihad vs. McWorld*. New York: Ballantine.
Bhaskar, R. (1989). *Reclaiming reality: A critical introduction to contemporary philosophy*. New York: Routledge.
Bhaskar, R. (1994). *Plato, etc.: Problems of philosophy and their resolution*. New York: Routledge.
Bhaskar, R. (2008). *Dialectic: The pulse of freedom*. New York: Routledge.
Bhaskar, R. (2012). *The philosophy of metareality: Creativity, love and freedom*. New York: Routledge.
Collier, A. (2004). *In defence of objectivity*. New York: Routledge.
Donati, P., & Archer, M. (2015). *The relational subject*. Cambridge: Cambridge University Press.
Foucault, M. (1988). *The history of sexuality: The care of the self*. New York: Vintage.
Frankl, V. (2006). *Man's search for meaning*. Boston: Beacon.
Fukuyama, F. (2006). *The end of history and the last man*. New York: Free Press.
Gorski, P. S. (2013). Beyond the fact/value Distinction: Ethical naturalism and the social sciences. *Society, 50*, 543–553.
Haidt, J. (2013). *The righteous mind: Why good people are divided by politics and religion*. New York: Vintage.
Hartwig, M. (2007). *Dictionary of critical realism*. New York: Routledge.
Ignatieff, M. (2003). *Human rights as politics and idolatry*. Princeton: Princeton University Press.
Joas, H. (2013). *The sacredness of the person. A new genealogy of human rights*. Washington, DC: Georgetown University Press.
Keat, R., & Urry, J. (1975). *Social theory as science*. New York: Routledge.
Maritain, J. (1973). *Person and the common good*. South Bend: University of Notre Dame Press.
Norrie, A. (2012). The scene and the crime: Can critical realists talk about good and evil? *Journal of Critical Realism, 11*(1), 76–93.
Norrie, A. (2015). *Critical realism and the metaphysics of justice*. Paper presented at 2015 meetings of the International Association of Critical Realism, South Bend, Indiana.
Pinker, S. (2012). *The better angels of our nature. Why violence has declined*. New York: Penguin.
Porpora, D. (2001). *Landscapes of the soul: The loss of moral meaning in American Life*. New York: Oxford University Press.
Porpora, D. (2004). The human project. In M. Archer, A. Collier, & D. Porpora (Eds.), *Transcendence: Critical realism and God* (pp. 155–167). New York: Routledge.
Porpora, D. (2015). *Reconstructing sociology: The critical realist approach*. Cambridge University Press: New York.
Sayer, A. (2011). *Why things matter to people*. New York: Cambridge University Press.
Sidgwick, H. (1981). *The methods of ethics*. New York: Hackett.
Smith, C. (2009). Does naturalism warrant a belief in universal benevolence and human rights? In J. Schloss & M. J. Murray (Eds.), *Scientific, philosophical and theological reflections on the origin of religion* (pp. 293–317). New York: Oxford University Press.
Smith, C. (2010). *What is a person? Rethinking humanity, social life, and the moral good from the person up*. Chicago: University of Chicago.
Smith, C. (2014). *The paradox of generosity: Giving we receive, grasping we lose*. Oxford University Press: New York.

Smith, C. (2015). *To flourish or self-destruct: A personalist theory of human goods, motivations, failure, and evil*. Chicago: University of Chicago Press.
Taylor, C. (1967). *Neutrality in political science*. http://www.mercaba.org/SANLUIS/Filosofia/autores/Contemporánea/Taylor,%20Charles/Neutrality%20in%20political%20science.pdf
Taylor, C. (1994). *Sources of the self: The making of the modern identity*. Cambridge: Harvard University Press.
Turner, B. (1993). Outline of a theory of human rights. *Sociology, 27*(3), 489–512.

Chapter 4
Reflexivity in a Just Morphogenic Society: A Sociological Contribution to Political Philosophy

Ismael Al-Amoudi

Introduction: Reflexivity, Side-Lined in Public Debates and Political Philosophy?

Late Modernity's morphogenic tendencies bear on people's ability to flourish in various, and ambiguous, ways. In particular, morphogenesis unbound presents agents with contextual incongruities, that is, novel configurations and associated problems for which tried and tested solutions are of little avail (Archer 2012). Whenever exemplars and traditional sources of normativity are of limited help to solve novel problems, the onus for solving the latter is placed on agents' personal powers of reflexivity. Late modernity thus entered the scene with a threat: individuals can either be reflexive and stand a chance to flourish, or they must accept they will not thrive.

This reflexive imperative comes in various guises. As a case in point, citizens of twenty-first century liberal democracies – especially young adults – face a treble injunction if they wish to fit in as mature members of society. Firstly, they ought to take personal responsibility for their 'employability', though in terms defined by employers. Secondly, they ought to participate in democratic political processes, though mainly by voting through established channels. And thirdly they ought to look up to those who display 'leadership' in various spheres of life, though especially so in lucrative activities. All three injunctions seem, on the surface, to value autonomy and reflexivity. But their *ad nauseam* repetition also indicates that those enjoined are not automatically able to exercise adequately those reflexive powers needed to sustain a satisfactory social trajectory or to participate in their communities' governance.

I. Al-Amoudi (✉)
Cardiff Business School, University of Cardiff, Colum Drive, Aberconway Building, Cardiff, CF10 3EU, UK
e-mail: al-amoudii@cardiff.ac.uk

M.S. Archer (ed.), *Morphogenesis and Human Flourishing*, Social Morphogenesis, DOI 10.1007/978-3-319-49469-2_4

Yet, there is scant philosophic, or even public, discussion of the distribution of effective reflexive powers or of the organisations and institutions that may ensure these reflexive powers are fairly distributed.[1] Instead, public discussions of 'employability' focus on the curricula of educational institutions that should provide training valued by for-profit organisations whereas discussions of 'democratic participation' usually evoke either the opacity of political institutions or the deficiencies of electoral marketing strategies that ignore groups deemed to be politically disengaged. In all cases, the disengagement from professional and political life is explained as lack of professional skills, information and interest. And the proposed remedies include a combination of enhanced marketing communication (identifying and manipulating citizens' desires efficiently) and inspirational leadership (enthusing electors with a sense of purpose to achieve pre-defined ends). By focusing attention on professional skills, information and 'leadership', these discussions obscure, however, the distribution of effective human reflexive powers that are nonetheless essential to the organisation of just societies and to the flourishing of those humans who live in them. I borrow Archer's (2012) modalities or modes of reflexivity (fractured, communicative, autonomous and meta-reflexivity).[2] Moreover, my argument relies on the significant assumption (developed in the section "Injustice resulting from unequal social reflexivity in morphogenic society" below) that intensified morphogenesis bears on the effectiveness of these modes of social reflexivity.

While a satisfactory discussion of the omission, or downplaying, of how unequally effective modes and powers of reflexivity are distributed[3] in the public debate would require more resources than I have, it might nonetheless be instructive, and achievable, to examine their omission in influential works of political philosophy. Firstly, because such works do influence the conceptions of policy-makers, journalists and educated citizens. But secondly, and more fundamentally, because a discussion anchored in political philosophy can clarify which (missing or inadequately supported) institutions and organisations should be mandated by the state, and publicly funded, to help foster and attenuate unequal distributions of, citizens' reflexive powers.

The following chapter undertakes this task by taking a lead from the influential theories of justice developed first by John Rawls and then by Amartya Sen and

[1] I base my argument on the assumption that powers of reflexivity can vary between persons, according to their dominant modes. By doing so, I do not imply that there exist uniform or perhaps even precise ways of measuring differences in reflexivity.

[2] Of course, other modes of reflexivity may be forthcoming (see Carrigan in this volume).

[3] In section "Injustice resulting from unequal social reflexivity in morphogenic society" below, I discuss the unequal effectiveness, in a morphogenic society, of fractured, communicative, autonomous and meta-reflexivity. Note that the discussion leaves open the question of the relation between various forms of reflexivity and the conditions for a given mode becoming dominant for particular persons.

Martha Nussbaum.[4] It attempts to trace to what extent, why and how two types of human reflexive powers that are nonetheless essential to the organisation of just societies and to the flourishing of those humans who live in them have not been considered in political philosophy.

While reflexivity can broadly be defined as '*the regular exercise of the mental ability, shared by all normal people, to consider themselves in relation to their (social) contexts and vice versa*' (Archer 2007: 4, italics in original), I concentrate in this paper on two types of reflexive powers. The first type is *social reflexivity* which can broadly be defined as each person's capacity to formulate, respond and act on the question: 'how should I make my way through the social world?' This is the form of reflexivity which Archer (2003, 2007, 2012) has studied over more than a decade and discussed over 1000 pages.

The second reflexive power I discuss could be termed *political reflexivity*. It can broadly be defined as each person's capacity to formulate, respond and act on the question: 'how can we steer society together?' To my knowledge, this type of power has not been as fully addressed as social reflexivity by realist social theory. We find, however, important and relevant ideas in the writings of Donati on relational steering (Donati 2013) and in Donati and Archer (2015) on relational subjects.

For each of these powers, I discuss why they matter all the more in the context of a morphogenic society. To what extent do they seem to be missing from key theories of justice? What other personal powers are required for the realisation of these forms of reflexivity? And what (currently missing) institutions and organisations might be conducive to fostering these powers?

Before engaging with these themes, some conceptual clarification is required first on the contribution of sociology to political philosophy. And second on the nature and currency of morphogenic society as well as its significance for citizens endowed with differing abilities and propensities to engage in communicative, autonomous and meta-reflexivity.

The Contribution of Sociological Theory to Political Philosophy

This chapter establishes a discussion between two academic domains defined by distinct objects of study. On the one hand, sociological theory investigates the nature and basic mechanisms through which social relations are sustained and transformed.

[4] Note that an intermediary draft attempted to discuss the absence of social and political reflexivity in the works of Alasdair MacIntyre. While the analysis was ultimately side-lined to preserve the chapter's consistency, two considerations might be worth salvaging. First, MacIntyre makes a contribution to moral rather than political philosophy in the sense that he does not intend to establish which institutions ought to be mandated by law in a just, or otherwise good, society. Second, how social and political reflexivity map into the Aristotelian and Thomist virtues is not straightforward, though we might venture that reflexivity holds much in common with phronesis and prudence.

On the other, theories of justice (and, more generally, political philosophy) examine the principles according to which one set of social relations ought to be preferred over another. Since 'political power is always coercive' (Rawls 1993: 68), political philosophy contributes to clarifying which institutions should be enforced by the state's coercive powers and/or publicly funded in a just society.

These two domains are, at least in principle, complementary. Indeed, sociological theory remains largely uncritical if it lacks an implicit or explicit political philosophy (Callinicos 2006, esp. pp. 217–43, see also Gorski 2013, Sayer 2011, Smith 2015). Conversely, political philosophy provides shallow, uninformed and ultimately misleading critiques if it is not informed by sociological theory (Bhaskar 1998; Collins 1988).

In practice, social theory and political philosophy intertwine with varying degrees of felicity. Chernilo (2014) reminds us for instance of a tradition of philosophical sociology, that is, of sociology that draws from philosophy's reflection on the good, the just and the human. Unfortunately, positivist currents of sociology seem to be dominating many an academic department, not least in the hegemonic USA. In the worse cases, sociology distances itself not only from political philosophy but also from social theory as it retreats into quantification and computation, two practices that provide illusory safeguards against normative commitment. In slightly better cases, sociology recognises the value, and some of the findings, of social theory but relies only implicitly and cursorily on normative considerations whose systematic study it leaves to political theory.

The present paper is located in the tradition of philosophical sociology. But with a twist, as its main contributions are addressed directly to political philosophy and rather indirectly to social theory. Although I base my arguments on a social ontology that would arguably displease Randall Collins, we could perhaps borrow his expression *sociological philosophy* to describe my intended contribution (Collins 1988). Yet, Collins' position deserves to be nuanced when he claims that.

> philosophy has not made the transition from the social to the sociological. Philosophers invoke the social in a general and taken-for-granted way, while their use of actual sociology is meagre and often uninformed. (Collins 1988: 669)

Indeed, I would like to argue briefly that political philosophy's 'meagre and often uninformed' use of sociology constitutes a conscious and to some extent justified, accomplishment. My point is not that sociological theory should have no input into political philosophy, including theories of justice. It is rather that we need to be careful to avoid restricting the commendably universal scope of political philosophy when we add considerations drawn from sociological theory.

Political philosophers rely, usually implicitly or cursorily, on assumptions about the nature and functioning of societies that are systematically studied by social theory. However, they also go at great length to rely on as meagre a use of sociology as they can. I believe this stance is justified by political philosophers' willingness to extend the validity of their argument to the widest possible, ideally universal, range of possible social configurations.

John Rawls's *Theory of Justice* provides a useful lead. I find it admirable in many respects but the one that fascinates me most is the care with which Rawls draws the boundaries of his discussion: the basic structure of society is the sole focus of enquiry; the discussion is limited to drawing realistic utopias under the assumption that people comply with principles of justice and with arrangements agreed according to these principles; the discussion is restricted to the level of a single nation in a pluri-national world (Rawls 2001: 14–5). Rawls's parsimony is pursued in his minimalist anthropology as he bases his theory of justice on only two moral powers: people's sense of justice and their ability to form a conception of the good (Ibid.: 18–9).

I view this parsimony of specific moral and empirical facts as a great strength for a theory that claims relevance in any social or cultural context. In other words, through careful delimitation of scope, Rawls achieves pan-historical relevance. In this chapter, however, I will introduce two additional sociological considerations with a view to develop, without disfiguring or undermining, liberal egalitarian theories of justice.

The first concerns human reflexivity. I believe we can enrich Rawls's theory of justice without restricting its ahistorical relevance by adding social theoretical considerations on *social reflexivity*, (Archer 2003, 2007, 2012). I further add a (tentative) conception of *political reflexivity* understood as humans' reflexive capacity to engage in collective action to steer society together. These additions are analogous to Sen's well-known argument (Sen 1992: 73–87) that primary goods are not automatically converted into satisfactory human functioning, and that such conversion is necessarily mediated through human capabilities that may themselves be unequally distributed in terms of their efficacy. I argue in this chapter that the powers of human reflexivity do matter for achieved fairness. I also argue that they are not included in Rawls's list of primary goods. Finally, I argue that, while reflexivity is ontologically a power of the same sort as the capabilities discussed by Sen and Nussbaum, the latter have not taken into account its central importance for matters of social justice. Note that the claims I will make about human reflexivity are themselves generically ahistorical. Therefore my introducing human reflexivity does not restrict the ahistorical validity of the normative discussion of justice. I might be wrong about human reflexivity and my overall argument should then be rejected. However, if I am right, the resulting claims do not restrict the scope of validity of the theories of justice of Rawls, Sen and Nussbaum.

The second sociological consideration I introduce to theories of justice concerns morphogenic society. And this consideration is certainly historical in nature as we should distinguish between the philosophical theory of social morphogenesis and the substantive theory of morphogenic society. The explanatory framework of social morphogenesis is philosophical and claims universal validity across societies: every human society is deemed to comprise human agents, social structures and cultural systems, and these are deemed to evolve through processes that can usefully be traced as morphogenic/morphostatic cycles, and so on (Archer 1995). However, the concept of *morphogenic society* (which I discuss further below) refers to one particular, or rather potential social configuration. Whether a society is morphogenic or not is an empirical, historical, fact. It follows that by introducing the concept of morphogenic society into a philosophical discussion of the just society I am restricting my claims' scope of validity to include societies that exhibit social morphogenic features while excluding those that do not.

Before examining the implications of refined conceptions of human reflexivity for just morphogenic societies, I unpack the nature and significance of morphogenic society in light of reflections held in the Centre for Social Ontology over the past 7 years or so.

Morphogenic Society: What It Is and Why It Matters

This section examines the nature of morphogenic society. It discusses the dimensions of social morphogenesis, examines to what extent we can say we are currently living in a morphogenic society and signals contemporary normative problems attributable to morphogenesis unbound.

What Morphogenic Society Is and What It Is Not

Archer (2013) refers to morphogenic society, as opposed to morphostatic society, as a form of society in which mechanisms generating social transformation overwhelm mechanisms maintaining social stability. However, abrupt social change is NOT sufficient to characterise morphogenic society. Indeed, morphostatic societies may, and actually did, change abruptly because of foreign invasion or because of biological disasters such as plagues or famine. What is characteristic of morphostatic society is rather the fact that transformational mechanisms are exogeneous rather than endogeneous. Change results from another nation entering in war or an exceptional innovation or natural disaster. On the other hand, morphogenic society is defined by the endogeneity of change when morphostatic mechanisms are weaker than morphogenetic ones. Change in a morphogenic society results from people performing the practices and respecting the rights and duties associated with their roles. They do so, however in changing ways conducive to the elaboration of new roles.

Not only is morphogenic change endogeneous rather than exogeneous; but it is also tendential rather than actual or phenomenal. Indeed, if we view societies as open systems (Bhaskar 1998), it should not surprise us that the existence of morphogenic mechanisms may be disconnected from their actual realisation. Think for instance of the role of public and private debt in maintaining wealthy lifestyles in the last quarter of the twentieth century. Actually, a whole generation of workers in First World countries lived in relative opulence. They also lived under an illusory impression of economic and political stability when relations of power were actually shifting in favour of large private corporations and to the detriment of workers and states.

There is, finally, the question of the use of the singular or the plural. I may have, in my own writings, oscillated between referring to 'morphogenic societies' and 'morphogenic society'. The use of the singular can be interpreted in two ways. First as referring to a species of society, second, and more significantly, as signalling the advent of a single global society. Mentioning plural 'societies' signals, however, that human culture entails remarkable diversity. It may also express a political will of the author to refrain from contributing to excessive homogenisation and destruction of cultural specificity. In the fourth volume of the *Social Morphogenesis* series I examined the globalisation of norms and suggested that while simple, straightforward cultural and normative arrangements (e.g. using a toothbrush regularly) were increasingly homogeneous, complex norms were, on the contrary increasingly fragmented (e.g. hackers contesting intellectual property). Overall, the use of singular or plural should not be problematic as long as the above distinctions are held in mind.

The Dimensions of Social Morphogenesis

Morphogenesis is not synonymous with perception of acceleration (Lawson 2014). And neither is it synonymous with actual acceleration. But is it reducible to a tendency to acceleration? In other words, is the intensification of morphogenetic mechanisms equivalent to tendential acceleration?

I examined this question in Al-Amoudi (2014) and developed it further in Al-Amoudi and Latsis (2015) and Al-Amoudi (2016). My argument was that morphogenesis entails several dimensions. Acceleration of social change is one of these dimensions, which I termed, for want of a better expression, *sequential morphogenesis*. There is, however, another dimension to morphogenesis: the production of coexisting institutional variety which may also be referred to as *concurrent morphogenesis*. Technological acceleration provides an example of sequential morphogenesis while diversification of normatively acceptable familial arrangements provides an example of concurrent morphogenesis.

The intensification of sequential morphogenesis produces a significant emergent mechanism examined in Al-Amoudi and Latsis (2015). We argued that intensified morphogenesis does not only create novel social forms but, in many circumstances, it is also conducive to the obsolescence or death of social forms.

Are We Currently Living in a Morphogenic Society?

To say that society is morphogenic certainly does not entail that morphogenic mechanisms overwhelm morphostatic ones 'everywhere'. As I argued in the second volume of the *Social Morphogenesis* series (Al-Amoudi 2014), morphogenic society differs from Liquid Modernity (Bauman 2012). Some, though by no means all social institutions incur intensified morphogensis. Crucially, those institutions that resist morphogenesis are endowed with exceptional normative influence. Think for example of the growing importance of the very resilient principle of private property of the means of production (Al-Amoudi 2014). Another example of a mechanism deeply entrenched and resisting significant morphogenic pressures is provided by Graeber's remark that the principle according to which 'one ought to pay back debts' overwhelms humanitarian considerations (Graeber 2011), often with disastrous consequences for human flourishing.

But social morphogenesis is also unequally distributed as morphogenic societies are characterised by heterogenous social and institutional landscapes. As Maccarini puts it, morphogenic societies entail enclaves and vortices (Maccarini 2015). That is, zones of relative institutional stability that coexist with zones of intense and even turbulent social change.

On these bases, I believe we can reasonably affirm that we are currently living in a morphogenic society. But is this configuration likely to last? Realist theorising has always been wary of future prediction, and rightly so (Bhaskar 1998; Lawson 1997, 2003). We have reasons to say, however, that, in our current state of knowledge, we have no reason to expect a reversal to morphostatic societies in the foreseeable future (for a full argument, see Archer 2014 on the stabilisation of morphogenic societies).

Normative Problems in Morphogenic Societies

If the analyses I proposed in the second volume of the *Morphogenic Society* series (Al-Amoudi 2014) are not too mistaken, normativity appears to be fragmented along a number of dimensions. The effects of this fragmentation are not always negative for human flourishing. For instance, many previously unproblematized ethical questions have been brought to light precisely because of the multiple memberships enabled by a morphogenic society. These categorical ambiguities have led in turn to struggles for recognition and have arguably resulted in the increased awareness of most members of society about the specific needs of the least favoured members of society.

On the other hand, scrutiny of normativity in contemporary morphogenic society points to a worrying dilution of norms relative to solidarity. This dilution is observable both at the level of the nation-state – the withering of the Welfare-State – and at the level of the private sphere with the increasing commodification of relations of care. Moreover, the fragmentation of normativity is manifested in the appearance of novel mundane problems for which past wisdom is of little help and which require, therefore, the discussion and the (typically emergent) establishment of novel norms. These discussions are also complexified by the fact that those arguments accepted without question in one group can be seen as problematic in another group with which discussion is nonetheless necessary in order to reach a collective *modus vivendi*. The elaboration of mutually acceptable norms is further complicated by the fact that those traditional institutions in charge of settling disagreements are themselves increasingly contested. This contestation has not (yet?) led to violent outbursts but has generated a proliferation of anormative regulation (Archer 2016) and increased reliance on novel arbitrators operating in parallel with the more conventional ones. In the juridical domain, an increasing number of cases are being treated in the margins of the juridical system and, while the confidentiality of arbitration makes it impossible to measure these numbers precisely, strong indications are provided by the proliferation of training courses for arbiters and the establishment of arbitration associations that set their own standards at the margins of national or international juridical systems. In the familial sphere, the right to judge and decide, traditionally attributed to parents, seems to be increasingly shared with a number of others, including professional parenting advisors, mass media and, more recently, parental networks.

Moreover, it is significant for the present paper that intensified morphonecrosis (Al-Amoudi and Latsis 2015) presents people both with contextual discontinuity (a consequence already noted in Archer 2003) but also with contexts that encourage power struggles whose stake is institutions' death or survival (morphonecrosis' *agonies*). Contexts of morphonecrosis and social agony affect people's ability to engage in social and political reflexivity in ways that the sections "Social reflexivity: how should I make my way through the world?" and "Political reflexivity: steering society together" below will attempt to clarify.

Finally, morphogenesis unbound encourages novel forms of social inequality stemming from differential powers to interpret and act upon codified rules (Al-Amoudi 2016). These arguments provide a background for the present paper. Not only because they characterise Modernity, late or otherwise, as a form of inegalitarian liberalism (a characterisation that is rather common knowledge for anyone familiar with Marxist scholarship). But, more importantly, because these investigations highlight the centrality of interpretive powers and examine the social and economic inequalities resulting from unequal powers of interpretation.

In sum, the problems of normativity in morphogenic society matter if we are interested in contemporary obstacles to Eudaimonia and intend to re-examine reflexivity in relation to normative questions of political philosophy.

Social Reflexivity: How Should I Make My Way Through the World?

Recent realist social theory has explored the human powers of social reflexivity to some depth. I build on the works of Archer (2003, 2007, 2012), Donati (2013) and Donati and Archer (2015) to offer a contribution to theories of justice. I argue in particular that in a morphogenic society, social reflexivity becomes necessary to people's satisfactory functioning and flourishing. Social reflexivity should therefore be listed among the central human capabilities that Nussbaum (2003) uses as a standard to assess a given society's level of fairness or to compare across different social models. Moreover, realising the moral importance of social reflexivity indicates new directions for egalitarian philosophers interested in discussing realistic utopias (Rawls 2001: 4–5). If my argument that social reflexivity should be considered as a central human capability is accepted, then future political philosophical reflection should also consider which institutions are most capable of fostering social reflexivity for equal citizens.

Modes of Social Reflexivity: A Very Brief Refresher

The conception of social reflexivity on which I base my argument has been developed to some length in Archer (2003, 2007, 2012). I now present only those aspects which are vital to this chapter's intelligibility. Social reflexivity is conceived as a personal emergent power through which people conduct internal conversations in which they attempt to relate their concerns with their social contexts and vice versa, with a view to taking appropriate courses of action.

Of direct relevance to this chapter's argument, powers of social reflexivity are not evenly distributed among persons. Different persons are differently equipped with the capability to ask and act upon the question: 'how should I make my way through the world?' and its corollaries: 'what matters to me?' and 'what should I do about it?' Indeed, by collecting first-person accounts of life-stories, Archer identifies four distinct modes of reflexivity.

Meta-reflexivity consists in being capable of critical reflexion about one's own internal conversations and about effective action in society. This mode of reflexivity attends particularly to the question 'what matters to me and my view of the good society?'.[5]

Autonomous reflexivity consists in being capable of sustaining self-contained internal conversations leading directly to action. This mode of reflexivity attends particularly to the question 'what should I do about it?'

Communicative reflexivity consists in being able to initiate an internal conversation but not to conclude it and take appropriate action without help from other interlocutors who complete and confirm initial thoughts.

Fractured reflexivity consists in being incapable of attempting to use one's reflexive powers without incurring intensified distress and disorientation, to the point of interrupting the internal conversation before a course of action is elaborated.

[5]My own understanding is that meta-reflexivity and autonomous reflexivity are not necessarily exclusive of one another.

Of particular importance for my overall argument, powers of reflexivity can, to some extent and as may any other personal emergent power, be nurtured or destroyed. Archer's interviews indicate, for instance, that communicative reflexivity can be fractured following severe contextual discontinuity. But they indicate too that fractured reflexivity can also mend in an appropriate social context. And I can think of no reason why autonomous and meta-reflexivity could not be developed through appropriate social relations and practices.

The Morphostatic Assumptions of Theories of Justice

Why do Rawls, Sen and Nussbaum ignore unequally effective powers of social reflexivity? It does not suffice to say that Archer's works were not written by that time as other authors did investigate, though in different terms, similar phenomena. For instance, Bandura's studies of self-efficacy point (in their own terms) to differently shared capacities of autonomous reflexivity. And Kohlberg's works on moral development point (also in their own terms) to differently shared capacities of meta-reflexivity. I would suggest, rather, that the downplaying of unequally distributed powers of social reflexivity is in great part explainable by the fact that John Rawls, Amartya Sen and Martha Nussbaum *reason in the implicit context of a morphostatic society*. In such a society, mechanisms of stabilisation are sufficiently powerful to grant contextual continuity. As a result, social reflexivity is not essential to people's satisfactory functioning.

Similarly, human reflexivity is not listed among the primary goods to be secured by an adequately designed basic structure of society (Rawls). These primary goods are: basic rights and liberties; freedom of movement and occupation; powers and prerogatives linked to positions; income and wealth; social bases of self-respect. Reflexivity is not reducible to any combination of primary goods, yet it is an essential capability for their acquisition and production in a morphogenic society. Indeed, in a morphostatic society agents are not significantly penalised, and are quite often rewarded, if they follow the advice of well-defined figures of authority for their important choices. There are therefore premiums, or at least no significant penalties, associated with communicative reflexivity in morphostatic societies. This is why, for instance, communicative reflexives who seem functional and happy in morphostatic societies often suffer from reflexive fracture in the ever-changing contexts of Late Modernity (Archer 2012: pp. 125–65).

Moreover, in a morphostatic society, the premiums and penalties associated with autonomous reflexivity seem to depend on the person's social position. In a society where social relations and hierarchies are stable, where social trajectories are limited and where normative frameworks are both homogeneous and compelling, the opportunities for bargain hunting and calculative innovation are necessarily limited and the premiums associated with them are limited too. Note however how, in inegalitarian morphostatic societies, autonomous reflexivity is encouraged and developed in the education of ruling classes but not in the education of commoners.

Machiavelli's *The Prince* and Louis XIV's *Le Metier de Roi* contain advice for rulers that encourage autonomous reflexivity. Meta-reflexivity seems notably absent, however, from these treatises.[6]

The Meagre Assumptions of Theories of Justice on Social Reflexivity

Social reflexivity is only very partially addressed by Rawls's minimalist philosophical anthropology. It is covered by the second moral power, that is, people's capacity to formulate a comprehensive conception of the good. This capacity is taken for granted and operates as a boundary for political philosophy as Rawls conceives it. Basically, people are capable of formulating conceptions of what a good life worth living is. They are also capable of engaging in actions through which their conception of the good is realised. However, the discussion of these powers belongs to the domain of moral and ethical philosophy and not to political philosophy as Rawls envisages it. As a result, Rawls attempts to outline his theory of justice while remaining uncommitted to any specific conception of the good. The only restriction imposed on conceptions of the good is that they should be 'reasonable' in the sense of being compatible with other people's comprehensive conceptions of the good.

Rawls's theory of moral development draws significantly on the works of Kohlberg. Although Rawls's *Theory of Justice* only mentions Kohlberg in a couple of footnotes, the whole Chapter VIII (The Sense of Justice) mirrors very closely Kohlberg's three-step development of moral consciousness.[7] However, Rawls emphasises the acquisition of a sense of justice over the acquisition of the power to examine, criticise, and subsequently adopt, reject or refine possible courses of action by comparing them with ultimate concerns. The resulting conception is, on the one hand, one that goes beyond the *morality of association*[8] and that could perhaps be described as meta-reflexivity. But on the other, it is also a conception that downplays the role of social structures and of socio-cultural interaction in the formation of human moral powers.

At this point, we might note an ontological slipping that operates within *Theory of Justice* and that might partly explain Rawls's inattentiveness to the

[6]I leave open the question of whether the use made of the works of Aristotle, Augustine and Aquinas encouraged meta-reflexivity or whether it encouraged lucid self-examination while shielding pre-defined values from critical assessment.

[7]Habermas's philosophical anthropology too is heavily influenced by Kohlberg (c.f. Habermas 2007: 116–94).

[8]The morality of association is defined as a relatively early moral stage in which moral standards are impressed by the dis/approval of those in authority. The dependence of Ego's reflection on Alter's validation draws this power close to communicative reflexivity.

formation of moral powers qua powers and the resulting lack of interrogation of the social conditions of the possibility of their development. Indeed, while Rawls mentions the two moral *powers* of citizens in a well ordered society, the section of *Theory of Justice* that exposes his conception of moral development focuses on the development of moral sentiments. Moral sentiments are understood there as entrenched dispositions rather than mere feelings. I believe that Rawls is right to avoid identifying moral sentiments as feelings, but by relying on the category of disposition or sentiment he also ends up losing sight of moral powers being in essence reflexive *powers*. I wonder if, had Rawls consistently evoked moral powers, whether Sen and Nussbaum might have investigated more thoroughly the social injustices resulting from, or indicated by, the unequal distribution of moral powers and, more generally, of efficient human reflexivity?

Should Social Reflexivity Be Listed as a Central Human Capability?

When Martha Nussbaum (2003) draws up a list of 'central human capabilities' that are deemed to be fundamental entitlements in the context of a just society, human reflexivity appears on the list in a fragmented and partial way. Nussbaum's list features: life; bodily health; sense imagination and thought; emotions; practical reason; affiliation; concern for other species; play and control over one's environment. Reflexivity, social or political, does not appear as a capability in its own right. Yet, it is not entirely absent from the list as it is partially covered by practical reason.

Nussbaum defines 'Practical reason' in the following succinct terms: 'Being able to form a conception of the good and to engage in critical reflection about the planning of one's life.' Nussbaum adds, between brackets: '(This entails protection of the liberty of conscience and religious observance).' I take it that she envisages 'practical reason' as synonymous, or at least very close to the second moral power Rawls attributes to people, i.e. 'a capacity for a conception of the good: it is the capacity to have, to revise, and rationally to pursue a conception of the good.' (Rawls 2001: 19) Rawls further specifies that 'such a conception is an ordered family of final ends and aims which specifies a person's conception of what is of value in human life or, alternatively, of what is a fully worthwhile life.'

While both Nussbaum and Rawls view 'practical reason' (Nussbaum's terminology) as a power or capability, they differ about the question of its prevalence. Rawls recognises the existence of people who are less capable of practical reason than others. Their case is treated as a sub-case of those citizens who are not capable of acting as 'fully cooperative members of society' for some reason. The case of these persons is not viewed as a significant central feature of every society, however, but rather as a 'difficult complication' that can be studied at a later stage of reflection. That is, after we first develop a theory of fairness populated exclusively with fully cooperative, and assumedly morally reflexive, agents. As Rawls has it: 'it is sensible to lay aside certain difficult complications. If we can work out a theory that covers the fundamental case, we can try to extend it to other cases later.' (Rawls 1980: 546, cited in Nussbaum 2003: 53).

Nussbaum, however, attempts to include persons who are not fully cooperative members of society into her philosophical reflexions on the just society. She refuses to treat persons who are less, or insufficiently, endowed with practical reasoning abilities as marginal cases. She reminds us rightly that in every society people are incapable of such powers for the first 10 or perhaps 20 years of their lives. And those lucky enough to live into old age can expect periods, sometime extending to 20 years, during which their moral capabilities might be limited.

Nussbaum draws several conclusions from the above observation. First, care during periods of extreme and asymmetrical dependency deserves to figure as a 'primary good' (Rawls) or, more precisely, as a 'central human capability' (Nussbaum). Second, the contractualist Kantian justification of care is less coherent than an Aristotelian/Marxist justification based on an understanding of the human as a being in need of a rich plurality of life activities to be shaped by affiliation and practical reason.

What strikes me, however, is that neither Rawls nor Sen nor Nussbaum seem to care for the position of those agents who are relatively less equipped than others with effective reflexive powers even though they are not in vital need of constant care. Yet, I believe that this inequality is very significant. First, because it concerns a large number of persons and can't be treated as an exceptional 'difficult complication', second, because it affects significantly the life chances of people, third, because reflexivity (as most powers) can be trained or, when fractured, repaired to some extent (cf. Archer on fractured reflexives on the mend). Fourth, because distribution of dominant modes of reflexivity bears structural effects and contributes to reproducing inegalitarian social structures.

Injustice Resulting from Unequal Social Reflexivity in Morphogenic Society

I have argued so far that the theories of justice of Rawls, Sen and Nussbaum presupposed morphostatic contexts and that they downplayed powers of social reflexivity. I now argue why social reflexivity matters in a morphogenic society. None of the arguments I present below is novel. Most are drawn from Archer's trilogy, especially Archer (2012). Some are additions or refinements I made in the context of the *Social Morphogenesis* series.

Social morphogenesis generates both novel opportunities and novel threats. Since agents are not automata moved by hydraulic forces, the way they reflect on their circumstances and the way they take action matters both for their own social trajectories and for the elaboration of subsequent social structure.

Archer (2012) judiciously accentuates that social morphogenesis is particularly harmful for communicative and fractured reflexives. On one hand, morphogenesis is conducive to a decline (Archer 2012) or a fragmentation (Al-Amoudi 2014) of authoritative sources of normativity. On the other hand, intensified morphogenesis implies significant contextual discontinuity or incongruity over a lifetime. The result is not only a world that looks odd to the older generation (Halbwachs 1992, 1997), but also a world that may and does change significantly over a decade (Archer 2012). Two consequences follow for communicative reflexives. First, the networks of advisors on which they rely can disperse. Think for instance of the banality of parents remarrying or of friends moving into another city for familial or professional reasons. Second, the experience of persons constituting these advisory networks is rapidly obsolete in a morphogenic society. This fact has been thoroughly investigated in Archer (2007) and Archer (2012). Think, for instance, of the career advice and example provided by miners to their children in post-Thatcher Britain. Archer (2012) ventures a plausible hypothesis: many communicative reflexives who could have lived reasonably good lives are so distressed by morphogenetic contextual discontinuity that their communicative reflexive powers are fractured as a result.[9]

At a general level, those same unbound morphogenetic processes that fracture communicative reflexivity also impede fractured reflexivity from mending into communicative reflexivity (Archer 2012: 249–91). We can specify further this abstract and general consideration by tracing the deleterious effects on fractured reflexives of the current lib-lab version of morphogenic society (Donati and Archer 2015). My point here is not only that Late Modernity impedes fractured reflexivity from mending, but also that Late Modernity is conducive to heightened suffering for those who fall-through 'the system'. First, many of the Welfare State institutions that developed post-WWII are declining. And while I have defended elsewhere the idea that workplace participation could, from a Rawlsian perspective, compensate for this decline (Blanc and Al-Amoudi 2013), we see scant signs of this happening. Second, as Dean's Foucauldian analyses (Dean 2007, 2010) rightly points out, contemporary neo liberal societies tolerate and even encourage violence upon those persons who are deemed to lack autonomy. Third, while I remain extremely sympathetic to the forms of third sector associations called for by Donati (Donati and Archer 2015), the emergence of such associations is limited in current morphogenic society based on relative stability of the mechanisms most fundamental to capitalism (i.e. rights of private property and obligation to pay financial debts, see the section "Are we currently living in a morphogenic society?" above). My impression is that these associations remain parasitic on the public sector to the extent that they depend on

[9]I am still hesitant about the nature and worth of communicative reflexivity. On one hand, it is construed by Archer as incomplete or lacking autonomous and meta-reflexivity. But on the other, it could perhaps be symptomatic of a beautiful democratic imaginary. A reflexive yet humble person might appreciate the value and diversity of others' points of view and thus refrain from taking action without thorough consultation. In this regard, it might be a sign of humility, open-mindedness and ultimately superior reflexivity to consult Alter and offer her a significant role in the conversation.

grants. And, in the absence of public funding, they also depend on the private sector to the extent that benevolent participants rely on salaries obtained from for-profit organisations.

That autonomous reflexivity is rewarded in a liberal inegalitarian morphogenic society should not be surprising. In terms of social trajectories, social morphogenesis produces a continuous array of novel opportunities and threats, and autonomous reflexives are particularly well equipped to analyse these unprecedented situations and engage in unconventional courses of action that best match their specific situation. In terms of norms, morphogenic society sends mixed messages that autonomous reflexives are particularly well equipped to pick and mix. Archer seems therefore justified to conclude that 'the autonomous reflexives find a ready home and feel thoroughly at home in these institutions of late modernity.' (Archer 2012: 205).[10]

Meta-reflexives are perhaps those who correspond most closely to the minimalist anthropology on which Rawls, Sen and Nussbaum base their theories of Justice. They are indeed the only group capable of forming, rather than merely adopting, a comprehensive conception of the good. And they realise that contemporary society does not allow them to live this life adequately and that perhaps no society, even a just one, will ever allow them to live up fully to their ideals.

Whether the development of meta-reflexivity is worthy depends on our conception of worth. In contemporary society, meta-reflexives seem to have trajectories that are more volatile than autonomous reflexives. However, I can think of no reason why in a more just society their social trajectories should become less changeable. At most, it could be argued that contemporary society causes particularly acute suffering to meta-reflexives as those individuals who do not follow a career in the private sector or who do not set up their own business are particularly penalised by unbridled capitalism in comparison with those who do. Yet, even in a well-ordered society, I would expect autonomous reflexives to obtain more primary goods than meta-reflexives – if anything because the former spend their energy pursuing goods recognised by the ambient ideology while the latter also evaluate them.

---

[10]This conclusion should come, however, with reservations. First, while Archer's investigations study the effects of modes of reflexivity on social trajectories, these effects are also encountering other countervailing mechanisms. In inegalitarian liberal morphogenic society, social class defined in terms of the economic capital possessed by parents might matter more than reflexivity. Moreover, if Picketty (2014) is correct, then contemporary Western societies witnesses levels of economic inequality unseen since the nineteenth century, and current tendencies point to widening gaps. Second, while Late Modernity is certainly beneficial to large corporations and particularly wealthy individuals (the infamous 1 %) it is not necessarily so for small entrepreneurs (see Al-Amoudi 2016) or even middle-class individuals. In this context, it might be expected that growing numbers of autonomous reflexives might become disillusioned with the promises of inegalitarian liberalism as they realise they will not benefit from inequalities. Third, reflection in terms of social trajectories obscures the importance of goods that are irreducible to wealth or social status. Yet, the rising sales of self-help books and of expensive coaching for middle-class professionals provides anecdotal evidence of the malaise produced by consumer society (for a critique of the materialistic wellness ideology, see Cederstrom and Spicer 2015).

In other words, if the situations of autonomous and meta-reflexives were compared either through Rawlsian primary goods or through Nussbaum's list of Central Human Capabilities, I could expect fractured reflexives to score less than communicative reflexives who would themselves score less than autonomous reflexives. And I am not sure where meta-reflexives would score, though my expectation would be that their group should display the highest variance.

There are, however, two very important reasons for encouraging or facilitating the development of meta-reflexivity in a just society. The first is that meta-reflexivity is a good in itself. That its exercise may not be conducive to maximisation of material and social goods enjoyed by the individual does not make it less of a good.[11] Agreed, meta-reflexives are likely to follow zig-zaging rather than ascending social trajectories, and agreed they are exposed to feeling continuously disappointed with themselves as much as with the people and institutions they encounter who fail their moral ideals. But whether meta-reflexivity brings happiness depends precisely on our conception of happiness. Under a conception of happiness-as-feeling-happy, meta-reflexivity is certainly a recipe for unhappiness. However, under either an Aristotelian conception of happiness as eudaimonic cultivation of powers (*arete*), meta-reflexivity is constitutive of true happiness.

The second reason why meta-reflexivity is important, and perhaps even crucial, in a just society is that of all forms of reflexivity, meta-reflexivity is the only one that can both challenge the status quo efficiently and at the same time proceed out of a sense of justice rather than following self-serving interests. In other words, it covers both Rawlsian principles. Its development is thus called for as a necessary condition of possibility for a liberal egalitarian society that corresponds to the theories of justice put forward by Rawls and after him Sen and Nussbaum.

Organisations Fostering Social Reflexivity in a Just Morphogenic Society

Neither social theory nor political philosophy can design in detail the institutions needed in a just society. Political philosophy's primary role is to draw realistic utopias (Rawls 2003: 4) and offer criteria for comparing different possible societies. It can help us, however, to identify institutions that are currently missing and it can also help us draw justifications for these institutions.

I have argued so far that unevenly distributed and effective modes of social reflexivity matter in a morphogenic society. It follows that a just morphogenic society should comprise institutions and organisations that help fostering social

[11] Acknowledging the goodness of meta-reflexivity does not disturb the liberal separation of just and good dear to Rawls. I do not specify which values meta-reflexivity should uphold, I just propose that being able to criticise values is good in itself. Again, there is a homology with the second moral power.

reflexivity. What I have not done is to propose concrete institutional arrangements that can contribute to a less inegalitarian distribution of effective reflexivity across society. In what follows I provide just a few directions.

Archer's investigations among University students indicates the importance of the family in the cultivation of social reflexivity (2012). Families generating relational evils seem either to impede the full development of reflexivity, resulting in fractured reflexive children, or they seem to 'enforce' instrumental rationality at the expense of moral considerations. On the other hand, families generating relational goods tend, according to Archer, to generate either communicative reflexivity or meta-reflexivity – depending on the normative dissonance children had to face.

What this means is that the familial context matters as it provides conditions of possibility for the growth of social reflexivity. And indeed, social reflexivity is to an extent one of the many relational goods generated by families.

However, what Archer's study does *not* mean is that family should be the sole point of action of public policy aiming to favour the development of reflexivity. First, because social inequality precisely affects families, since families can fail and children cannot be held accountable for their family's ills. Second, because families are never sufficient. Archer's study of reflexivity indicates indeed that strong familial consensus is not necessarily conducive to the development of powers of moral reflexivity. This result might be surprising for the most conservative members of society as it breaks a number of right-wing myths: first that the ability to make autonomous ascending career choices are best fostered in happy families and second, that moral powers are best fostered in homogeneous normative environments.

Very fortunately, the family is not the only organisation through which children develop their powers of social reflexivity. Schools, sport clubs, religious communities and informal groups of friends matter too. These organisations might be subsidiary to family and might help fostering social reflexivity.

How can they do so? Well, I can only be very brief and tentative here. One possibility could be to provide children with opportunities to converse with people from a broad range of horizons in a context that encourages civility. Another could be to provide efficacious counter-discourses to the largely anormative messages conveyed by the market (have you thought of your employability?) and by the State (have you voted and have you followed the procedures?) A third direction is to consider people all of ages and not only children. If reflexive powers evolve during a person's life, then organisations fostering reflexive powers should also be accessible to adults. In particular, the workplace seems particularly anormative, in spite of calls for the creation of moral spaces in corporations (Blanc 2014). A fourth direction might be to replace 'couselling' and 'coaching' with groups akin to the associations studied by Donati (Donati and Archer 2015: 229–62).

Political Reflexivity: Steering Society Together

I use the expression *political reflexivity* to refer to the human powers involved in judging society's worth and, equally importantly, in initiating collective action to govern and transform society. To my knowledge, realist social theory has dedicated more energy to studying social reflexivity than political reflexivity. Rawls examines, as we have seen in section "The meagre assumptions of theories of justice on social reflexivity" above, the formation of moral sentiments. He does not study, however, the capacities needed to steer a just society by equal participants. This omission is problematic as liberal egalitarian philosophy thus supposes implicitly either that political reflexivity is equally distributed or that its unequal distribution is unproblematic. In this paper, I attempt to argue exactly the reverse: (a) political reflexivity is unequally distributed; (b) this is problematic in a morphostatic society and even more so in a morphogenic society; (c) this unequal distribution can somewhat be remedied; and (d) finding such remedies is a project that should matter both to realist relational theorists and to liberal egalitarian philosophers.

What Is Political Reflexivity?

Political reflexivity can broadly be defined as the personal emergent power through which people reflect and act on the question 'how can we steer society together?' The metaphor of steering connotes both the idea of governing society and the idea of changing its trajectory purposefully, that is, towards a destination that is preferable to where the ship would go without its crew's continuous efforts. It should immediately be noted that, while in principle the whole global society might perhaps be steered, the expression 'steering society' also and mainly refers to the steering of parts of global society: coalitions of states, states, as well as large and small organisations and human groups. That is, the object of steering is constituted by sets of social relations constitutive of society.

The nautical metaphor reaches a significant limit, however, when we consider that, while steering a ship transforms or purposefully maintains its trajectory, steering society is about transforming or maintaining society itself. Thus, steering society is at once a matter of maintaining the relations and activities necessary for society's continuous reproduction and it is a matter of transforming social relations and activities with a sense of direction. I now compare and contrast political reflexivity with two notions resembling it, first with social reflexivity and then with leadership.

Political Reflexivity vs Social Reflexivity

Political reflexivity has in common with social reflexivity that both are personal emergent powers. Indeed, it is never society that steers itself (a structural deterministic fantasy), nor is it ever culture that steers it (a cultural deterministic fantasy), but people who do the steering, albeit through processes that presuppose the existence of social structures and cultural systems.

Moreover, political reflexivity is, like social reflexivity, a *reflexive* power. Firstly because the action of steering – be it a ship or a social organisation – is open to unintended consequences and unexpected contingencies. And second because there are always multiple directions in which a social organisation can be steered.

Like social reflexivity, political reflexivity does not operate in the absence of internal conversations held by participants. Indeed, subjects of political reflexivity have to consider their own concerns, their understanding of their social context and the likely responses of other persons. I would like to venture, however, that *the structure of the reflection at play in political reflexivity is different from the structure of the reflection at play in social reflexivity*. Especially, whereas social reflexivity considers the subject's social position as its point of departure and as its point of destination, i.e. the subject's social position, political reflexivity takes the social relations in which the subject (may) engage as its point of departure and destination.

Several significant implications follow from this difference between social and political reflexivity. Firstly, steering a set of social relations is by nature a collective action. A single subject may decide to abandon or ignore a set of social relations, but she can only steer them in collaboration with other subjects. Thus, the 'together' clause is not tautological in the question 'how can we steer society together?'

Secondly, political reflexivity supposes a certain degree of maturity on part of the subject. Since steering implies collective action it presupposes that the subject has already entered some form of corporate agency and that a realistic sense of 'We' has formed through anterior cycles of socialisation. The expressions 'how can we steer society together?' and 'how can I contribute to steering society?' are not interchangeable, and a moment's thought indicates the latter is open to uncoordinated actions (actions that are neither understandable nor held desirable by others) unless it is reformulated in the plural. Moreover, since steering social relations implies transforming the rights and obligations of those entering these relations, political reflexivity necessitates some (realistic) sense of current roles and how they may be transformed for the greater good. Finally, since steering social relations implies anticipating (even by guessing) how the steering will affect the distribution of resources, the subjects of political reflection must orient their reflections towards some (fallible though founded) understanding of the positions of primary agents affected by the relational steering under consideration.

Thirdly, because political reflexivity attempts to mobilise a collectivity of agents, it must be justifiable in conventional terms, understandable by those whose collaboration is required. There is in political reflexivity an external or public moment that is not necessary to social reflexivity. Private rumination may help to a point but it fails without the ability to publicise ideas convincingly.

Political Reflexivity vs Leadership

The discourse of 'leadership' marks one of the ugliest cultural evolutions at the turn of the twenty-first century. This trend affects middle classes grooming their children into 'leadership' as well as would-be corporate managers and, more recently, professionals and civil servants. Leadership precludes however, both meta-reflexivity and a democratic imaginary. The contemporary discourse of leadership insists very heavily on the 'values' and 'norms' of leaders. However, these values and norms are meant to be taken for granted rather than continuously questioned as meta-reflexivity would. Moreover, the expression 'leadership' presupposes an asymmetry between the leader and the led. It presupposes that the leader knows better what is good and how it can be achieved. Her role is therefore to manipulate the led into following her plan. The manipulative dimension of leadership is mystified by the open rejection of coercion: leaders are expected to mentor, inspire, explain, show, convince, and so on. As an enthusiastic commentator has it:

> After crafting an image of what the leaders want the organization to achieve, they [the leaders] charismatically communicate their vision to their followers... Moreover, transformational leaders connect followers' self-concepts to the organization's mission and vision through idealized influence, inspirational motivation, intellectual stimulation and individualized consideration. (Hartnell and Walumba 2011: 232, cited in Alvesson 2013: 173).

Behind its enthusing rhetorics, the relation leader/led is unidirectional to the extent that the led are not expected to reflect critically, let alone answer back, to the vision formulated by the leader. I surmise, however, that a relationship based on political reflexivity rather than leadership would instead be at best symmetrical and at worst asymmetrical, though it would never be unidirectional. Even when the balance of power is skewed, each participant in the relation is ready to revise her concerns and her beliefs in light of the other's arguments.

Some of the Capabilities Needed for Political Reflexivity

My interest in alternative forms of governance and in political reflexivity developed when I started contributing to a social movement. I discovered, not only that effective participation into public life requires a broad set of skills or powers but also that these powers are unequally distributed in society. While some of these inequalities might be attributable to natural differences, and while some of these natural differences might only be compensated for up to a point, it also appeared that through the formation of propitious human relations and through adequate experiences, most people, including myself, could improve these skills.

The difficulties faced by such movements as *Indignados* and *Occupy* (and many others before them) are particularly revealing about the political powers required for militantism in particular and from participation in public life in general. It is especially when these powers were missing, or when they were progressively and painfully acquired after initial mistakes, that their importance became salient. Among these powers, we could list:

(a) *Developing a sense of the common good*: participants in a political movement are prompted to justify their claims, and they have to do so by referring to a conception of the greater good rather than to egoistic interests. Many incidents occurred (from conversations breaking down to participants engaging in physical intimidation) whenever claims were made with reference to too narrow interests.

Moreover, while in some political movements the common good may be restricted to its members' common good, claims are more influential when they address a common good that extends beyond the relatively narrow circle of participants. I understand the theories of justice developed by Rawls, Nussbaum and Sen as attempts to formulate universal conceptions of the common good that extend across generations and across social positions.

(b) *Developing a democratic imaginary*: not bossing people around, refraining from imposing one's views, seeking consensus, etc. While the ethics of discussion constitute a crucial topic and have been substantially theorised by writers such as Habermas, it is noteworthy that the full exercise of political reflexivity encompasses activities that suppose powers ranging beyond those covered in theories of justice or in discourse ethics.

(c) *Turn taking in conversations*: avoiding monopolising the conversation or interrupting others but also, and equally importantly, knowing when to jump in and speak. Since there are no formal rules in conversation turn-taking, this capability is largely based on tacit knowledge acquired through practice rather than on explicit knowledge of the sort that can be conveyed by ethical, moral or political philosophy.

(d) *Speaking in public*: public speaking with clarity and eloquence, but also knowing how to stop, seemed difficult to some participants, especially those for whom the activity was new and those who felt these occasions were the sole ones they had been offered to voice their concerns.

(e) *Interpreting the news*: several participants felt suspicious about the mainstream press. Their suspicion was not so much directed towards the authenticity of released information as much as towards the selection of news publicised and the (neo-liberal) interpretations provided by journalists.

(f) *Discipline in honouring commitments*: the movement went through disappointments when deadlines were missed and commitments were not honoured. More generally, many members were not used to organise their time or workload.

(g) *Ability to engage in a meaningful discussion with existing authorities*: in particular, some members wrote letters to the local authority that were qualified by the head of the municipality as 'delirious'.

(h) *Developing a sense of compromise*: in group discussions, members were using hand signals to express agreement or disagreement. Yet the most important signal was neither 'I agree' nor 'I disagree and veto' but rather 'I do not fully agree but am ready to live with this proposed amendment'.

The above powers constitute a non-exhaustive list. But we can note from it that political reflexivity's constitutive powers do not overlap exactly with the powers constitutive of social reflexivity. The skills allowing people to make their way through the world are not exactly the same that allow them to steer society. But why do these skills matter? Why are they essential to a just society? To this question I now turn.

Why Political Reflexivity Matters

Why does the ability to participate in the governance of the organisations with which one is involved a matter for justice? Rawls's identification of self-respect provides an important argument for self-governance, not only at the level of the state, but also in the context of various organisations which bear on our lives, including work places in contexts of weak welfare-States (Blanc and Al-Amoudi 2013). There is, however, much more to participating in governance than acquiring the bases of respect and self-respect. Similarly, Nussbaum's notion of affiliation provides but a limited approximation. It is also striking that, while Tocqueville identifies political associations as a fundamental mechanism of democracy in America,[12] he has very little to say about the powers necessary for participating actively in such associations.

At heart is the question of the realisation, or negation, of real freedom and of positive liberties (Berlin). Indeed, the Aristotelian principle (Rawls 1971: 424–33) and the view of wo/man as a 'political animal' (Aristotle) suggest that wo/man flourishes by participating actively in the governance of the city. Thus, political reflexivity is at once a human power or virtue and it is a good in itself whether in a morphostatic or in a morphogenic society.

Moreover, in light of my activist experiences, I am tempted to reinterpret Jo Freeman's (1972) classic short text on the tyranny of structurelessness as indicative of a lack in contemporary democracies. Indeed, a realist approach to social structure reveals that the tyranny lamented by Freeman does not result from the absence of structure but rather from the presence of informal yet real and inegalitarian structures. The inequalities she discerns are not due to an absence of structures but rather to their very presence and asymmetry. Some agents are better equipped with social and political powers than others. Her account mixes two forms of inequalities. Those that result from unequal power and those that result from wide

[12]'The most natural privilege of man, next to the right of acting for himself, is that of combining his exertions with those of his fellow-creatures, and of acting in common with them. I am therefore led to conclude that the right of association is almost as inalienable as the right of personal liberty. No legislator can attack it without impairing the very foundations of society. Nevertheless, if the liberty of association is a fruitful source of advantages and prosperity to some nations, it may be perverted or carried to excess by others, and the element of life may be changed into an element of destruction. A comparison of the different methods which associations pursue in those countries in which they are managed with discretion, as well as in those where liberty degenerates into license, may perhaps be thought useful both to governments and to parties.' (Tocqueville 2013: Chap. XII)

social prejudice against certain social positions. Yet, even the solution she proposes, which consists in maintaining some formal structure in social movements, also presupposes that members are capable of political reflexive powers such as those listed above.

Why Political Reflexivity Matters All the More in Morphogenic Society?

Why is the uneven distribution of powers necessary to political reflexivity particularly problematic in the context of a morphogenic society? Firstly, in a morphogenic society, human organisations are prone to face heavier environmental changes and to go, themselves, through particularly intense transformations in order to thrive or, at least, survive. Yet, in the absence of adequate checks and balances and in situations of concentration of power, each organisational change provides those governing the organisation with opportunities to accentuate inequalities in their favour. Moreover, the formal systems of checks and balances are, as the History of twentieth and early twenty-first century suggests, insufficient to keep accumulation in check. Keeping decisions in check necessitates more than formal procedures, it also necessitates powers of political reflexivity. These powers need not be exercised by everyone at every time. But they must exist as real capabilities that might be exercised should doubts arise. Yet, today, how many can read a balance sheet? Or speak at a public assembly? Or start a petition? And equally important, how many know when to 'let go' and to prioritise those battles worthy of citizens' time over those that are secondary?

Secondly, the temptation in a complex and seemingly perilous environment is to entrust the helm to those who know or pretend to know how to govern. The effect is the rise of technocratic management that is increasingly disconnected from the ethos and local knowledge of those affected by decisions. The contemporary distrust of elites provides a historically contingent, yet all the more urgent, reason to consider political reflexivity and its real structural bases. The twenty-first century rise of populism, both under its authoritarian and its direct-democratic forms, indicates growing distrust of elites and the severe dysfunctions of indirect democracy. On one hand, we witness a willingness to follow leaders who do not seem to have been corrupted by the temptations of public life (the Fascist *Front National* party's slogan was for a long time: 'la tête haute et les mains propres') and whose character and understanding of everyday affairs has not been blunted by bureaucratic or technocratic mentality (cf. M. Le Pen and N. Farrage's crusades against European bureaucracy). On the other, we witness relatively large, though ephemeral, political formations that display an appetite for direct democracy as well as unequal individual abilities to contribute to the movement's governance or to furthering its causes.

What Organisations May Help Fostering Political Reflexivity?

Just as with social reflexivity, political reflexivity is fostered through myriad organisations. We can identify, however, some organisations that play a particularly important role:

(a) *The family* certainly plays an important part and is arguably the principle setting where the child learns the basic skills constitutive of political reflexivity. Yet, we must go beyond the imagery of the family as a microcosm of society and acknowledge that, while the first rudiments of political reflexivity might be acquired in familial settings, the maturation and full development of political reflexivity necessitates relations and interactions with members of other families. That is, political reflexivity can fully flourish only by crossing the family's boundaries.

(b) *The school* constitutes another crucial institution for the development of political reflexivity and associated skills. It is so whenever it offsets the potential deficiencies of the least politically reflexive families to some degree. But equally importantly, the school is also a place where the child is confronted with members belonging to the same community but to different families. Through discussion with peers, she can learn to confront views and understand differences of outlook with members of different families that may hold different concerns and differing visions of the world (including society). Moreover, teachers offer important counter-points to the authority of the parents as they provide the child with authority figures whose values and world-views, while compatible with those of the wider community may also differ from the specific values and world-views of the child's parents.

    In this light, the school is (or at least can be) a site where children are prepared for democratic political life. Note, however, how this conception of the school is different from those aspirations, held for instance by extreme right group *Collectif Racine*, which purports to restrict the school's activities to 'instruction' while claiming that 'education' is the exclusive prerogative of the family. It is not surprising that movements such as *Collectif Racine* and others also propose to ban the League of Human Rights from performing activities in and with members of (high) schools.

(c) *Societies and clubs* also provide propitious organisational spaces in which subjects can exercise their powers of political reflexivity. These societies and clubs may encompass a wide range of activities ranging from sports to boy scouts and from chess clubs to drinking societies. However, because such institutions are rarely financially self-sufficient (unless they treat their members as customers and thus pervert their relationality), they are unfortunately prevalently mainly accessible to middle and upper class agents. This elitism is all the more damaging as it contributes in turn to the unequal distribution of powers of political reflexivity among members of society. Indeed student societies are particularly prevalent in elite institutions such as Ivy League universities, Oxbridge or the French Grandes Ecoles. In French Grandes Ecoles, there is a common understanding that these societies equip future 'elites' with basic social and political skills. Yet, in spite of their current elitism, these organisations might serve as exemplars for more accessible ones that would benefit from public subsidies and be located in less privileged areas.

(d) *Work organisations* are perhaps the most significant organisations where adults can exercise their political reflexivity for the greatest part of their life. Yet, most work organisations, especially lucrative ones, are structured as nepotistic or autocratic rather than democratic organisations. In spite of philosophic arguments calling for considering a wider range of corporate institutions in the basic structure of society in the context of the Welfare State's decline (Blanc and Al-Amoudi 2013) and calls for the creation of moral spaces in private corporations (Blanc 2014), there is to date, little political interest in considering the democratic potential of well-ordered work organisations in a just society.

(e) *Social networks* such as Facebook thematic pages have the potential to contribute to the flourishing of human political reflexivity just as they also hold the potential of intensifying narcissistic individualism. In Italy, for instance, Internet pages dedicated to a street or neighbourhood are reported to have enhanced the social bonds among its users.[13] The latter meet online but also offline and engage in discussions relative to their common relational good (their neighbourhood) that mobilise and exercise political reflexivity (New York Times: 2015).

Moreover, while social media can and often are used as passively as television or reading the *Sun*, I have personally found they provided interesting fora to exchange views on significant news and social and political developments. Particularly beneficial were the views of distant 'friends' whom I could not meet regularly and who would interpret the same piece of news from a very different perspective. The structure of FB allows for responses and responses to the responses, that is, a dialogue. Indeed, FB can provide a public agora that is severely missing from contemporary society. Contrary to a political club, however, it gathers 'friends' and 'friends' of 'friends' with differing political sensitivities. In many cases heterogeneous political views are conducive to unsocial behaviour (aka flaming), however, when the capabilities necessary to political reflexivity are properly employed (see the section "Some of the capabilities needed for political reflexivity" supra) the resulting discussion can enrich, rather than narrow or frustrate, the views of all participants.

[13] I am grateful to Pierpaolo Donati who pointed this important example to me.

Conclusion

This chapter has attempted a sociological contribution to political philosophy. It took stock of the normative problems arising from intensified social morphogenesis and addressed their political implications on the effective functioning of two human powers of reflexivity, social reflexivity and political reflexivity, that have been sidelined in the theories of justice of Rawls, Sen and Nussbaum, largely because these philosophical works presuppose morphostatic rather than morphogenic societies.

I have argued that both effective social and political reflexivity are unevenly distributed in contemporary societies. This uneven distribution matters all the more in the context of intensified morphogenesis, to the point of prompting the inclusion of social and political reflexivity, as well as the powers essential to their functioning, among other basic human capabilities.

Social reflexivity can be conceived as people's ability to reflect and act on the question: 'how should I make my way through the world?', a question that can be subdivided into 'what matters for me?' and 'how do I get it?' In times of intensified social morphogenesis, people able to reflect autonomously on the question 'how do I get it?' are at a competitive advantage, though with a catch as this (sub) question alone does not guarantee that the concerns they pursued are really those that matter most for them.

People able to reflect (meta-reflexively) on the (sub) question 'what matters most for me?' are, on their side, penalised if their ultimate concerns are not compatible with the values implicit in careers within large corporations or starting a for-profit enterprise. This penalty stems less from morphogenesis unbound than from capitalism unbound. It is, however, all the more damaging to the prospects of a just society if we consider that meta-reflexivity is a good in itself and that meta-reflexives are those most inclined to challenge the status quo and proceed out of a refined sense of justice rather than self-serving interest. It is, however, those unable to initiate (fractured reflexivity) or conclude their social reflexions without the help of others (communicative reflexivity) who suffer most from the contextual discontinuity and increased variety brought by intensified morphogenesis.

Political reflexivity can be conceived of as people's ability to reflect and act on the question: 'how can we steer society together?' This form of reflexivity does not operate without individual subjects holding internal conversations. The latter are oriented, however, towards the set of social relations to be steered rather than towards participants' personal social trajectories. They must take into account the roles and resources of both Ego and the many Alters whose collaboration is sought. They thus suppose a certain maturity of the subject and, equally importantly, her ability to justify her projects vis-à-vis Alter. Contrary to 'leadership', political reflexivity is democratic as all participants are expected to be ready to revise their concerns and their beliefs in light of others' arguments.

Social and political reflexivity are both personal emergent powers, and they can only be operational if subjects possess a range of distinct personal emergent powers. Although they are arguably subject to natural variations, these powers can be fostered through a number of organisations including families, schools, societies, work organisations and even social media.

If the theses above are accepted, it follows that in well-ordered societies, the state should encourage, transform, and when appropriate subsidise organisations that can foster social and political reflexivity rather than encourage, and sometimes fund, organisations that enjoin people to improve their employability, cast voting bulletins or respect leadership under its various guises.

References

Al-Amoudi, I. (2014). Morphogenesis and normativity: Problems the former creates for the latter. In: Archer MS (Ed.) Late modernity: Trajectories towards morphogenic society. Cham: Springer.

Al-Amoudi, I. (2016). In letter & in spirit: Social morphogenesis and the interpretation of codified social rules. In M. S. Archer (Ed.), *Morphogenesis and the crisis of normativity*. Dordrecht: Springer.

Al-Amoudi, I., & Latsis, J. (2015). Death contested: morphonecrosis and conflicts of interpretation. In M. S. Archer (Ed.), *Generative mechanisms transforming late modernity*. Cham: Springer.

Alvesson, M. (2013). *The triumph of emptiness. Consumption, higher education & work organization*. Oxford: Oxford University Press.

Archer, M. S. (1995). *Realist social theory: The morphogenetic approach*. Cambridge: Cambridge University Press.

Archer, M. S. (2003). *Structure, agency and the internal conversation*. Cambridge: Cambridge University Press.

Archer, M. S. (2007). *Making our way through the world*. Cambridge: Cambridge University Press.

Archer, M. S. (2012). *The reflexive imperative in late modernity*. Cambridge: Cambridge University Press.

Archer, M. S. (2013). Social morphogenesis and the prospects of morphogenic society. In M. S. Archer (Ed.), *Social morphogenesis*. Dordrecht: Springer.

Archer, M. S. (2014). Introduction: Stability or stabilization – On which would morphogenic society depend? In M. S. Archer (Ed.), *Late modernity: Trajectories towards morphogenic society*. Cham: Springer.

Archer, M. S. (2016). Anormative social regulation: An attempt to cope with social morphogenesis. In M. S. Archer (Ed.), *Morphogenesis and the crisis of normativity*. Dordrecht: Springer.

Bauman, Z. (2012). *Liquid modernity*. Cambridge: Polity.

Bhaskar, R. (1998). *The possibility of naturalism*. London: Routledge.

Blanc, S. (2014). Expanding workers' 'Moral Space': A liberal critique of corporate capitalism. *Journal of Business Ethics, 120*(4), 473–488.

Blanc, S., & Al-Amoudi, I. (2013). Corporate institutions in a weakened welfare state: A Rawlsian perspective. *Business Ethics Quarterly, 23*(4), 497–525.

Callinicos, A. T. (2006). *The resources of critique*. Cambridge: Polity Press.

Cederstrom, C., & Spicer, A. (2015). *The wellness syndrome*. Cambridge: Polity Press.

Chernilo, D. (2014). The idea of philosophical sociology. *The British Journal of Sociology, 65*(2), 338–357.

Collins, R. (1988). For a sociological philosophy. *Theory and Society, 17*(5), 669–702.

Dean, M. (2007). *Governing societies: Political perspectives on domestic and international rule*. Maidenhead: Open University Press.

Dean, M. (2010). *Governmentality: Power and rule in modern society*. London: Sage.

Donati, P. (2013). Morphogenesis and social networks: Relational steering not mechanical feedback. In M. S. Archer (Ed.), *Social morphogenesis*. Dordrecht: Springer.
Donati, P., & Archer, M. S. (2015). *The relational subject*. Cambridge: Cambridge University Press.
Freeman, J. (1972). The tyranny of structurelessness. *Berkeley Journal of Sociology, 17*, 151–164.
Gorski, P. (2013). Beyond the fact/value distinction: Ethical naturalism and the social sciences. *Society, 50*, 543–553.
Graeber, D. (2011). *Debt: The first 5000 years*. New York: Melville House.
Habermas, J. (2007). *Moral consciousness and communicative action*. Cambridge: Polity Press.
Halbwachs, M. (1992). *On collective memory*. Chicago: Chicago University Press.
Halbwachs, M. (1997). *La Memoire collective*. Paris: Albin Michel.
Hartnell, C., & Walumba, F. (2011). Transformational leadership and organizational culture. In N. Ashkanazy et al. (Eds.), *The handbook of organizational culture and climate* (pp. 225–248). Thousand Oaks: Sage.
Lawson, T. (1997). *Economics and reality*. London: Routledge.
Lawson, T. (2003). *Reorienting economics*. London: Routledge.
Lawson, T. (2014). A speeding up of the rate of social change? Power, technology, resistance, globalisation and the good society. In M. S. Archer (Ed.), *Late modernity: Trajectories towards morphogenic society*. Cham: Springer.
Maccarini, A. M. (2015). Turbulence and relational conjunctures: The emergence of morphogenic environments. In M. S. Archer (Ed.), *Generative mechanisms transforming late modernity*. Cham: Springer.
New York Times. (2015). *Italian neighbors build a network*. First online, then off. Article by Gaia Pianigiani. Published 24 Aug 2015. http://www.nytimes.com/2015/08/25/world/europe/italian-neighbors-build-their-own-social-network-online-and-off.html?_r=0. Accessed 8 Apr 2016.
Nussbaum, M. C. (2003). Capabilities as fundamental entitlements: Sen and social justice. *Feminist Economics, 9*(2–3), 33–59.
Picketty, T. (2014). *Capital in the twenty-first century*. London: Belknap Press.
Rawls, J. (1971). *A theory of justice*. Oxford: Clarendon Press.
Rawls, J. (1993). *Political liberalism*. New York: Columbia University Press.
Rawls, J. (2001/3). *Justice as fairness: A restatement*. Cambridge, MA: Harvard University Press.
Sayer, A. (2011). *Why things matter to people*. Cambridge: New York.
Sen, A. (1992). *Inequality reexamined*. Oxford: Clarendon Press.
Smith, C. (2015). *To flourish or self – destruct: A personalist theory of human goods, motivations, failure, and evil*. Chicago: University of Chicago Press.
Tocqueville, A. (2013). *Democracy in America*. Available via Project Guttenberg. http://www.gutenberg.org/files/815/815-h/815-h.htm. Accessed 8 Apr 2016.

Chapter 5
The Morphogenic Society as Source and Challenge for Human Fulfillment

Andrea M. Maccarini

'Good Life' After Modernity? A Missing Link and the Semantics of Decadence

In the Introduction to their edited volume *The Quality of Life*, Martha Nussbaum and Amartya Sen agree that to think about human thriving 'we seem to need a kind of rich and complex description of what people are able to do and to be' (p. 2). Moreover, they insist that such an account must not only be a *plural*, but also an explicitly *multidimensional* one:

> We need, perhaps above all, to know how people are enabled by the society in question to imagine, to wonder, to feel emotions such as love and gratitude, that presuppose that life is more than a set of commercial relations, and that the human being [...] is an 'unfathomable mystery', not to be completely 'set forth in tabular form'. (Nussbaum and Sen 2009, pp. 1–2).

This statement involves two distinct, though related claims. The former is that human beings and human relations are essentially something that exceeds utility or functionality, the second is that not only society in general, but the particular shape a given society takes – '*the society in question*' – can have an enabling or constraining influence upon their thriving. Taken seriously, this formula not only refers to the obvious, generic fact that social conditioning constrains or enables individuals in various ways, but entails that different *types* of societies have *specific* implications for the meanings of 'good life' and the very possibility for people to live it, due to their structural and cultural features.

Both claims are important. But while the former has been articulated in complex and systematic theories, the latter seems to remain relatively unexamined. It is to

A.M. Maccarini (✉)
University of Padova, Padua, Italy
e-mail: andrea.maccarini@unipd.it

M.S. Archer (ed.), *Morphogenesis and Human Flourishing*, Social Morphogenesis,
DOI 10.1007/978-3-319-49469-2_5

this issue that the present chapter is devoted. The missing link I want to address concerns the factors fostering human flourishing and the 'good life',[1] on the one hand, and the principal features of contemporary global society, on the other hand.

Arguably, the fact that such a link has been missing – or at least poorly examined – also explains something about the socio-cultural processes which are currently affecting the ideas and practices of human flourishing. In Western late modern societies, happiness is apparently a big deal. There is currently an extended literature on this topic, so overwhelming in quantity as to make references meaningless. From scientific research down to popular magazines, happiness is a tremendously fashionable theme. There is, above all, a vast literature concerning the psychological dynamics of happiness, that is of the processes through which human individuals come to develop their personalities and life course in ways that are subjectively rewarding. Popular culture is quite generous with handbooks suggesting ways to be happy and remain in unfailingly good spirits – including such brilliant ideas as eating good food, slowing down one's pace of life, having good conversations, taking some time off for ourselves, going shopping, doing meditation, and so on. Ideas and practices concerning what makes human beings flourish could be traced in various social processes, organizations and institutions.

But although 'happiness' is everywhere, our society seems rather uncertain about how to define and measure it – let alone achieve it. For one thing, welfare systems do not seem to be very effective in this respect.[2] In a broader perspective, there are indexes such as the OECD's 'better life', which mainly consist of material variables (e.g. housing, services, income, education, health, pollution, safety), and place most immaterial aspects under the label of 'life satisfaction'.[3] Other indexes, like the funny 'iHappy' one, are based on people's spontaneous reactions to world events as found on the media. In further cases, spontaneity is superseded by training. At Sacred Heart School, Tipton, Birmingham (UK), 'happiness' is a class among others

[1]Words are important. Although happiness, *eudaimonia*, good life, flourishing, (self)fulfillment, thriving, and more are all being used in analyses revolving around similar problems, they have different, sometimes even incompatible meanings and implications. Beyond the quick and basic clarifications offered in this section, I will articulate my own word choice in the section "Skills, cooperation, and transcendence: emergent forms of the human good in the morphogenic society". Until then, I will use the above expressions as uncommitted synonyms.

[2]This sweeping generalization might raise some eyebrows. Besides the well-known 'crisis of the welfare state', the robustness of such a statement can be tested by criss-crossing the extension of welfare systems with some available index of 'happiness'. Such an operation is likely to reveal that the connection between 'more welfare' and 'more happiness' is less than strong at the international level. I must forego pursuing the technicalities involved in the way such indexes are constructed. Furthermore, in the context of welfare literature it is increasingly difficult to find systematic views articulating any kind of 'new promise' for future society. See e.g. Esping-Andersen (2002), in which the neo-liberal and the Third Way approaches are mentioned as emerging blueprints for welfare reform and criticized for not articulating a sound principle of social justice.

[3]See www.oecdbetterlifeindex.org

(like math, history, etc.), designed to learn resilience and deal with anxiety.[4] Does happiness have to be taught and learned like Latin?

These scattered examples are just meant to show that popular as well as scientific interest for our topic is ubiquitous. An exhaustive study of human flourishing in contemporary society, then, would have to deal with multifarious cultural trends (from sources as different as academic ethics and the cultural industry), intentional collective actions and policies, emergent social forms and lifestyles, and more. In addition, definitions – i.e. explicit notions – as well as actual practices meant to nurture human flourishing should be considered. The result would probably be fascinating, but the enterprise requires a book-length treatment. Therefore, this chapter will follow a much more modest program. The present reflections are guided by the assumption that the emerging societal constellation displays the hallmarks of a 'morphogenic society' – the societal formation whose emergence represented our working hypothesis throughout this series of volumes. Thus, the specific issue I want to explore in this chapter is the relation between human flourishing and the morphogenic society (hereafter MS). I will argue that this particular macro-social framework presents a special kind of environment, which involves specific challenges as well as opportunities for living a 'good life'. After a brief overview of current mainstream views of human thriving, and some elaboration on the relevance of the missing link which served as the starting point of the chapter (the section "'Good Life' after modernity? A missing link and the semantics of decadence"), I will outline some of these challenges, and the responses articulated by social actors and their cultures (the section "The morphogenic society and its challenges to human flourishing"). I will then highlight the place where I believe the crucial challenge lies, and finally spell out some consequences of different strategies and choices in facing such a challenge (in the section "Skills, cooperation, and transcendence: emergent forms of the human good in the morphogenic society"). This will lead me to conclude with a few suggestions as to what conditions of existence we should expect to be inherent to human flourishing in the horizon towards which we are bound – both as individual persons and as collectivities. This whole argument may be usefully outlined through two guiding distinctions: *flourishing/calling* and *flourishing/enhancement*. Hopefully, the meaning of this will become clear in the section on "Skills, cooperation, and transcendence: emergent forms of the human good in the morphogenic society."

As regards the causes fostering human happiness, modern political thought has conceived of it as the natural outcome of progress, which in turn consisted of the continuous advancement of *science and technology*, coupled with increasingly rational political *institutions* and steady *economic growth*. The emergent effect of these dynamics would build a world where human beings could flourish. True, the two divergent branches of Western modernity – namely European and American liberal democracies versus the Soviet model – widely differed in the role they

[4]The same thing is reported as happening at the Wellington College, Crowthorne (UK), and in some US schools – up to the 'positive psychology' class at Harvard.

attributed to individual freedom and to political planning.[5] However, both models pointed to an 'end state' – albeit hidden in the mist of the historical 'long term' – where human individuals would finally be materially wealthy and free to develop their 'pure' individuality, satisfying their natural needs.

As to the cultural content of such a 'good life', diversity allowed for various equilibria between different notions. For present purposes, these may be summarized (and perhaps overly simplified) through two distinctions: *subjective/objective* and *material/immaterial*. Human flourishing may be held to result from the pursuit of purely self-defined goals or from the fulfillment of a given 'nature', which involves universally valid needs and ends. Furthermore, such human needs may be mostly material – health, wealth, safety, physical pleasure – or essentially immaterial – i.e. psychological and/or spiritual. The tension between these alternatives generated various combinatorial games, resulting in more or less unstable equilibria. Western modernity, in its successful moment, managed to strike a balance among such configurations, finding relative compatibilities and establishing forms of social life which were generally tolerable for human personalities. For example, material wealth consistently increased, requiring systematic, but relatively bearable effort for the average worker-citizen, and providing safety through economic and political institutions. At the same time, individual self-determination was unchained, whilst the bulwarks of the cultural heritage were kept reassuringly, if precariously, in place. This provided some sense of social belonging, while decreasingly setting real limits to behavioural variety – as if individuals could become emancipated without really 'leaving home' (or destroying its fabric). As we will see, the MS constitutes a societal environment that prompts the radicalization of extremely unstable combinations, thereby disrupting what may be called the 'modern compromise of happiness'.

Such an articulation in subjective, objective, material and immaterial dimensions also appears in most analytic models about human well-being. Evidence from big survey projects like OECD's 'How's Life' framework has long shown how different well-being can be in countries with very similar levels of GDP per capita. Therefore, the relevance of the factors beyond GDP has been emphasized in the related models. Individual well-being thereby adds up to the aggregation of material conditions and the quality of life In turn, the sustainability of such well-being over time requires preserving different types of capital, namely economic, human, social and natural capital.[6]

These models and approaches are illustrative of a wide-ranging intellectual and policy oriented movement leading to a multidimensional understanding of human thriving. However, what they still miss is (i) the connection with specific *societal*

[5]On the Soviet model as a particular variation of Western modernity see Arnason (1993).

[6]See OECD (2015a), where the quality of life is made up of a list of elements from work/life balance to education and skills to social connections, to the quality of the environment and subjective well-being. Other national surveys gave been developed in recent years on the basis of the OECD framework. In the case of Italy see for example the 'BES' index of just and sustainable well-being (Istat 2015).

challenges, and (ii) an idea of what *generates* well-being, unifying and giving human meaning to that vast array of factors. And because the relationships between society and conceptions of the good life is not being itself examined, this literature often represents more an *expression of* a given society and culture than a *reflection upon* it.

The missing link remains unexplored. Thus, such a highly developed awareness of the relevance of individual well-being is accompanied by a growing malaise held to characterise the macro-social framework of individual lives. Western modernity has unfolded under the sign of progress. And the idea of progress, as it was articulated in Europe between the middle of the sixteenth and the end of the eighteenth century, has always involved an *inner*, generally assumed to be an *unproblematic* connection, with personal happiness. The self-representation of Western modernity – with its cultural program and institutional complex – as a *eudaimonistic* machine is too well-known to need further discussion. In his famous 'Digression on ancients and moderns' (1688), Fontenelle was referring both to scientific progress and to human happiness when he drew his self-evident, categorical conclusion: « il est évident que tout cela n'a point de fin». Since then, and even through recurrent crises, this has been the fundamental faith of all moderns.

But in our days, this proud certainty would hardly be shared by the Western public, which is now experiencing the painfully sharp edge of social and historical contingency. After the Second World War, it was said that fear was behind us, while hope lay before us. Although Western citizens are still by far those who get the best life chances in the world, something is clearly changing. Fear is everywhere, and hope seems to be declining. At the end of the 1980s, after the increasing awareness that we were 'growing to the limits',[7] 1989 and the fall of the Berlin Wall inspired many to expect an age of regeneration and world peace. Such hopes lasted one decade, and burned in the Twin Towers explosion. There is now the feeling of a 'change of season', that feeds both on structural data and on people's perception. In cultural terms, Western societies are increasingly unable to imagine a future, unless in the form of ecological, technological, or political catastrophes.[8] Both in terms of material wealth and of life satisfaction, we are witnessing the first generations since World War II who believe things are getting worse, not better, and are rather pessimistic about future prospects. Fifty-two percent of American voters are reported to feel that America's best days are in the past, while belief that the nation's best days are still to come (35 %) hovers near its lowest level.[9] In economic

[7]And this applied to the great institutions of European welfare systems.

[8]Illustrating this point in an empirically exhaustive way would require more space than we have here, and it would make a paper in its own right. Suffice it to note that *utopian* thinking has now been silent for decades, while most imaginative work – e.g. books as well as movies – has taken on a *dystopic* form. For a social scientific interpretation of our incapacity to articulate a positive vision of the future, which emphasizes the inherent limits of the so-called 'knowledge society', see Willke (2002).

[9]According to the Rasmussen Reports' national telephone survey, 20–21 October 2015, the question was: «When you think about our nation in the context of history, are America's Best Days

terms, the International Monetary Fund is on record as saying that the United States has just five more years until they are no longer the world's largest economy. Europe, with its slow economic growth, its identity crisis and its demographic winter, is not doing any better. Whatever its multiple causal factors, the demographic decline of European peoples makes it difficult to believe that life itself is regarded as a good. And whatever the most plausible interpretation of such a social fact may be, it does not witness to happy peoples who share a confident outlook for the future. This somehow parallels the intellectual movement which heralds the necessity of 'degrowth', paving the way for the West to settle for some kind of collective 'active ageing'.[10]

To sum up, the Western public manifests decreasing belief in the capacity of their countries to tame complexity and face the major challenges of our times. Decadence is becoming our *Zeitgeist*.[11]

It is in this historical context that we start our reflection upon the meaning and hopes of a 'good life'. While most indexes of happiness, human development, and the like, are usually oriented to individuals and their closer spheres of interaction, it is the macro-societal, even civilizational framework that is being radically called into question. Because its stability and vitality cannot be taken for granted, its once undisputed connection with human flourishing is becoming increasingly puzzling. Our question then concerns how anyone can flourish – and what flourishing may mean – given our specific societal predicament. My point is that such an issue has hardly been studied beyond rather generic statements. In the face of most present challenges, both popular culture and the intellectual élites either miss their meaningful connection with our 'lifestyles' or tend to reassert the beauty of the Western 'way of life' as something we should root for. Little work seems to focus on what goods it is possible for people to achieve and which ones, instead, are being disrupted or made increasingly arduous to obtain in this kind of society.

Thus, a renewed reflection upon eudaimonia and the 'good life' is in order. But what kind of reflection is involved? One way to qualify my personal contribution is to say I intend to treat the problem in question from a sociological perspective. This certainly draws a distinction. However, referring to social science is not enough, since there are at least two different ways in which sociology could deal with human flourishing. One is to work out a meta-theoretical framework that allows us to ask questions about the good life, both at an individual and a collective level, within sociological theory. This is the approach most social theorists take. Some of

---

in the future or in the past?». The percentages indicated mark the highest level of voter pessimism in two years and is up 13 points from the days when Barack Obama was elected president. The percentage of voters who feel the nation's best days are still to come (35 %) is down 13 points since President Obama's inauguration in January, 2015.

[10]If one looks at the pictures used to promote the notion and practices of active ageing for European elderly populations, one often finds them pathetically mimicking young attitudes and behaviours. I cannot dwell here on what would probably be an interesting piece of visual sociology – as a socio-cultural interpretation of icons and images.

[11]For refined and empirically robust formulations of such a mood see Ferguson (2011, 2012).

them have made a compelling case for a non-positivist approach to social science, and convincingly argue about the necessary mutual relationships between various disciplines. Their main point is to assert the relevance of ethics and values to real life problems, which in turn prompts social science to shed its deceptively neutral or dismissive attitude to such issues. Criticism of Hume and the facts/values distinction is clearly a crucial point in this context.[12] As anticipated above, the issue I will tackle in this chapter is a different one. I agree with most of the meta-theoretical arguments, but I want to address the substantive connection between human flourishing and some of the current societal trends and conditions. What can sociology say about this? One possible research agenda involves the following steps:

(i) studying what is being elaborated within our cultural system, what symbolic variety is emerging as regards the ideas and practices constituting, or leading to, a 'good life';
(ii) examining their internal relationships with structural dynamics;
(iii) finally, drawing some implications from this structural and cultural landscape in terms of what human good is made possible, is fostered or hindered, through these socio-cultural processes.

Of course, the two approaches I have briefly sketched above are not mutually exclusive. In fact, they are internally related, for a substantive study of human flourishing within a given societal domain only makes sense once a conceptual framework is in place that allows us to ask the relevant questions and to conduct the related analyses.

Linked to all this is an anthropological issue: the ontological challenge and the shifting meaning of being human is an essential element to be considered, if we want to make sense of the symbolic and practical alternatives which are going to appear on the stage of the MS.

I'll leave it for readers to determine whether my approach could fall within the range of concrete utopianism. The latter, ultimately deriving from such authors as Ernst Bloch, has found a definition within critical realism, according to which it amounts to 'constructing MODELS of alternative ways of living on the basis of some assumed set of resources, counterbalancing ACTUALISM and informing hope'.[13] Its function is precisely to 'pinpoint the real, but non-actualised, possibilities inherent in a situation, thus inspiring grounded hope to inform emancipatory praxis' (...)'.[14] And it may be true that 'in many areas of our everyday lives we already act in 'the way social utopians have believed we could act' – in terms of reciprocity, non-egoism, trust and reconciliation (...)'.[15] What I intend to do is simply to use the resources of sociological theory, in order to sketch an outline of

[12] See for example Gorski (2013), Sayer (2011) and Smith (2015), as some of the best examples of this stream of sociological work.

[13] Hartwig (2007), p. 74.

[14] Ibidem, p. 75.

[15] Ibid.

what could possibly happen. And I deem it very important to remember that even if we act in certain ways in our everyday life, this should not be treated as immediate evidence that social life could be qualitatively different at the macro level. Moreover, for most of us everyday life itself may well be as ambivalent as it gets, while we still have reasons to regards it as 'good'.

The Morphogenic Society and Its Challenges to Human Flourishing

The defining features of what we call a 'morphogenic society' (MS) have been clarified before. In a nutshell, let us just remember that the MS involves a particular institutional configuration, in which structures and cultures tend to stand in relationships of contingent complementarity, thereby producing a situational logic of opportunity.[16] Such a societal formation issues a fundamental challenge to the meanings and possibilities of human flourishing.

In considering how societal frameworks generate-and-entail different ideas of eudaimonia, and what consequences the MS is going to have in this respect, two main theses will emerge. The *first* is that the current situation requires us to call into question the meanings of what used to be two major bulwarks of Western 'successful modernity',[17] i.e. (i) science and technology, and (ii) individual autonomy (in its expressive as well as instrumental dimension). These have been the very spearhead of (positivistic) 'progress', modelling the (alleged) inherent historical trend to perfection and happiness of humanity. The *second* says that one key point to discern among the various forms of eudaimonia that are developing in the MS concerns the ways to cope with transcendence – both on the individual and collective level.

As noted above (in the section "'Good Life' after modernity? A missing link and the semantics of decadence"), techno-science and individual autonomy are pivotal points around which the challenge ultimately revolves.[18] These two points touch upon essential features of the great utopias of the Twentieth century. Therefore,

[16]See for example the first volume in this series (Archer 2013). The theoretical framework including the concepts of contingent complementarity, situational logic, and more was laid down in Archer (1988).

[17]It is perhaps time to note that my continuous, boring addition of 'Western' to qualify my every reference to 'modernity' is not just a reflex, but wants to do justice to the notion of multiple modernities , which might be particularly important while discussing ideas of the good life, but lies far beyond the scope of the present essay – and of my own competence. Within the now extended literature on multiple modernities, it will be enough for present purposes to refer to the seminal work of Eisenstadt (2000).

[18]This statement somehow echoes Charles Taylor's well-known thesis about the 'malaise of modernity', which has to do with individualism and instrumental reason. See Taylor (1991), especially pp. 1–12. However, although the background is certainly similar, my own argument develops in a rather different direction.

they are crucial to explaining their outcomes and failures, as well as to study how the cultural system of the MS is working to articulate new ideas of happiness and human fulfillment.

The emergence of the MS obviously entails massive social change along many different dimensions.[19] Three sets of phenomena are especially important for our present argument:

(a) the explosion of possibilities for action and experience;
(b) the acceleration of social life;
(c) the saturation of social and symbolic space.

Let us briefly outline all of them, and explain how they represent a challenge to the modern formula of human flourishing.

(a) The *multiplication of possibilities for action and experience* lies at the core of the MS and of its 'engine', i.e. the logic of opportunity. Scientific and technological innovation are clearly supporting this process. The related transformations of the economic sphere, particularly of work and working environments, the increased centrality of human resources (represented in the semantics of personalization, creativity, problem solving skills, etc.), and deep cultural change (e.g. concerning values), coalesce to generate new personal lifestyles and forms of social life.
(b) *Social acceleration* theory has been proposed as a particular perspective from which modernization theory can be reinterpreted. In a previous essay, I maintained that it should not be (too ambitiously) treated as a 'prime mover' of social morphogenesis, but as an empirical generalization that keeps together a large set of empirical evidence concerning the temporal structures of society. I also argued for its connection with the generative logic of the MS.[20] The basic idea is that 'large' social dynamics, meso-level processes, and interactions in everyday life are increasingly accelerating, changing the individual and collective 'rhythm of life', disrupting old equilibria in temporal structures as well as in our personal use of time – e.g. the work/family balance, the shape and trajectory of personal biographies, etc.
(c) There is another element to be added, although its inherent relationship with the MS would need more explanation than I can offer in this chapter. It may be called the *saturation of social and symbolic space*, and it is really the emergent effect of three different factors:

    (a) One is the enormous growth of relational and communicative networks – increasingly consisting of virtual relationships – that fill every gap of silence and claim a growing amount of our time.[21]

[19] Some of the most relevant dynamics are explored in Archer (2014). My own chapter in that volume (Maccarini 2014) may also be taken as setting the stage for my present argument.

[20] See Maccarini (2014). For a recent formulation of the theory see Rosa (2013).

[21] Such a phenomenon was effectively described, among others, by Kenneth Gergen (1991).

(b) The other might be introduced by a quote from Karl Jaspers: 'A total metamorphosis of history has taken place. The essential fact is: *There is no longer anything outside*. The world is closed. The unity of the earth has arrived'.[22]

(c) Coupled with its increased impact, which technology allows human intervention to have on every level of the social and natural world, these factors add up to what Archer (in this volume) has called 'finitude' as a morphogenetic feature of contemporary global society.

Despite the obviously suspicious nature of such grand and sweeping declarations, this is a very consequential point, about which sociologists would probably have to reflect more systematically than they have done so far. What I want to emphasize here is that these big 'social facts' converge in generating a saturated communicative, symbolic, and physical environment for people to inhabit.

The outcome of these trends can be summarized as an intensified *pressure upon human beings*, which is the other face of the coin of the now fashionable 'centrality of the person'. We already know that the MS involves the crisis of routine action and the rise of the *reflexive imperative.*[23] We might now venture to extend such a hypothesis, considering the widening and intensification of reflexivity to be covering one aspect of a more complex phenomenon, namely a *multidimensional pressure on the human*. Such a pressure surely includes reflexivity and the 'selective imperative', in the related issue of decision making. However, the trends of social change outlined above also push towards flexibility, adaptation, and above all are increasingly demanding in terms of the *personal effort* required to participate in social processes of any kind – from education to work, down to health, civic life, and so forth. Performance is no more confined to the sphere of the market economy. Activation, mobilization, investment, initiative, have become keywords in social life, as well as passwords to get services – e.g. welfare benefits.

The idea that people must be enabled to help themselves, learning to protect themselves from risks, and that this requires their wholehearted mobilization, is now rather commonsensical, e.g. in most literature about the transformations of the European welfare systems. As a result of this, education has achieved a central position in lifestyle and the life course, while new, hybrid policy mechanisms arise that are centered on education and training. While this situation is quite clear, few seem to have seen its consequences in terms of the personal stresses and strains these social dynamics bring about. And while concern-oriented reflexivity is the response to the choice-and-decision making issue, it is more unclear how people can cope positively with the rest of the problem.

In other words, the present situation could be described as a crisis (indeed, the end?) of *Entlastung*. The concept of *Entlastung* (literally 'exoneration') must be traced to Arnold Gehlen (2007, 2013). Basically, his point is that humans

---

[22]K. Jaspers (1953, p. 127). The italics is mine.

[23]M. Archer (2012).

as vulnerable, flawed beings, need help in what are crucial dimensions of their surviving and thriving. This is the task of institutions. Now, what I am arguing here is that the capacity of institutions to perform such a task might be sharply declining.[24] Participating in institutions and their organized forms of life, making one's way through them and their consolidated paths (e.g. successfully completing a 'curriculum') ultimately makes less sense than ever. The human person is becoming central in global society, but this means she must increasingly fall back on herself. And she needs a broader range of skills than she once used to.

All of this has important consequences for the meanings and hopes of human flourishing in the MS. Both the above distinctions – subjective/objective and material/immaterial – are going to be affected by the new predicament. The old equilibria are being pushed beyond their limits, towards more extreme solutions. More precisely, the set of factors I have indicated is having an influence upon (i) the will to empower (or enhance) oneself, to achieve more skills and powers; (ii) the temporal duration and intensity of attachment people can display towards ideals, institutions or other people; (iii) the way to conceive of transcendence, both in one's own existence and in the historical context. These three points are crucial to the idea of human flourishing. I will now try to outline how they are embodied in some ongoing sociocultural trends, which represent empirically existing responses to the ever present human need for happiness. At the same time, such an argument should convey some evaluative considerations about what (concrete) utopias or ideals are still conceivable in the current societal conditions.

Skills, Cooperation, and Transcendence: Emergent Forms of the Human Good in the Morphogenic Society

Let us now turn to examining different ways to cope with the logic of opportunity that is typical of the MS. As we will see, the chosen themes around which my analysis revolves have to do with the points identified above, namely the will for empowerment, the capacity of attachment, and the push to transcendence. Arguably, these are the major *foci of tension* in the cultures of human fulfillment within the MS. The way they are socially and culturally constructed, interpreted, and lived out could be decisive for human good. And reciprocally, such different paths to human good will deeply affect the 'human' quality of the MS.

One first focus has to do with education. This evokes the problem of skills. In some, increasingly mainstream lines of scientific and policy related thought, the basic idea is that given the pressure on the human being prompted by the explosion

[24] Some authors would counter that institutions are simply switching to 'enabling institutions', and that the related 'malaise' can be explained away as a peculiar characteristic of some particular countries (see e.g. Ehrenberg 2010). For what merits such studies may have, it remains true that institutions are now bound to take on a different function.

of the possibilities for action and experience, we can learn our way out of such a predicament through the *acquisition of skills* and the building of a *skills society*. Such a notion is obviously complex, but its core lies in the range of skills individuals are said to need in order to meet the challenge. The emphasis falls on learning. But what shall we learn, and how?

A vast educational and psychological literature provides endless lists.[25] On the cognitive side, we could summarize it as follows: the whole curriculum should be redesigned, emphasizing such competences as (i) pattern recognition, memory and rapidity of information processing; (ii) accessing, extracting, and interpreting knowledge; (iii) conceptualization, arguement, and reflection. The huge quantity of the knowledge we should acquire, and the extent it should be functional to some practical goals, remain pretty contested issues. However, a more recent trend stresses the importance of social and emotional skills. These are very interesting in that they mark the rediscovery of a more integral approach to human characteristics that exceed cognitive performance. They revolve around the following fundamental points:

(a) achieving goals: perseverance, self-control, passion for the goals;
(b) working with others: sociability, care, respect;
(c) managing emotions: self-esteem, optimism, trust.

In other words, social and emotional skills should allow people to (i) react against challenges and face life's hardship; (ii) support the increase of personal effort and the capacity to work; (iii) promote one's social engagement.

Finally, 'happiness' and fulfillment are supposed to come as an emergent effect of these practiced attitudes and of the effective coping with the world's complexity they make possible. It can be easily observed that such skills imply a reactive, a pro-active, and an integrative dimension, while nothing constitutive comes into the picture. Identity and meanings do shape the learning environments, but apparently find no way into the profile of the 'global citizen' (and worker). This is the product of a semantics of skills that merges economic and psychological frameworks, shoving complex, multidimensional constructs, such as for example trust, optimism, and care into the funnel of 'skills'. In this context, critical thinking is defined as the ability for strategic calculation and the openness to new solutions to problems. Thus, critique is redefined as competence and performance. Indeed, lifestyle or a successful governance of life itself becomes a matter of competence and performance. The educational ideal, and indeed what makes a successful life, approaches the idea of

[25]See OECD (2015b) for a review and the attempt at an integrated approach. The following summary draws upon this text, as it provides both a good literature review and the concrete plan expressed by a global institution. As far as global policy actors are concerned, the OECD can serve as a good example. This institution has been, and currently is one of the heralds of the so-called skills society. 'Better policies for better lives' is its defining slogan, and skills development is part of such 'better policies' that are supposed to talk to the first challenge outlined in section "The morphogenic society and its challenges to human flourishing."

pure exercise. Its subject, therefore, will be the *practising person*.[26] Now, these skills are important for people to sail through turbulent societal waters, and to participate in various social spheres. Given the decline of *Entlastung*, this is increasingly a personal task. However, human goods and skills are not the same thing. One may well have a concern, and care about some good, but s/he also needs to *be able* to do what must be done to pursue such a concern. On the other hand, someone may well be able to care for other people, but could choose not to display this capacity in certain cases, if s/he believes it's not worth doing it. And in turn, only through the actual practice of care that one may come to discover the good that lies in a given relationship. This inner relationality involves more than a skill.

Such a critique might be dismissed as a humanistic interference with a more dependable scientific approach. However, the whole point of these studies lies in their capacity to predict some given life outcomes – such as a successful marriage, a fulfilling working life, civic engagement, social cohesion, and so forth. And all these enterprises entail a motivational energy and a meaning which will hardly come from the fascination of practice itself. We could say that skills' development can only work as the *practical* companion of concern-oriented reflexivity, through which people's identification, attachment to and pursuit of meaningful goals is effectively sustained.[27]

Given the relevance of education, it is instructive to introduce the issue of cooperation, as something related to the above notion of skills and a skills society. If well-being, and indeed collective prosperity and thriving in the MS lie in skills' development, an aspect of this whole scenario has to do with the respective role of competition and cooperation in that very process of skills' development. We must carefully distinguish this issue from that which has already been tackled by Archer (2014), when explaining that the generative mechanism of late modernity is constituted by market competition and the diffusion of applied science needing to 'work together'. Such a synergy is quite different from the idea of cooperation, by which is meant a logic of mutual help in learning processes and in the development of one's professional capacities. A big divide separates essentially individualistic and competitive views of skills' development from the idea of cooperative learning, which involves 'doing things together', collective effort, and mutual support. The original case here has been made by those who claim that flexible capitalism, with its competitive logic and the reduction of once lifelong careers to short term commitments, is resulting in the decline of skills and the loss of human capital. As a consequence, the process of skills development should be made less competitive, putting a premium on cooperation. Cooperation must itself be treated as a 'craft',

[26]This expression intentionally refers to Sloterdijk's (2013) notions of practice and anthropotechnics. More on this below.

[27]This means, the social and emotional skills approach can only work within the overarching framework of a concern-oriented theory of reflexivity (Archer 2000, 2003). In Sloterdijk's anthropotechnic terms, this answers the crucial question about «what keeps the rope tight». On the issue see also Maccarini (2016b).

to be fostered through a politics of time and space,[28] and obviously goes beyond the social skill of 'being nice and respectful' of others, that is of just being able to *function with* others. The point here is that the potential of each needs the cooperation of others to be developed. The times, spaces, and social environments that would be adequate to such a goal must be further specified.

So far, I have been arguing that human fulfillment in the MS requires the capacity to pursue meaningful goals in conditions of high pressure. This involves embracing an active attitude and developing a broad range of skills to build an adequate, continually evolving coping structure. At the same time, the capacity to cooperate must be cultivated as a craft in its own right.

Now, these capacities correspond to the needs of self-empowering and of meaningful belonging. However, as we have seen, the skills approach can be overly reductionist as regards the motivational force and the meaningful purpose that keeps people wanting to learn – and ultimately, to work on self-improvement. Further, finding the right balance between the logic of competition and the logic of cooperation requires a complex approach, which involves a politics of relationships, times and spaces. A distinction between *flourishing* and *calling* can make sense of these points. Throughout the text I have been using the term 'flourishing' as a synonym for the 'good life' or even 'human good'. But the meaning of 'flourishing' can be specified referring to its opposite within particular distinctions, one of which is that between *flourishing* and *calling*. In this context, flourishing is taken to mean purely mundane success, that is, a successful life in purely immanent terms (health, professional success, wealth, etc.). Here flourishing amounts to sheer self-assertion, and opposes any idea of a 'mission' human beings should 'accomplish', although this might mean putting one's well-being in jeopardy. This meaning – which is the one that resonates with Douglas Porpora's critique – appears in Charles Taylor, who distinguishes flourishing from 'Axial' notions of the human good, as were articulated within Christianity and Buddhism.[29] That said, in this context the problem ultimately consists of keeping flourishing and calling together. Unilateral formulations would either forget where the light of meaning comes from into the personal life course, or dismiss the pressure and the change in the role of institutions human beings must face in the MS. This also explains the meaning of my own word use. I do not consider flourishing to be necessarily opposed to an idea of 'calling'. One proposal might be to use the term '*fulfillment*' as a relational term connecting flourishing and calling. More precisely, it would mean the *type and 'quantum' of flourishing that is required to respond to a personal calling*. Such a word use is justified by the fact that both nature and missions can be said to be *fulfilled*. Moreover, it would have the advantage of avoiding the questionable opposition of calling and personal happiness, and in fact to hint at the possibility that fulfilling one's calling is what really paves the way to *true* and *complete* happiness – however

[28]This argument has been consistently made by Richard Sennett (2007, 2012).

[29]See Porpora's chapter in this volume. Taylor's use of the word is to be found in various parts of his work. Here I refer to the clear statement in Taylor (2007), pp. 150–151.

sometimes in rather counterintuitive ways.[30] More generally speaking, my thesis is that human good in the MS depends on a delicate balance between all these symbolic elements.

These themes call out a more general one, which I have called the issue of transcendence. In a sense, this can be said to epitomize the ultimate challenge of the MS, insofar as it calls into question personal and collective identity in a radical way.

But what do we mean by transcendence, and why do we mention it here? Within a sociological discourse, transcendence refers to the sense of being overcome and overwhelmed by something that exceeds one's limits in time and space. Such a sense of 'being transcended' may be experienced in positive-joyful as well as in negative-painful events of life. The result is usually the opening of one's identity boundaries and often deep changes in one's personal identity. Nature, art and the *sublime*, death and the keen sense of life's finitude, love, are examples of this.[31] In turn, human persons are not only passively undergoing such experiences. Transcendence may also be understood as a *typically human need to 'go beyond'*, i.e. to overcome given contexts and situations, exceeding what one has been, done, and experienced. Such a definition draws a distinction between transcendence and religion. However, religious cultures are obviously among the most important interpreters of such a human feature, elaborating symbolic codes which define how a given collectivity copes with such an experience, and makes sense of the world as an exceeding entity as well as of the ways people act for self-transformation.[32] The specific type of symbolic elaboration concerning the idea of transcendence, and its relational distinction from immanence, is highly consequential for the way societies articulate their identity, meaning not just what their past history was, but even more what they intend it to be in the future.[33]

Both on the individual and the collective level, then, it is quite clear that the idea of transcendence influences the notions of personal and social good. My point here is that the sense of transcendence is not being left untouched by the processes characterizing the MS. So, what is happening with that basic need in the MS? We might say that the MS has an ambivalent relationship with the sense of transcendence. Once again, the modern equilibrium reached in the cultures of

[30]In Charles Taylor's words, like "dying young on a cross". Taylor 2007, p. 151.

[31]This part of the definition is due to Joas's contribution (2008). My own take on the concept also involves the following. Note that such a notion of self-transcendence does not entail any strong hypothesis as to what causes the experience to happen, nor does it work only on the individual level. Finally, it is also important to note that experiences are not self-interpreting, but people must draw upon culture to make sense of them.

[32]See for example Shulman and Stroumsa (2002). On the societal relevance of the distinction immanence / transcendence see Donati (2010). From a different perspective, Hartmut Rosa's argument about religion as the vertical axis of 'resonance' plays a similar tune (Rosa 2016, pp. 435–453). The whole literature on the Axial Age, and its recent revival, is also a witness to such an interest. For a recent review with an extended referencing apparatus see Bellah and Joas (2012).

[33]Donati (2010) draws attention to this point.

society is made unstable. New formulations of the relational distinction of immanence/transcendence tend to emerge. On the one hand, intensified morphogenesis triggers new social imaginaries, and prompts new ways to (try to) overcome the present predicament. On the other hand, social acceleration and even more the saturation of social space make it more likely for transcendence to collapse upon immanence.[34]

This is where another distinction becomes helpful, namely that between *flourishing* and *enhancement*. Here, the difference lies in conceiving of the human good in one of the following ways: flourishing means the accomplishment of one's natural potential, i.e. to develop one's full strength, to 'bloom' according to the qualities inscribed in our nature – which does not eliminate the element of personal effort or autonomy of will, but involves a specific direction and some idea of limits. The other term – enhancement – conveys the idea of grafting 'powers' on a 'platform' which has no principled 'form' – i.e. no 'nature' – and therefore can be 'empowered' with no inherent 'limit'. In this sense, the idea of flourishing is meant to think of human good within the limits of human reality. That is to say, it involves a realist concept of human (personal) ontology to contrast 'morphological freedom'.[35]

Projecting the distinction immanence/transcendence upon the ideas and practices of flourishing makes clear we find ourselves at the crossroads of two diverging cultures.

(a) One defines the act of transcending as a recognition of one's limits and of the irreducible transcendence of otherness. The relationships multiply and magnify the difference, unity generates other differences and differences call for relationships. The more ego approaches alter, the more s/he remains in his/her difference, and the more this prompts ongoing exploration. Transcendence involves reaching out to someone or something *external*, changing oneself in the process – i.e. leaving previous states to acquire new ones over (life)time;
(b) an alternative sense of transcendence occurs when ego tries to *include* everything *within* him/herself, whose depth must be continually nourished through the swallowing of other experiences and alterity. The individual has no principled *limit*, but lives of the continuous effort to live different states *simultaneously*, without letting go of any previous way of being.[36] The self is continually

[34]As I will try to explain: social acceleration may be regarded as a companion of secularization – and more generally, the change of the temporal structures of society has deep implications for the idea of transcendence – as was noted, among others, by Blumenberg (1986).

[35]Morphological freedom refers to the will of human beings to 'give themselves a form' beyond 'natural' limits. Western cultural systems now tend to translate such a will into a right. On morphological rights see the discussion in Maccarini (2016a).

[36]As Simmel would say, translating temporal consequentiality into spatial coexistence.

enhanced in his/her 'component powers'. The selective imperative is rejected, as well as the idea that one's life must have a definite shape.[37]

All these are not just lexical details. Such distinctions can serve as tools to interpret the various cultures of the human good which take center stage in the MS. These rather abstruse formulations could be said to distinguish between alternative lifestyles, and should be illustrated at length by reference to such social phenomena as the couple and the family, the experience and the cultural construction of adulthood, life course trajectories, lifelong education, the ethics of generative succession, genetic engineering, and more.

If culture (a) above follows a neo-humanistic track, in culture (b) the idea of a 'good life' conceived as immanent self-enhancement clearly opens the door to a brand new different way to make sense of one's place in the world. Here anthropology is superseded by anthropotechnics (Sloterdijk 2013).

It is crucial to add that each of these cultures articulates a particular idea of *perfection*.[38] In the former case, it consists of spending one's lifetime in ongoing cultivation of foundational relationships and in endless discovery of the landscapes encountered along the path of one's calling. This involves a continuous possibility of making one's *exit* (heteroreference). In the latter, it has to do with the capacity to include every 'virtue' and to actualize every potential *within* oneself (self-reference). Which culture will prevail in terms of the practices of identity building among younger generations, given this symbolic variety, is a matter for empirical study – as well as for educational commitment.[39]

In a similar vein, deep symbolic changes may be taking place at the collective level. As briefly anticipated in the section "'Good Life' after modernity? A missing link and the semantics of decadence" above, modernity had its views of how to exceed the given order of things. And here too, an idea of perfection has often been articulated through an appeal to 'transcendence', i.e. through reference to 'another time' or 'another place'. Table 5.1 presents a simplified scheme of the ideological alternatives in this domain. It is interesting to note that the utopian way to solve the problem of the relationship with perfection resembles the self-referential, enhancement-oriented pole of self-identity.[40]

Most of the crimes and misdemeanors of the twentieth century were committed in the name of secular ideologies, which interpreted this drive to build 'the good

---

[37] I am referring to Archer (2012) and her theory of reflexivity, where the selective imperative comes as the necessity to give one's life a *shape* through the exercise of prioritization between concerns and the related life plans.

[38] Reference to Michael Sandel (2009) is here intentional, although we're not making this very case here.

[39] Self-reference in this sense comes close to what Rosa defines a 'dumb relation to the world' (2016).

[40] For example, utopian kingdoms are usually set apart from other lands; they involve no progress or decline over time, but live in some sort of 'eternal present'; they are systems which are complete in themselves and do not need amendment, and so forth. For a still useful, very scholarly source in this field of studies see Rizzardi (1984).

Table 5.1 Exceeding space and time

	Immanence	Transcendence	
Past	Arcadia	Eden	Primitivism
Future	Utopia	Heaven	Millenarism

Adaptation from H. Levin (1969), quoted in Rossi (1976), p. 43

society' in a purely immanent sense. In the Cold War era, an equilibrium emerged that we had (wrongly) come to regard as almost 'natural'. One atheist geo-political entity confronted another one, in which the religious heritage had become conveniently 'functionalized' and individualized, i.e. tamed but still lingering in the background. At the same time, all non-modern forms of religion were simply pushed to the margins of the bipolar world.

In the present day, that constellation has exploded, and the MS is generating new variety. Only a rough sketch can be drawn here, for which I find it useful to refer to Madsen's image of an emerging contrast between an archaic paleo-durkheimian submersion of the self into politically organized communities versus a post-durkheimian exaltation of the self in an expressive spirituality.[41] The latter process intertwines with another trend: hyper-complexity prompts semantics that are 'religious' in that they give up rational discourse, which is held to be inadequate to shed light upon the divine as a dimension of pure 'mystery'.[42] In the process, certain branches of post-modern culture tend to reevaluate some kind of archaic wisdom, which is claimed to provide an access to the underlying mystery of the world. This explains the odd mix of hyper-modern scientific language and archaic myths and symbols to be often found in the narratives of various 'new age' cults.[43]

If there is some truth to this image, could we talk of a post-durkheimian West vs. a paleo-durkheimian 'Rest' – particularly where political turmoil and nation- or empire-building processes still look for a theological legitimation? Such trends could well be described as 'Axial catastrophes', in that they involve radical 'exits' – in the opposite directions of religious fundamentalism and radical secularization – from the mediation formulas between immanence and transcendence.[44]

In the reconstruction of such formulas by cultural, religious, and political élites – in different ways according to different cultural and religious traditions – lies the hope that collective life in various regions of the MS develops a 'humane' or 'good' form of dynamic vision of the future, and of the ways to get there.

[41]Madsen's interpretation (2012, p. 432) can be traced back to Charles Taylor (2007, pp. 455 ff., 487ff.), to which he makes explicit reference.

[42]A similar case is made by Donati (2010, ch. 2, especially pp. 45–49).

[43]This sort of breakup between '*fides*' and '*ratio*' – and the resulting awkward *contaminatio* between archaic myths and scientific knowledge – as part of popular culture finds an easily observable expression in the cultural industry – e.g. in science fiction movies and television series.

[44]Elsewhere I called these 'formations of the secular', borrowing an expression from Talal Asad but fundamentally changing its meaning (Maccarini 2010).

Conclusion. Being (Fulfilled as) Human in the Morphogenic Society

I have been trying to spell out some conditions for human fulfillment in the present morphogenic societal context.

To sum up, the main argument may be outlined as follows:

(a) the MS challenges the modern ideas of human fulfillment because of the explosion of possibilities for action, social acceleration, and the saturation of social and symbolic space;
(b) this results in an unprecedented pressure upon human personalities, of which the reflexive imperative is a factor (concerning the aspect of decision-making), and in the crisis of the modern function of institutions;
(c) the emergent needs of self-empowering, cooperation craft, and new forms and possibilities to 'exceed' the current predicament can be interpreted and institutionalized in different ways, whose guiding principles may be grasped through the distinctions flourishing/calling and flourishing/enhancement;
(d) the hopes of 'good life' depend on a balanced combination of these polarities, without 'catastrophic' exits from the relational pull towards radical conceptions. In this sense, human fulfillment can be said to appear as the emergent effect of flourishing and calling, more precisely of flourishing within, and oriented to, a given sense of calling. This entails the emergence of new sources of the self, whose decisive feature lies in the relation individuals entertain with transcendence and the related notion of limit;
(e) ultimately, a sense of transcendence, and its mediation with the secular sphere, interweaves all the major dimensions of the big issue of human fulfillment in the MS. This is because some specific features of the MS call transcendence into question in their own special way. Thus, a renewed reflection on transcendence ultimately constitutes the core of the good life in a MS. In this sense, the future is religious, or it won't be human at all.[45] This does not involve any myth of cultural integration, but our capacity to conceive of a future that exceeds our individual lifetimes and that can still make sense to other generations.

This prompts a more general conclusion. Beyond the notions of well-being as long lists of factors, the challenge of the MS leads to precisely the understanding that it is *a certain quality of our relations to the world* that must be changed, if hopes of a good life are still to be cultivated. My argument has tried to specify at least a few conditions that would make such relations not alienating, but humanly fulfilling. In a nutshell, the deepest need is to live within a relation of concern – involving the ability to become strong evaluators, to engage with symbolic systems that can give meaning to one's life. Such a relation must be articulated throughout all spheres of

[45](Donati 2010, 30).

human life and activity, it has an individual and a collective dimension, and entails horizontal and vertical axes.[46]

The provisional character of these reflections is all too apparent. However, if they are at least provisionally acceptable, I may try to draw a few corollaries. Although they derive from the main argument above, such a connection is not immediate. The reason to spell them out here is merely to lay the ground for future inquiries into very concrete matters.

(a) In the same way that people cannot speak 'language' in general, but only one particular language, so they can practice one religion, not 'religion' *tout court*. In other words, human persons only flourish within an horizon. Therefore, it is necessary to guarantee that cultural particularities may continue to live and thrive, while also learning to interact in a reciprocally enriching relationship. So, the MS must make (social and symbolic) space for particularities and promote networks to facilitate their connection – for travelling from one to the other. Multiple stories should be allowed to coexist, traditions and collectivities should be able to live on, to continue with their own narrative – even removing obstacles to relationships and to personal choice. The MS should nurture the mutual discovery, recognition, and exchange of gifts between civilizations, beyond multicultural illusions and misplaced nationalistic nostalgia.
(b) It is also crucial to develop a culture of non-disposability and gift, which guarantees the respect of human dignity beyond instrumental rationality. A related point is that people should not be kept apart from experiences that may lead to self-transcendence, and thereby to commitment. It is important to avoid the impoverishment and even mutilation of experience. In other words, if a sense of calling must be recalled, we should also create the right conditions for people to be able to hear such a calling. This point has to do with the idea of 'teaching for commitment', i.e. to counter the cultural neutralization of education.

Finally, going back to the 'big picture', one may wonder what we have learned from the long history of the West in its struggle with the idea of personal and social perfection. Although it would be rather strange for a sociologist to engage in statements that sound dangerously close to the philosophy of history, I will venture to say this:

There is probably no 'progress', in the sense of a steady improvement of the human predicament. We are also not dealing with sheer contingency, leading to random, chaotic processes within an indifferent universe – which would prompt us to embrace Taylor's famous 'Victorian courage'. Human society is a complex entity, in which regular processes interweave to produce unpredictable actions. The least inadequate image I could think of is that of ever changing substantive challenges, while what is steadily increasing is human capacity, power and impact

[46]These formulations draw us close to Rosa's recent reflections on 'resonance' as a non-alienating relational mode (Rosa 2016). A systematic comparison with such a complex work lies beyond the limits of the present chapter.

on the world as such. Structural regularities and free agency therefore intersect within a scheme of spiralling challenge-and-response. What we need to know is what our specific challenges are. Such challenges are always connected with specific ages, within which efforts make sense and human life can take a meaningful 'good form'. Tension is permanent, but situations are unique. Victory and defeat are never definitive, but fighting makes sense because it allows 'better lives' to reach their goal. Combining cyclicity and linearity, instrumental rationality and non-disposability, relationality and individuality, openness and closure, all seems to me to summarize the best of Western wisdom. If some of the latter can still be useful in global society, it may lie in this ability to build mediations, combinations, and relationships.

References

Archer, M. S. (1988). *Realist social theory. The morphogenetic approach*. Cambridge: Cambridge University Press.

Archer, M. S. (2000). *Being human. The problem of agency*. Cambridge: Cambridge University Press.

Archer, M. S. (2003). *Structure, agency and the internal conversation*. Cambridge: Cambridge University Press.

Archer, M. S. (2012). *The reflexive imperative in late modernity*. Cambridge: Cambridge University Press.

Archer, M. S. (Ed.). (2013). *Social morphogenesis*. Dordrecht: Springer.

Archer, M. S. (Ed.). (2014). *Late modernity. trajectories towards morphogenic society*. Dordrecht: Springer.

Arnason, J. P. (1993). *The future that failed. Origins and destinies of the soviet model*. London/New York: Routledge.

Bellah, R. N., & Joas, H. (Eds.). (2012). *The axial age and its consequences*. Cambridge, MA/London: The Belknap Press of Harvard University Press.

Blumenberg, H. (1986). *Lebenszeit und Weltzeit*. Frankfurt: Suhrkamp.

Donati, P. (2010). *La matrice teologica della società*. Soveria Mannelli: Rubbettino.

Ehrenberg, A. (2010). *La société du malaise*. Paris: Odile Jacob.

Eisenstadt, S. N. (2000). Multiple modernities. *Daedalus, 129*(1), 1–29.

Esping Andersen, G. (2002). Towards the good society, once again? In his. (with D. Gallie, A. Hemerijck, J. Miles). *Why we need a new welfare state* (pp. 1–25). Oxford: Oxford University Press.

Ferguson, N. (2011). *Civilization. The West and the rest*. New York: Penguin Books.

Ferguson, N. (2012). *The great degeneration. How institutions decay and economies die*. New York: Penguin Books.

Gehlen, A. (2007). *Die Seele im technischen Zeitalter. Sozialpsychologische Probleme in der industriellen Gesellschaft (1957)*. Frankfurt: Klostermann.

Gehlen, A. (2013). *Der Mensch. Seine Natur und seine Stellung in der Welt (1940)*. Graz: AULA-Verlag.

Gergen, K. (1991). *The saturated self. Dilemmas of identity in contemporary life*. New York: Basic Books.

Gorski, P. (2013). Beyond the fact/value distinction: Ethical naturalism and the social sciences. *Society, 50*(6), 543–553.

Hartwig, M. (Ed.). (2007). *Dictionary of critical realism*. London/New York: Routledge.

Istat. (2015). *BES 2015. Il benessere equo e sostenibile in Italia*. Roma: Istituto nazionale di statistica.
Jaspers, K. (1953). *The origin and goal of history*. New Haven: Yale University Press.
Joas, H. (2008). *Do we need religion? On the experience of self-transcendence*. Boulder/London: Paradigm Publishers.
Levin, H. (1969). *The myth of the golden age in the renaissance*. Bloomington: Indiana University Press.
Maccarini, A. (2010). Il prisma della religione: mediazioni, ri-velazioni e controversie nella società globale. In D. Arasa & J. Milàn (Eds.), *Communication, the church, and the culture of controversies* (pp. 107–164). Roma: Edusc.
Maccarini, A. (2014). The emergent social qualities of a 'morphogenic' society. Cultures, structures, and forms of reflexivity. In M. S. Archer (Ed.), *Late modernity. Trajectories towards morphogenic society* (pp. 49–76). Dordrecht: Springer.
Maccarini, A. (2016a). The normative texture of morphogenic society: Tensions, challenges, and strategies. In M. S. Archer (Ed.), *Morphogenesis and the crisis of normativity*. Dordrecht: Springer.
Maccarini, A. M. (2016b). On character education: Self-formation and forms of life in a morphogenic society. *Italian Journal of Sociology of Education, 8*(1), 31–55. doi:10.14658/pupj-ijse-2016-1-3.
Madsen, R. (2012). The future of transcendence. A sociological agenda. In R. N. Bellah & H. Joas (Eds.), *The axial age and its consequences* (pp. 430–446). Cambridge, MA: The Belknap Press of Harvard University Press.
Nussbaum, M. C., & Sen, A. (Eds.). (2009). *The quality of life*. New York: Oxford University Press.
OECD. (2015a). *How's life? 2015: Measuring well-being*. Paris: OECD Publishing.
OECD. (2015b). *Skills for social progress: The power of social and emotional skills, OECD skills studies*. Paris: OECD Publishing.
Rizzardi, L. (1984). Il fascino della perfezione: questioni preliminari ad una interpretazione psicologica dei significati politici dell'utopia. In A. Quadrio (Ed.), *Aristarchi (a cura di), Questioni di psicologia politica* (pp. 171–269). Milano: Giuffrè Editore.
Rosa, H. (2013). *Social acceleration. A new theory of modernity*. New York: Columbia University Press.
Rosa, H. (2016). *Resonanz. Eine Soziologie der Weltbeziehung*. Frankfurt: Suhrkamp.
Rossi, P. (1976). Sulle origini dell'idea di progresso. In E. Agazzi (a cura di), Il concetto di progresso nella scienza. Milano: Feltrinelli.
Sandel, M. J. (2009). *The case against perfection. Ethics in the age of genetic engineering*. Cambridge, MA/London: The Belknap Press of Harvard University Press.
Sayer, A. (2011). *Why things matter to people. Social science, values and ethical life*. Cambridge: Cambridge University Press.
Sennett, R. (2007). *The culture of the new capitalism*. New Haven: Yale University Press.
Sennett, R. (2012). *Together: The rituals, pleasures and politics of cooperation*. New York: Allen Lane.
Shulman, D., & Stroumsa, G. G. (Eds.). (2002). *Self and self-transformation in the history of religions*. Oxford: Oxford University Press.
Sloterdijk, P. (2013). *You must change your life*. Cambridge: Polity Press.
Smith, C. (2015). *To flourish or destruct. A personalist theory of human goods, motivations, failure, and evil*. Chicago/London: The University of Chicago Press.
Taylor, C. (1991). *The ethics of authenticity*. Cambridge, MA/London: Harvard University Press.
Taylor, C. (2007). *A secular age*. Cambridge, MA/London: The Belknap Press of Harvard University Press.
Willke, H. (2002). *Dystopia. Studien zur Krisis des Wissens in der modernen Gesellschaft*. Frankfurt: Suhrkamp.

Chapter 6
Does Intensive Morphogenesis Foster Human Capacities or Liabilities?

Margaret S. Archer

Introduction

To my knowledge this question has never been posed. Yet in this volume we are discussing the relationship between Morphogenesis and Eudaimonia on the assumption that the two are related in one way or another. If that is correct, then some causal process needs to be adduced for *how* it works, that is for *how* it makes the 'good life' attainable more readily and/or for more people, or the reverse. Therefore, such a process has to connect *features of societal change* with *characteristics of human subjects* (singular and collective), regardless of whether the outcome is viewed positively or negatively.

Potentially, the array of such 'features' and 'characteristics' is legion and could result in opposite conclusions about their relationship being positive or negative for Eudaimonia, so how is any theorist to choose? As ever, our propositions – ones that entail making or having made these choices – are theory-laden; this is necessarily the case and it is best to show explicit awareness of the fact. Hence, the title of this chapter deliberately reveals that it will draw upon two concepts germane to Critical Realism in responding to the question posed: does the intensification of Morphogenesis accentuate our 'liabilities' as human subjects' or expand our human 'capacities'? This does not prejudge the conclusion, if only because Realists are found on each side, nor does it preempt ethical discussion of what constitutes a 'good life' because these terms – capacities and liabilities – may be considered too thin. Lastly, it confines no-one to an either/or conclusion since there is nothing

M.S. Archer (✉)
Centre for Social Ontology, Department of Sociology, University of Warwick, Coventry, CV4 7AL, UK
e-mail: margaret.archer@warwick.ac.uk

M.S. Archer (ed.), *Morphogenesis and Human Flourishing*, Social Morphogenesis,
DOI 10.1007/978-3-319-49469-2_6

incoherent in maintaining that Morphogenesis might extend our 'liabilities' to suffering in new forms, whilst simultaneously expanding our 'capacities' in novel ways to do new and congenial things.

To get the discussion going, let me characterize briefly each of the diametrically opposed sides with the sole aim of showing that neither is unreasonable. On the one hand, why should anyone entertain the notion that intensified morphogenesis would or could promote the Eudaimonia or thriving for (more) human beings in global society through enabling the development or fuller use of their 'capacities'? The argument hinges on the new opportunities that are opened up (new experiences, novel jobs, newly recognized skills etc.) that elasticate existing 'capacities', develop networks, and acknowledge some forms of ability that previously gained no recognition and may not have been recognized even by their possessors. In other words, ascribed characteristics will diminish in importance and achieved ones increase as the notion of achievement itself diversifies. Furthermore, digitalization has opened up the cultural 'archive' for everyone (who is online) to explore the accumulated cultural heritage and the frontiers of new discoveries. Distances have shrunk in proportion to new modes of communication. New forms of social relationships have become optional. Thus, if more people can do more of what they do best – for remuneration, for pleasure, or for pro-social ends – this provides a stepping stone towards the 'good life', meaning that their flourishing will be enhanced. Of course, this is not automatically the case because subjects' doings and ends also include novel forms of damaging criminality, of torture and of harms, including self-harming; all new modes of viciousness, rather than virtue.

On the other hand, there are plenty of theorists – and some of them Critical Realists – who have maintained that we are creatures of routine, still guided in our aspirations and courses of action by habits or *habitus*, even when the contexts of our lives are changing dramatically (Archer 2010). Augment their ranks by those who make much less of routinized action but argue that the rapidity of change – the very fact of an increased 'variety' of opportunities becoming available to human subjects – is disorienting, destabilizing and a source of dissatisfaction because people can neither keep up with nor sample everything on offer. They are literally spoilt for choice, or by it, so 'acceleration theorists' claim (Rosa 2003 and our Vol. II 2014) for its critique). In short, to them, intensified Morphogenesis intensifies subjects' 'liabilities' to novel forms of suffering. The route to the 'good life' is no longer paved by traditional routines and subjects, whose reactions as 'distracted people' (Carrigan 2016) take the form of 'expressivism' and 'presentism' fit them extremely badly for designing their own *modus vivendi* in which they can thrive in contemporary society (Archer 2012). This, then is a very mixed choir of those mourning the demise of morphostasis in different keys.

The above are introductory sketches for setting the scene and are inadequate for pitting against one another. However, the key element that rarely features properly in ensuing debates is the nature of the scene itself. Social theorists in general are over-restrictive about the world in which we live. In other words, to them 'our human context' does *not* signify the whole natural world with its three orders; the Natural Order, our physical environment; the Practical Order, our material heritage, at any time, of tools, techniques and technology; as well as the Social Order. Instead, sociological imperialism increasingly accords primacy to the Social order and slides the Natural and the Practical under its hegemony. The effect is that singular subjects are cut off from direct contact with and influence by their interplay with the Natural and Practical Orders because these are mediated to them by the Social.[1] This will be the major theme of the present Chapter and it leads to some very different conclusions from those of the sociological imperialists and to some considerations that they cannot entertain.

At birth, human beings have a range of inborn *liabilities* and *capacities* in relation to the world they have entered. All of these exist only *in potentia* and *none* of them may be realized (walking, talking, loving) if the neonate does not survive (the sad fate of many migrant babies drowning in the Mediterranean or Aegean this year). In these cases, their *liabilities* succumbed to the combined influence of the three components of natural reality – the sea, ramshackle, unsuitable or overloaded boats, and a mélange of parental desperation and smugglers' greed. Human *capacities* are fragile and their development is demanding of time, care and propitious circumstances supplied by all three kinds of natural reality, working together without tension. The new opportunities furnished by intensified morphogenesis *can* only contribute to Eudaimonia provided that they enable enhanced development of our human *capacities* and reduce the import of our *liabilities.*

We all inhabit one world and the impacts of our various morphogenetic endeavors (intended, unintentional, unknown, aggregate or emergent) upon our three very different environments confront us all today with new threats, again working on our liabilities, the greatest of which is the extinction of humanity climatically through rendering the planet uninhabitable or nuclear warfare. As the first time that we live with the possibility of our species-extinction, so for the first time the entire population must choose between succumbing to its ultimate *liability* or collaboratively co-operating, using its combined *capacities*, to avert this conclusion. Facing finitude is an unprecedented (morphogenetic) feature that now outweighs our other concerns. Recognizing our shared finitude may prompt a higher collective regard for universal thriving, helping it for the first time collectively to override zero-sum competition by cooperation.

Human Thriving in the New Millennium

I take an essentialist approach to human thriving, like Sayer (2008) and O'Mahoney (2011) amongst Critical Realists, and hold, as they do, that it has an acceptable form.[2] In *Being Human* (2000) I grounded this ontologically in the fact that

---

[1]A similar slippage was the theme of Colin Campbell's excellent *Myth of Social Action* (1996), where he traced how the broader Weberian concept of 'action' was sedulously truncated into 'social action' by later theorists.

[2]As Sayer states, 'Whilst a strong and deterministic essentialism is always wrong and often dangerously misleading, a moderate, non-deterministic essentialism is necessary for explanation and for a social science that claims to be critical', (1997, 453).

	Natural Order	**Practical Order**	**Social Order**
Relationship	Object/Object	Subject/Object	Subject/Subject
Knowledge Type	Embodied	Practical	Discursive
Emergent From	Co-ordination	Compliance	Commitment
Relations Contributing to	Differentiating the bodily envelope from the environment	Distinction between subjects and objects	Distinguishing self from other people

Fig. 6.1 Three kinds of relations of human subjects with natural reality and their resultant effects (Source: Archer 2010)

constituted as we are and the world being as it is, every one of us has ineluctably to have some *concern* for their relationship with its three component orders. Each concern can vary in its personal prioritization by different human subjects, but relationally they cannot be totally indifferent to faring adequately in all of the three orders, if they are to survive and thrive. In other words, these are necessary relations that each newborn has to come to terms with ontogenetically as they grow up; the better they do so, the better they thrive.

Experientially, the Natural, Practical and Social orders may seem to have fuzzy boundaries, but they are phenomenologically indistinct only because they are often encountered simultaneously. The three orders are partially overlapping in the world and in the course of personal development (an overlap often encouraged by parents and teachers), and, most importantly, exert different causal powers upon different aspects of the human being. Were they merely analytically but not ontologically distinct, then the three orders just distinguished could exert no distinctive causal powers upon humans. In justifying that they do, let us examine the following summary diagram (Fig. 6.1).

The three orders are distinct – and not merely analytically so – because our direct encounters with nature are *object/object* ones (in relation to water, our bodies are floatables); with material artefacts they are *subject/object* relations where we, as subjects, encounter the resistances and affordances of objects and artefacts, acquiring skills in relation to them (children master holding and slowly tipping a full bottle of milk and drinking it at 3 months). Of course, this bottle was given to them 'socially', but a much later present of golf clubs never made anyone a good golfer; the skill of 'catching on' has to be *personally* acquired by everyone as does the embodied skill of swimming. If practical knowledge is the source of 'knowing how', the major contribution of linguistically encoded discursive knowledge, involving *subject/subject* relations, is 'knowing that'; through theoretical and authoritative statements not reliant upon experience (but on being told, for instance, that touching fire will hurt).

Humans necessarily have to sustain relationships with the natural world, with work relationships and with social relationships if they are to survive and thrive. Therefore, none of us can afford to be completely indifferent to the concerns that are embedded in our relations with all three natural orders. A distinct type of concern derives from each of these orders. The concerns at stake are respectively those of *'physical well-being'* in relation to the Natural order, *'performative competence'* in relation to the Practical order and *'self-worth'* in relation to the Social order.

Our emotional development is part of this interaction because emotions convey the import of different kinds of situations to us. In other words, the natural order, the practical order and the discursive order are the intentional objects to which three different clusters of emotions are related (Archer 2000). Because emotions are seen as 'commentaries upon our concerns' (Archer 2004), then emotionality is our first reflexive response to the world and what matters to us in it.

(i) In the world of Nature, the relational requisite for 'experience leading to a disposition' (say, to swim) is simply the co-ordination of a body with the properties of an environment (a watery one in the case of floating). This emergent skill (swimming) hinges upon the relationship between our physiological potentialities/liabilities and the positive/negative feedback received from the water. In nature human beings have the power to *anticipate* what the import of environmental occurrences will be for their *bodily well-being*. Anticipation is the key to affect. We know what the consequences of fire or icy water will be for our bodies and somatically this is projected as fear; were it not for anticipation, there would be nothing other than the pain of the event itself. It is from the interaction between environmental circumstances and embodied concerns that, because we are conscious beings, we can anticipate their conjunction and furnish ourselves with an emotional commentary. The relationship between properties of the environment and properties of our embodiment are sufficient for the emergence of emotions like fear, anger, disgust and relief.

(ii) In the Practical Order, tacit skills are emergent from the affordances and resistances presented by objects and the assimilation of and accommodation to them on the part of subjects. Activities such as competently playing tennis, a musical instrument, touch typing or driving all depend upon 'catching on' and, at more advanced levels (such as improvising at jazz or manoeuvring an articulated lorry), upon acquiring a real 'feel for the artefact'. In the practical order there is a distinct cluster of emotions which are emergent from our subject/object relations, which concern our *performative achievement*. These are the two strings made up of frustration, boredom and depression, on the one hand, and satisfaction, joy, exhilaration and euphoria, on the other. The task/undertaker relationship is quintessentially that of subject confronting object/artefact and what exactly goes on between them is known to the subject alone. Each task makes its own demands upon the undertaker if a skilled performance is to be produced. It thus carries its own standards which give the undertaker either positive or negative feedback. In other words, the sense of failure and the sense of achievement are reflected emotionally. Positive emotions foster continued practice and negative affect predisposes towards its cessation.

(iii) In the Social Order we cannot avoid becoming a subject among subjects. With it come 'subject-referring properties' (such as admirable or shameful), which convey the import of social normativity to our own concerns in society. Generically, the most important of our social concerns is our *self-worth* which is vested in certain 'projects' (in one's career, family, community, club or church) whose success or failure we take as vindicating our self-worth or damaging it. It is because we have invested ourselves in such social projects that we are susceptible of emotionality in relation to society's normative evaluation of our performance in their associated roles. Our behaviour is regulated by hopes and fears, namely anticipations of social approbation or disapprobation. Simply to be a role incumbent has no such emotional implications – pupils who vest none of their self-worth in their school performance are not downcast by examination failure nor, I argued in the last volume (Archer 2016), are penalties for infringing anormative regulations (such as collecting a parking ticket) met with feelings of shame.

Current Forms of Global Morphogenesis and Their Relationship to Human Thriving

Although the previous section, which built upon earlier work, was written in terms of persons in their concrete singularity, precisely the same points could have been made for collectivities or relational associations, from the dyad to macroscopic organizations, such as the UN. In this book, given constraints of space and our shared project of assessing the likelihood of the transition to a new social formation (Morphogenic Society), I will move to the other extreme and discuss the most macro-entity, the human race in its global context. By adapting the same diagram (used in Archer 2000, p. 162), the aim is to bring home the crucial point that all three orders of reality are themselves changing quite dramatically in our lifetimes, but that such morphogenetic changes are far from representing benign 'progress' in the sense of benefitting humanity or even introducing a better 'adaptive' fit between the social order and its environment; the tendency is in precisely the opposite direction as far humankind is concerned. In other words, I will argue that the *globalized context – for which humanity must take historical responsibility – is antipathetic to human thriving in all three orders of natural reality*. The obvious question is why the overall increase in opportunities should result in this perverse effect.

Moreover, although some of these threatening tendencies could be attributed to unintended consequences for a time, that time has passed. What humanity now confronts are un-natural transformations of nature itself, generalized commodification, including people, and the diffusion of ideationally distorted conceptions of 'presentism' that sap the capacity for people to shape a life reflexively for themselves. All of these result from the state of the world itself remaining the product of ruthless relational contestation.

I continue to maintain that 'we are who we are because of what we care about' (Archer 2000:10). Our personal identities are defined by our *precise constellations of concerns*, which significantly influence with whom each of us forms a 'we' (dyadic or associational) and the 'you' they aim to become as incumbents of social roles. Andrew Sayer stresses the same point about the importance of what matters to people: 'I argue that social science's implicit or explicit models of human beings as causal, meaning-endowing agents tend to overlook the fact that our relation to the world is not merely causal and interpretative, but are one of concern' (2011: 20). I have also underlined that our human concerns are not synonymous with high-mindedness but can be immoral, ignoble and illegal. In other words, concern[3] is a broader concept than Eudaimonia, which is usually translated as human flourishing, thriving, or doing and living well. Conversely, the pursuit of certain concerns is self-harming and harmful to others (as some cigarette packets remind us).

Lastly, although to have a concern may be applied to a particular person, its usage should not be exclusively 'personal' because it is common for the same concern to be shared by a couple and many voluntary associations come into being because the same issue matters to their members. More importantly still, our relations with others generate relational goods and evils that can only be produced together and enjoyed or suffered together and thus can never be reduced to the aggregate products of individual persons (Donati and Archer 2015). One of their causal powers is that as emergents they can prove particularly attractive or repellent to singular subjects who recognize that their own well being would be enhanced (or the reverse) by belonging to a couple or a community enterprise. This is one of the drivers towards 'we-ness', but also what prompts dissociation from particular 'we's.

The main point I want to make in this Chapter is that today, meaning the period roughly since 1980, relationships between these three orders of natural reality have been drastically transformed. New contradictions have emerged between them, some of which are objectively unsustainable in ways that were unpredictable and are unprecedented. Each affects human agents (singular or collective) and does so by *accentuating their liabilities and restricting their capacities*. In brief, I will argue that the current state of the world, meaning the relationship between its three orders, is unconducive to the thriving of the global population as a whole. This is something new; historically there has never been an era whose social formation did not depend upon intensifying the liabilities of some to the benefit of others. But what are the consequences if Eudaimonia becomes beyond the reach of all?

---

[3]This term translates with difficulty into many European languages.

(a) The Natural Order

Nature used to be described and sometimes defined as self-subsistent, that is following its own laws with virtual immunity to human doings.[4] This is inscribed in its etymology with the Latin *natura* signifying essential qualities or an innate disposition, and deriving from the Greek *physis* referring to the intrinsic qualities of plants, animals and geographical features that had developed of their own accord. Although some locate an injunction to human mastery over nature in the book of Genesis, contemporary Biblical scholars tend to interpret this rather as being made responsible for stewardship of the earth. The notion of full-blooded 'mastery' was articulated during the Enlightenment (and is embodied in Faust), but more as an encouragement to throw off theological fetters than to engage in any technological exploit or exploitation – 'science' was still inadequate to the mission. (Only Saint- Simon had a glimpse of its potential when writing about his 'ship of knowledge').

For example, even crop rotation, which had been practiced in the Middle East since 6000 BC, took place on no scientific basis at all, but was a matter of trial and error. It remained such during Charles Townshend's four-crop rotation (the Norfolk System) that became the foundation of the British agricultural revolution, which still lacked a developed theory of nitrogen fixation and replenishment; it simply paid off to do it in terms of yield. Even in 1817, Ricardo reserved a special category of Rent for 'nature's bounty' in the form of land, which itself involved no costs of production because it was not produced by humankind. Similarly, mining, whose origins are dateless, did involve labour costs that encouraged indentured workers, as it still does in parts of the world today. However, payment by the load mined (the equivalent of piecework in textiles), had already allowed the first industrial revolution to take-off on the basis of owning or acquiring land with coal below it and a tight-fisted mine owner seeing a better gain to be made from it than by arguing over protectionism in the wool trade. 'Modernity's Man', as I called him in *Being Human* (2000 Ch. 2) had begun to come into his own. Yet, Nature, though increasingly raped and pillaged (and romanticized), still had more than two and a half centuries to run before confronting the Anthropocene.

The paradoxes of the Anthropocene are numerous. Those that I will briefly explore are the effects of Climate Change signalling the millennial switch from 'Man's mastery of Nature' (a phrase previously intended to celebrate something very positive to human well-being) to its opposite, the repercussions of destructive human interventions in Nature upon themselves. The paradoxes in question are intended to warrant the following conclusions: (i) that in so far as scientific publications shape the outlooks of those they study, various disciplines are responsible for exculpating humanity from responsibility; (ii) that the consequences of

[4]Of course some animals were hunted and some encouraged to proliferate; some land was rendered infertile and other tracts came under cultivation but these were small scratches on the face of the earth.

unmitigated Climate Change exacerbated global inequalities by falling most heavily on the poorest and excluding them from sharing in any of the benefits of global morphogenesis; (iii) that the self-designated 'beneficiaries' of continued denial, nevertheless experienced negative effects in terms of climatic emergencies that did not enhance their well-being; (iv) that the resistance of the BRICS (and the USA) to UN Agreements for reducing carbon-emissions, seriously diminished social integration in international relations.

(i) Quite reasonably in the 1980s, research and publications on global warming came from the natural sciences. Rather less understandable was the marginal role assigned to 'Human Activities'. In the NASA sponsored report (1986), which first published the Bretherton model, these social activities were confined to a small black box on the outer periphery. The implication was not that 'we humans had created this problem; so we must solve it' and neither did the general public in the developed world take it that way. More depressing was the silence of the sociologists. Bibliographical analysis revealed that a mere 3 percent of items dealing with global environmental change had been produced by sociologists nearly 20 years later (ISSC 2013, 493–496). Instead, mainstream economics represented the social sciences with its familiar individualistic approach that ignored structures and endorsed market mechanisms through the approval given to 'emissions trading' between nations. If 'cap and trade' could fix matters, no-one need feel their Eudaimonia was at stake.

(ii) Consequently, the structured injustice whereby the consequences of global warming fell most heavily upon the poorest in marginalized nations, who used considerable less fossil-fuel energy than those in developed countries, were largely ignored in the academy. Yet, almost 75 % of the annual carbon dioxide emissions are released by the Global North, with its mere 15 % of the world's population (Holdren 2007). Since one wealthy person could emit as much CO_2 as 70,000 of the poor in the poorest countries (Roberts and Parks 2007), the injustice was hard to deny. Equally, the consequences did not seem to affect us in developed countries; our well-being was not damaged by loss of our livelihoods through desertification, deforestation, water acidification and contamination; we were not victims of enforced migration to escape rising sea-levels, flooding or droughts; we did not become the inhabitants of shanty towns on the peripheries of the nearest settlement, without shelter or employment and prey to recruitment into the drugs trade or resorting to selling our bodily organs (Scheper-Hughes 2016). Did we have moral responsibility for the harms sustained by distant others? At least the question began to be asked (Daniel Finn 2014).

(iii) At last the data about the unfriendly relations between the social order and the natural order were marshalled into comprehensive books rather than left on scattered websites. But that was not until 2015, meaning just months before the successor to the Kyoto agreement (that the US never signed) and the Copenhagen stalemate (2009) was to take place in Paris (December 2015).

Credit goes to the ASA's Task Force on Sociology and Global Climate Change for the publication of *Climate Change and Society: Sociological Perspectives* (Dunlap and Brulle 2015), to the two Pontifical Academies who worked together to produce *Sustainable Humanity, Sustainable Nature, Our Responsibility* (Dasgupta et al. 2014), and the Pope's Encyclical *Laudato sí*, all warning a global threat was upon us and that its structural injustices were our responsibility as was protective action to preserve our 'common home'. Virtuous action is integral to Aristotle's Eudaimonia; in late Modernity, no virtue had been shown by the West towards 'the rest'. Was it about to pay for this, or to act collectively and commit to contributing less than a 2C degree rise in temperature and to achieve de-carbonization by 2050?

(iv) Prolonged structural injustices have repercussions too. The Indian delegation to the UN COP21 meeting spelt these out without holding their punches. The message was that you, the developed countries, still beneficiaries of your 'dirty' industrial revolutions, now want to deny us the right to be 'filthy' in the same way to the same end. In honesty 'we' have to accept that this is the case, but 'our' counter-justification is serious, if unfair. Unless the BRICS do accept to restrict emissions, then the whole global world faces *finitude*; *for the first time the natural order and the social order are locked in mortal combat in which we will all be losers*. But that may not render the BRICS speechless. The cumulative emissions from developed societies remain in the atmosphere for a minimum of a hundred years. Why should they not bear the burden of more extensive cuts in order for some of the fastest developing countries to 'catch-up' and thus be reimbursed for past structural injustices? That would seem to be at least a reasonable response in terms of *phronesis* or practical wisdom; the trouble is that of regress. If the BRICS are permitted to be 'dirtier' for a period, how are they going to compensate much less developed countries for committing the identical injustice towards them? To characterize the process of social change as a matter of *relational contestation* (and neither self-government nor self-organization) had never seemed more appropriate.[5]

Each aspect described above is the product of morphogenesis, yet instead of yielding a 'win-win' outcome, their combined result may make us all terminal losers because there will be no posterior social formation. Perhaps these are over-gloomy thoughts induced by concentrating upon our natural human *liabilities* rather than our human *capacities*. Thus I will introduce Fig. 6.2 from which to discuss the other relationships between the three orders of natural reality to balance the picture.

[5]Of course there are alternatives that thankfully were endorsed in Paris, December 2015; namely funding (probably inadequate as yet) to assist them in adapting their energy sources towards 'cleaner' ones.

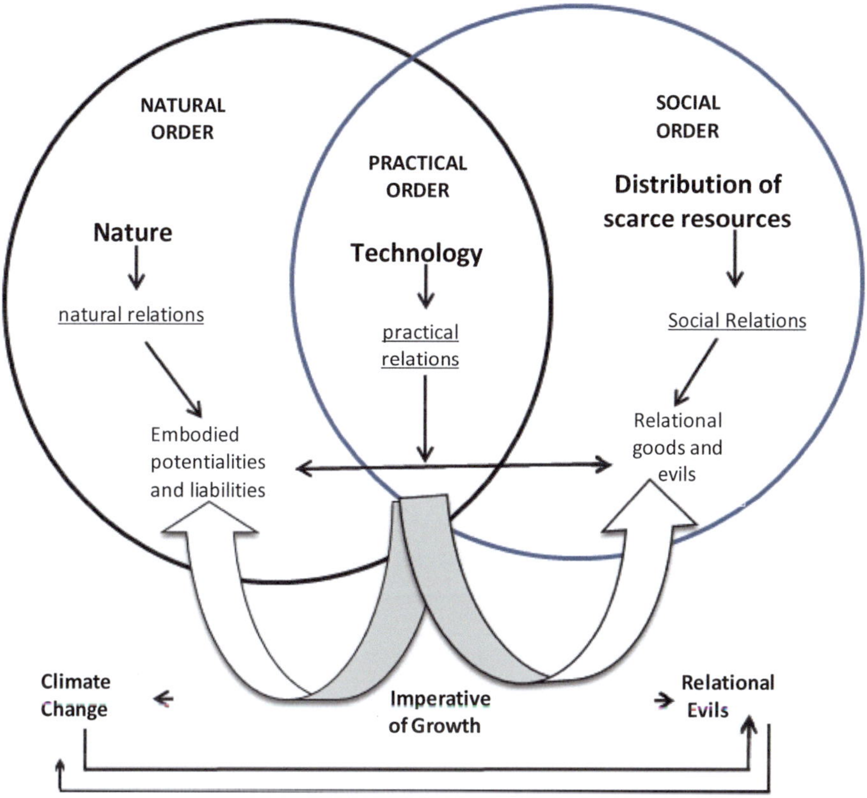

Fig. 6.2 Relations between the three orders of natural reality

(b) The Practical Order

When I first wrote in general terms about the Practical Order in relation to the two other orders of natural reality, it was held to be the pivot between Nature and the Social (Archer 2000 Ch. 5). Hence the intermediary position assigned to it on the above diagram, which it retains. In a nutshell, the Practical Order as pivotal derives from it playing the role of a 'translation medium' between the Social and the Natural orders and vice versa.

'Translation' is both constrained and enabled by the different human interests that are vested in the three orders and their forms of knowledge. Thus, (i) Embodied and Practical knowledge are wedded to an instrumental concern ('does it work?'), which is both challenged and extended by theoretical knowledge that abstractly explicates the causal powers involved ('this is what makes it work'). The hiatus is more than the psychological resistance of agents who will not trade well-tied practice for new tentative (and fallible) theorising. Rather the onus is upon scientific theories to prove themselves by enhancing practice. Science has to show its applications in the practical order before it can uproot established practice and underpin the elaboration of better practice. For example, the science on which the Industrial Revolution depended was available two centuries before it was applied. Similarly, (ii) working in the opposite direction, the new possibilities opened up by theoretically informed applied practices and their novel artefacts confront agents with a new phenomenal domain, which, with every technical advance, sets a new challenge to embodied incorporation.[6] Working from the middle, (iii) innovations in practical knowledge set the same problem of whether or not they can be mastered in an embodied fashion by naturalizing an artefactual process (such as knitting or computing) and, equally, (vi) whether the new skilled 'feel for' doing something can be conveyed in a manner sufficient for eventual theoretical illumination ('what we are doing when we have a sense of this is . . . ').

The impact of (new) scientific knowledge on practice is both indirect and delayed. The initial effect of a new theory is to undermine the old theoretical bases underpinning established practices. What it does is to show that the premises of some practice are ill-founded. However, although the theoretical import is that the practice should be abandoned, because the new theory does not tell us what to do instead, it is a poor pragmatic reason for jettisoning an established practice whose practical utility remains unassailed. Thus, for scientific theory to act as the growing point of practice, a second stage is involved, where new theories enter the practical order, but only through their application as successful additions to material culture. This pays their admission fee. Applied science and technology are the artefactual modes of translation and transition from theoretical to practical knowledge.[7] The main historical engine principally though not exclusively responsible for these transfers has been the material advantages derived from them and has thus lain in the hands of the economy. Yet if what is transferred is materially advantageous, this could sound like an account for developmental complementarities, without losers. That is where the metaphor of 'translation' can be as misleading as any other for it deflects attention from who conducts the enterprise, for which motives and interests, under what conditions and *cui bono*.

The last thing we can do is to take the protagonists' rhetoric at face value, be they entrepreneurs or economists, for who would oppose 'growth', 'development' or 'progress', the terms recommending change? Yet they were as deceptive as the glass beads colonial adventurers had proffered in exchange for land. As far as the natural order was concerned, 'growth', which sounded the most innocent of these recommendations, turned out to be the most sinister because it concealed the ensuing contradiction. Whatever subsequent forms were assumed by capitalism or neo-liberalism, *the imperative of growth* was always paramount and to their own advantage (see Porpora 2014 Ch. 4). Nature, with its capacity to feed the

[6]When desktop computers arrived at the University of Warwick in 1990 some secretarial staff felt unable to rise to this challenge, yet had previously mastered Pitman's shorthand and then the electronic typewriter, but now sought other employment or took retirement.

[7]Whereas Bourdieu endorses an epistemological break between forms of knowledge, I only insist upon their different ontological origins. Consequently, Bourdieu's position then precludes 'translatability' between knowledge domains: mine does not, which is precisely why I can venture the thesis that practice is pivotal to knowledge in general, whereas he cannot.

world's population, could reveal only its liabilities in the face of remorseless economic growth, because 'nothing grows faster in the growth society than energy consumption' (Anderson 1976: 153), with the consequences just examined.

In fact, as we all know, economic growth was enshrined in the metric of GNP/GDP that became the index of social development. Yet, as we also now know, infinite growth is environmentally unsustainable. How can this paradox be explained? In other words, how can it be that most consumers in the developed world more readily entertain the prospect of eco-disaster than the end of capitalism?

In turning to the effects of capitalism on the social order, I will simply summarize the analyses presented in previous volumes in order to draw out the contradiction between them. Competition is inherent to capitalist production and 'motors the technological innovation for which capitalism was praised even by Marx' (Porpora 2014); moreover, 'capitalism is healthy only when it is growing'. Growth is intrinsic to profit and both increase by shifting manufacturing to the 'extractive peripheries', where labour and raw materials are also cheaper, welfare minimal, toxic waste is a literal externality of production, and such countries represent a massive potential consumer market. This is the nub of the contradiction with the Natural Order: 'The pressures of capitalist competition produce the corporate predilection for 'externalizing' costs to the environment. In other words, unless there are rules fining corporate processes for pollution, then corporations, threatened by competitors, will opt to plough more earnings back into securing competitive advantage than into protecting the environment, especially where such spending offers no advantage competitively.' (Porpora 2014).

In the 1980s, market activities in the developed world shifted to finance capitalism, spawning innovative financial instruments (Morgan and Sun in this volume; Lim and Lim 2010) that were increasingly dependent on burgeoning new digital technology and could not have developed without it. What I want to accentuate here is that speedy digitalization enabled the capitalist market to override the loss of jobs and increase in income differentials in the population, to survive the financial crisis it had precipitated and the backlash to subsequent austerity measures. This was precisely because it had acquired the means to pull off the greatest scam of all time – that of artificially associating scarcity and hence purchase prices with cultural goods that could be freely exchanged without loss of value (see Archer 2014, 2015). This is what Hofkirchner rightly calls the enclosure of the Commons. It should rank as the world's greatest barefaced deception, but simultaneously the most profitable. Usually it is called 'commodification' and escapes censure because we are inoculated by decades of consumerism. Now there are simply more new products to acquire and to throw way because the commercialization of digital technology has in-built obsolesce built in to its scientific foundations.

Hence consumer competition for status symbols issued in a further paradox: 'when consumers are most hotly in pursuit of non-material meanings, their use of material resources is greatest' (Schor 2010: 41). This entails further negative impacts on the Natural Order, but ones just as conflictual with the Social Order and the eudaimonia of all within it. What you have defines who you are, and who you are has nothing to do with your capacities, merits or virtues but with the talentless 'celebrity lottery' or simply the lottery. As agents we are passive: victims of the people's roulette wheel, or willing to spend to gain a consolation prize from a scratch card offered at every supermarket check-out.

Increasingly, some have become less than passive, almost inert, because they are now 'disposable people', the largest category being the 'retired', with limited spending power but an increasingly expensive longevity. A further irony is the attempt made by the State to respond with rhetorical tenacity to maintaining their health care, whilst hospitals are run on the lines of Taylorism with through-put as their main target. (This is an illustration of Donati's argument about the oscillation between *lib and lab*). Equally disposable are non-working youth, especially those of ethnic origin, who make up the largest group in US gaols. Once again, economic morphogenesis has played on human liabilities rather than encouraging our capacities. Furthermore, Agential passivity has further causes and consequences arising from the 'mode of consumption', which will be examined in the next section.

(c) The Social Order

In 2012, I published a book entitled *The Reflexive Imperative in Late Modernity*. The thesis was extremely simple, namely that with the intensification of morphogenesis in all social domains, everybody, though especially the young, had to become more reflexive about themselves in relation to their social contexts and vice versa. Habit had long ceased to be a reliable guide to action and there seemed no justification whatsoever for claiming that current courses of action were built upon it (Archer 2010). Instead, the young (and the redundant and the old) had the increasingly difficult task of discerning their concerns and the more challenging one still of forging a satisfying and sustainable *modus vivendi* to which they could dedicate themselves. That was the only road now to personal and inter-personal flourishing. Donati and I ventured (2015) that it was also the route to producing 'relational goods' at the meso-level, which were good in themselves (trust, co-operation, reciprocity) but also served to stabilize the social order at these levels.

Instead, a very tiny category, almost possible to have neglected in the *Reflexive Imperative* (but see 2012, p. 277–290) were seemingly growing into what Carrigan calls 'distracted people' (2016). This trajectory began with the mobile phone (invented in the USA and largely made in China), shown in one experimental study to be the most prized possession of Junior High Schoolers, which they would 'rescue' in preference to their purses/wallets. Successively, the apps accumulated and with them, the false shame of not being seen on Facebook. I am often asked why I anathematise the latter shamelessly in print. The answer is not merely in terms of the fake, over-sexualized self-presentations that are encouraged, nor because of the blackmailing, 'outings', 'trollings' and even suicides recorded, and not (simply) because the photos and messages posted are the intellectual property of its founder – the latest recruit to Big Personalized Philanthropy. It is that if this banality is possible, then we are a failed global society in terms of Eudaimonia.

What it induces is a false 'presentism' in which today's doings have precedence over tomorrow's consequences, 'expressive' rather than purposeful responses to changing circumstances, and rejection of the quest for the 'unity of a life' that Charles Taylor (1997) saw as the keystone of personal Eudaimonia. All are sacrificed to a titillating voyeurism in the present tense. 'Expressivism' displaces any reflexive review of worthwhile commitment, which probably accounts for the ease with which street demonstrations can be whipped-together and the insurmountable difficulties of melding them into durable movements in support of a cause. Yet the consequences mount-up objectively. Growing millions are willingly paralysing their reflexive capacities (possessed by all normal people)[8] in favour of an ephemeral irrealism in which they have a thousand friends, a daily round of continual excitation, and where 'self-worth' is a matter of primitive attention getting.

I agree that this phenomenon cannot be attributed to the one source used for illustration. Yet if irrealist 'expressivism' is becoming global, then the realist response cannot avoid being that our foundational social institutions are not allies of Eudaimonia. At the personal level, the huge popularity attained by the social media in little more than 10 years testifies to the loneliness of people, particularly the young. They are neither comfortable with their own thoughts nor satisfied with the company they keep. Recently, I watched a father and his three late teenage children seat themselves for a five-course meal after the funeral of a close relative. All immediately placed their Iphones on the table, the father to talk to his latest girlfriend and the kids to scroll through recent text messages. None exchanged a word with the widow and none participated in any of the conversations that the remaining few of us tried to start. This says less about their (bad) manners than about their derogation of family life and preference for fictive virtual reality because the teenagers admitted that they knew few of those featuring among their networked 'friends'.

Given divorce and serial re-partnering, unemployment and jobs of short duration, uninterest in current affairs, un-involvement in voluntary causes, hobbies or sports, this lonely crowd had embraced the one role constantly available to them – that of consumers, in this case of ephemeral trivia. Social 'self-worth' consists in keeping up with it. Once again, this growing element of the social order had battened onto people's liabilities rather than exercising their capabilities. Another way of putting this is that the generation of Relational Evils had swamped Relational Goods and, in the vocabulary of youth, the former has globally 'gone viral'.

The Implications of These Contradictions Between the Three Orders of Natural Reality

This chapter began by maintaining that each and every human being needed to invest some concern in their relationship with Nature, with the Practical Order and with the Social as minimal conditions of their thriving, and alongside whatever

[8]This is my definition of reflexivity: 'Reflexivity is the regular exercise of the mental ability, shared by all normal people, to consider themselves in relation to their (social) contexts and vice versa' (2007:4).

other concerns mattered to them deeply. As a proposition, achieving satisfying and sustainable relations with all three orders does not itself result in flourishing, but can be regarded as a necessary but not sufficient condition of it. This is generally uncontentious because it coincides with needs that are almost unanimously agreed to be inscribed in our constitution as human beings. Thus, in his recent *To Flourish or Destruct* (2015), Christian Smith reviews 21 accounts of 'basic human needs', summarized in list form, among which he notes 'numerous substantive agreements and thematic repercussions among them' (p. 171). From these he synthesises or distils his own list of six 'basic human goods' that are 'natural, stable and universal' (p. 182). I am introducing this purely to underline the high degree of consensus that exists in relation to my proposition expressed in the first two sentences of this paragraph. Thus, Smith's six 'basic goods', held by him to represent our most fundamental interests and to produce our basic human motivations, do indeed include the three that have been under discussion here: in Smith's words, these are 'Bodily Survival, Security and Pleasure'; Knowledge of Reality (learning about the world and one's place and potential in it, including understanding material realities); Social Belonging and Love (pp. 181–2). Differences in our ways of formulating these goods are not important here.

Yet, something strange is at stake. In fact, I agree with his statement that 'Some specific things are by nature simply good for human persons, what constitute 'the good' for them. The basic interest of human persons is to realize those basic goods. Humans have the natural, real interest in achieving what for them is good' (Smith, p. 181). However, I have just devoted this chapter to arguing and illustrating the reverse. Namely, that each Order harbours a mega-problem – respectively, Climate Change, the Imperative of Growth, and the predominance of Relational Evils – that accentuates our *liabilities* rather than promoting our *capacities*. All of these have been traced to on-going morphogenetic processes, so should one conclude that morphogenesis is damaging to human thriving? That is too facile because for all that has been written about rapid change (acceleration) fostering 'destabilization', 'disorientation' and 'dissatisfaction' it would be only too easy to draw up parallel but equally negative lists of the consequences attending prolonged periods of morphostasis: famine, material inertia, slavery, frozen systems of social stratification, whole social categories deprived of human status etc.

Lists do not help because they condemn us to a flat ontology, to a 'variables' approach and, above all, to the inability to recognize that our liabilities (like our capacities) are not discrete but interactive, with the powers to exacerbate one another, thus compounding liabilities (or promoting capacities) into something with considerably greater malign (or beneficial) properties. Ontologically both are real but, as in basic banking, simple interest yields less than compound interest, although here we are not dealing with addition and multiplication. Nevertheless, a homeless person, without skills or friends is worse off than one who has the latter, although intersectionality is not a mechanical or mathematical process.

If we return to Fig. 6.2, it is clear that Climate Change and the Imperative for Economic Growth are both causally linked and mutually exacerbating to the detriment of the human race, though most detrimental to the poorest. If we think of late 2015 when the Paris Agreement was published, what had changed? In a nutshell, many of the previous Relational Evils had (potentially) been reversed. Although not a single one of the 165 participating nations declared itself suddenly uninterested in economic growth, all were persuaded by highly technical research (the Practical Order as pivotal) that any rise in carbon emissions above 2C degrees (using the Industrial revolution as the base line) would be disastrous for every country. Moreover, the continued economic development of all now depended on co-operative relations (with caveats) that mean the Agreement is a triumph over international relations at the previous Kyoto and Copenhagen meetings, without having reached complete consensus, (e.g. over 'compensation'). However, if followed up by appropriate action and legislation, the Paris Agreement would undoubtedly count as a Relational Good.

What would count as the equivalent, fostering Relational Goods rather than Evils in the current negative linkage between the Social and the Practical Orders – and thus representing a move towards Eudaimonia? What gives rise to the tension between these two orders is fundamentally that the neo-liberal Imperative to Economic Growth is reliant for its realization upon sustaining consumerism in the Social order. Currently, competition amongst consumers perfectly complements the growth imperative that advertising strains every sinew to maintain. What it sustains is a relational evil of competitiveness. In Michael Mann's diagnosis, 'the problem has been created by capitalism ably assisted by nation states and individual consuming citizens. These, unfortunately, are the three most fundamental social actors of our time' (2013: 362). Such exponential growth is 'bolstered by citizens unwilling to reduce consumption and politicians depending on GDP growth for re-election' (2013:368). This is an economical statement of the problem, but what can cut this vicious positive feedback between the two? Mann puts his faith in governmental regulation but, were measures severe (such as doubling VAT) they would flounder on the desire for re-election by those introducing them.

Most other suggestions hinge upon tax breaks and various forms of fiscal leverage. Their generic drawback is that they tie citizens even more tightly to the cash nexus. Suppose, instead, that we think of loosening this bond, diluting the bondage to capital by introducing alternative currencies that reward the cooperative generation of Relational Goods? Ethical, Time and Skill banks are already in operation, but could be generalized more boldly. Imagine the creation of Voluntary Credits for temporarily housing refugees and annulling Council Tax/*Taxe d'Habitation* for the period in question; consider making the payment of state pensions conditional (for the able bodied) upon the on-going accumulation of such Credits through voluntary pro-social activities, thus giving some point to the 20 years of active-life remaining to those retiring in their early sixties and also serving to reduce 'ageism'. Think of professionals extending their *pro bono* efforts for Voluntary organizations or parents of young children combining in collective childcare. All of these already exist; there is nothing utopian about encouraging the use of people's capacities. The above examples are obviously compromises because they retain links to material benefits, but they might serve to induce an appreciation of co-operation over competition that could lead further if gradually embedded as a normative expectation. As Donati summarized this state of affairs, ‘Only if we see the common good as a relational good, can we understand its inner connection with the human person’ (2008: 662 and 1991) and how s/he may approach Eudaimonia in the social order. After all, the market economy is a genus, of which capitalism is only one species (Zamagni and Zamagni 2010:11): markets *per se* do not entail the negative relationship between the Practical and Social orders under discussion.

Conclusion

Ultimately, the *good society* is one that promotes the Common Good. What makes it ‘good’ is that all contribute to generating it and without their cooperation it cannot exist. Thus, the Common Good entails a high level of *social integration* because without everyone contributing there would be a category of the ‘excluded’ or ‘self-excluded’ – of non-beneficiaries who cannot even be ‘free riders’ because to experience relational goods entails being in-relationship. What also makes it ‘good’ is that the relational goods produced in one sector do not conflict with those generated in any other, thus entailing a high level of *system integration* without which the goods in question would clash, damaging both – as I have sought to demonstrate in this chapter.

These are demanding conditions because although a potentially ‘good’ society *is by definition morphogenetic because relational goods are (new) emergent properties produced indefinitely*, it may well lose its claim to ‘goodness’ owing to the countervailing relational evils it is equally capable of generating, which can be just as morphogenetic (novel varieties of harm). Were the latter to predominate, both social and system integration would decline in consequence; the population in question (now global) would be re-divided into (temporary) winners and losers and the situational logic of opportunity would be indefinitely postponed as adversarial groups clung to the defence of their vested or objective interests – thus prolonging competition and tenaciously defending competitive advantages. This is roughly where humanity now stands. *Thus, intense morphogenesis alone, even when matched by parallel retreats in morphostasis, provides no warrant for announcing the advent of Morphogenic society as that of the Good Society.*

The most demanding of these conditions entails overcoming the lack of *system integration*, whose anatomy was laid bare during the current economic crisis, and of *social integration*, never clearer than in the European Union’s anti-humanitarian responses to the present migrant crisis and also in the proliferation of terrorism potentially making for a third world war. It seems essential to work in these sociological terms about the two forms of integration, whose referents are to emergent properties and powers, and to work to raise both in actuality. These are the ultimate conditions for kick-starting the universalization of Eudaimonia.

Otherwise, we are left merely with empirical observables, such as the ‘indignation’ of the ephemeral ‘Occupy’ movements, illustrated by the optimistic empiricism of Castells (2012), but lacking any account of how these could engage and integrate non-activists in the developed world, let alone in 'the rest'. In most ways, Graeber's advocacy of 'anarchism and democracy [which] are – or should be – largely identical' (2007: 330) differs mainly in his aim of eliminating the State's (legitimate Weberian) monopoly of violence and a genuine concern for building consensus. To him 'almost everyone agrees on the importance of horizontal, rather than vertical structures; the need for initiatives to rise up from relatively small, self-organized, autonomous groups rather than being conveyed downwards through chains of command; the rejections of permanent, named leadership structures; and the need to maintain some kind of mechanism – whether these be North American style "facilitation", Zapatista-style women's and youth caucuses, or any of an endless variety of other possibilities – to ensure that the voices of those who would normally find themselves marginalized or excluded from traditional participatory mechanisms are heard' (2007: 330). Although Graeber uses the term 'mechanism' above, this is precisely what is lacking. It is shown by the reference to those involved as 'autonomous groups' in the same citation. Thus, he bundles together a patchwork of protesting voices because together they will shout louder.[9] But volume does not unite or integrate or give direction; at best, it results in the book's title, *Possibilities.*

In policy terms, on the face of it, the recent popularity of the catch-phrase 'capacity-building' among INGOs, NGOs, professional bodies and a wide variety of voluntary associations, might appear as a counter-reaction against the remorseless play of macroscopic influences upon our human liabilities as analysed in this chapter. Generically, it seems to be so, but it is far too often not what it seems. Only too frequently its unit is taken to be the Individual and nothing beats Individualism for fostering competition and hierarchy, even when the referent is nominally to a collectivity (as in the 'capacity-building of women'). At most, such policies produce aggregate effects (for example, an n percent rise in computer literate women). These are improvements, but better is the enemy of best where human flourishing is concerned.[10]

Conversely, the Common Good, is the ultimate relational good, but without real relational goods – concern, trust and reciprocity with others – being generated from the bottom-up and interlinked with one another, there will be no chance for the Eudaimonia of all in a Morphogenic society. Human thriving, at all levels, has to be earthed in Relational Goods produced by Relational Subjects. Only given the

---

[9]In Andrew Sayer's words: 'this is where we live – between the actual and the possible, between present flourishing or suffering and future possible flourishing or suffering', (2011: 18).

[10]As a per-oration, consider the following reflection about limitations upon human capacities contained in Roy Bhaskar's posthumous book (2016: 81):

> Indeed for most people, for most of human history, the social has figured mainly as a source of constraint on, not enablement of human desires and possibilities. Not to acknowledge the constellational overreaching of enablement by constraint, the huge weight of the presence of the past, structural disembedding and structural sin (or sedimented, institutionalised master–slave-type relations of oppression) is idealistically to prioritise the personal over the social and slip back into individualism and misplaced voluntarism.

mutuality these embody can the benefits of extending the ‘capacities’ of every person and group prevail over the damaging consequences of preying upon their ‘liabilities’. After all, mutuality is nothing more than a modest name for win-win situations and ultimately for the Good Society.

References

Anderson, C. H. (1976). *The sociology of survival*. Homewood: Dorsey Press.

Archer, M. S. (2000). *Being human: The problem of agency*. Cambridge: Cambridge University Press.

Archer, M. S. (2004). Emotions as commentaries on human concerns. In J. H. Turner (Ed.), *Theory and research on human emotions*. Oxford: Elsevier.

Archer, M. S. (2007). *Making our way through the world: human reflexivity and social mobility*. Cambridge: Cambridge University Press.

Archer, M. S. (2010). Routine, reflexivity and realism. *Sociological Theory, 28*(3), 272–303.

Archer, M. S. (2012). *The reflexive imperative in late modernity*. Cambridge: Cambridge University Press.

Archer, M. (2014). The generative mechanisms transforming late modernity. In her (ed.), *Late modernity: trajectories towards morphogenic society*. Dordrecht: Springer.

Archer, M. S. (2015). How agency is transformed in the course of social transformation. In her (ed.), *Generative mechanisms transforming the social order*. Dordrecht: Springer.

Archer, M.S. (2016). Anormative social regulation: The attempt to cope with social morphogenesis. In her (ed.), *Morphogenesis and the crisis of normativity*. Dordrecht: Springer.

Bhaskar, R. (2016). *Enlightened common sense: The philosophy of critical realism*. Abingdon: Routledge.

Campbell, C. (1996). *The myth of social action*. Cambridge: Cambridge University Press.

Carrigan, M. (2016). The fragile movements of late modernity. In M. S. Archer (Ed.), *Morphogenesis and the Crisis in normativity*. Dordrecht: Springer.

Castells, M. (2012). *Networks of outrage and hope*. Cambridge: Polity.

Dasgupta, P., Ramanathan, V., & Sorondo, S. (Eds.). (2014). *Sustainable humanity, sustainable nature, our responsibility*. Vatican City: Vatican Press.

Donati, P. (1991). *Teoria relazionale della società*. Milan: FrancoAngeli.

Donati, P. (2008). Discovering the relational character of the common good. In M. Archer & P. Donati (Eds.), *Pursuing the common good: How solidarity and subsidiarity can work together*. Vatican City: Vatican Press.

Donati, P., & Archer, M. S. (2015). *The relational subject*. Cambridge: Cambridge University Press.

Dunlap, R. E., & Brulle, R. (Eds.). (2015). *Climate change and society: Sociological perspectives*. New York: Oxford University Press.

Earth Sciences Committee (Bretherton, F.). *Earth system sciences overview. A program for global change*. Report of the Earth Sciences Committee of the NASA Advisory Council, Washington, DC.

Finn, D. K. (Ed.). (2014). *Distant markets, distant harms*. New York: Oxford University Press.

Graeber, D. (2007). *Possibilities: Essays on hierarchy, rebellion and desire*. Oakland: AK Press.

Holdren, J. (2007). *Global climate disruption, What do we know? What should we do?* Presentation at Harvard University. Nov 2007.

International Social Sciences Council (ISSC). (2013). *World social science report: Changing global environments*. New York: UNESCO Publishing.

Lim, M. M.-H., & Lim, C. (2010). *Nowhere to hide: The great financial crisis and challenges for Asia*. Singapore: Institute of Southeast Asian Studies.

Mann, M. (2013). *The sources of social power* (Vol. 4). New York: Cambridge University Press.

O'Mahoney, J. (2011). Embracing essentialism: A realist critique of resistance to discursive power. *Organization, 1–19*, 723.

Porpora, D. V. (2014). Contemporary mechanisms of social change. In M. Archer (Ed.), *Late modernity: Trajectories towards morphogenic society*. Dordrecht: Springer.

Roberts, J. T., & Parks, B. (2007). *A climate of injustice: Global inequality and, North-South politics, and climate change*. Cambridge, MA: MIT Press.

Rosa, H. (2003). Social acceleration: Ethical and political consequences of a desynchronized high-speed society. *Constellations, 10*(1), 1–33.

Sayer, A. (2008). Essentialism, social constructionism, and beyond. *The Sociological Review, 45*(3), 453–487.

Sayer, A. (2011). *Why things matter to people*. Cambridge: Cambridge University Press.

Scheper-Hughes, N. (2016). Scars – Ruined lives and deaths of kidney trafficking victims. In M. Archer & M. Sanchez Sorondo (Eds.), *Human trafficking: Issues beyond criminalization*. Vatican City: Vatican City Press.

Schor, J. (2010). *Plenitude*. New York: Penguin.

Smith, C. (2015). *To flourish or destruct*. Chicago: University of Chicago Press.

Taylor, C. (1997). Leading a life. In R. Chang (Ed.), *Incommensurability, incompatibility and practical reason*. Cambridge, MA: Harvard University Press.

Zamagni, S., & Zamagni, V. (2010). *Cooperative enterprise: Facing the challenge of globalization*. Cheltenham: Edward Elgar.

Chapter 7
What Does a 'Good Life' Mean in a Morphogenic Society? The Viewpoint of Relational Sociology

Pierpaolo Donati

The Topic: Social Morphogenesis as Challenge to a 'Good Life'

The object of this contribution is not the concept or the ideal of the good life in itself, but which good life becomes desirable and possible in a morphogenetic society. My basic argument is that a good society, under conditions of radical morphogenesis, is feasible only through a particular 'politics of relationality'.

I propose to analyze the morphogenetic processes of morality prompted by the 'logic of opportunity' with a view to creating a good social life or, at least, a decent one. We have to address a plurality of normative logics that support different forms of social morphogenesis and, therefore, different moralities defining what constitutes the good life.

I am interested in highlighting the differences between the morality of opportunities according to *lib/lab* logic, on the one hand, and *relational* logic, on the other. To contest the *lib/lab* order of opportunities, a specific agonistic understanding of normativity may be necessary. The latter would be an emergent reality in a society after-modernity.

Since morphogenetic processes erode the dream of an 'unmediatedly human' society (i.e. a society in which what is peculiar to human agency is conveyed without mediations into social forms), I question the nature of what we call 'happiness', 'human good', 'the good life' from the viewpoint of its sociological constitution.

My argument is that in a society conceived as a field of opportunities, the distinguishing feature of 'living well' becomes the relational or non-relational nature of the good that is sought and realized by the acting subjects. It is necessary

P. Donati (✉)
Department of Sociology and Business Law, Università degli Studi di Bologna, Strada Maggiore 45, I-40125, Bologna, Italy
e-mail: pierpaolo.donati@unibo.it

M.S. Archer (ed.), *Morphogenesis and Human Flourishing*, Social Morphogenesis,
DOI 10.1007/978-3-319-49469-2_7

to clarify the modalities by which the good is generated and which effects follow from it. Substantiating this argument consists in giving evidence that there exists a specific logic of opportunities that is capable of realizing a 'society *of* the human', i.e. social forms that promote our humanity, whatever the (technological) means used to realize social relations. These latter can be generated only by subjects who are actively oriented to each other in a supra-functional sense (Donati 2009: 133). This is a society in which, from the standpoint of relational realism, the good life coincides with the creation of relational goods.

In short, this can happen in those social contexts that are capable of including new life opportunities within the social relations that orient the conduct of our lives toward an 'agonistic sociability'. This oxymoron alludes to the fact that, instead of encouraging citizens to bracket their moral and cultural disagreements, agonistic democrats cultivate oppositional yet respectful civic and political relations and practices (Deveaux 1999: 2). I argue that a flourishing civil society, on which a civil democracy needs to be grounded, can be fostered by those social networks that are able to generate competing relational goods.

Why the Problem of Human Happiness Is New

To simplify through synthesis, there are two alternative views on what human happiness might be, which have prevailed over the centuries: a *hedonic* idea of happiness and a *eudaimonic* one. For the hedonic conception, happiness is the result of avoiding pain and seeking pleasure, the key concept of all utilitarian schools of thought, in both its individual and aggregated forms. Social relations are considered as 'entities' that can bring pleasure or pain as other 'objects' do. On the other hand, we find the eudaimonic outlook, which, apart from being more theoretical and holistic, takes a different view of human relationality. It considers happiness as a more complex concept, not strictly limited to attaining pleasure and avoiding pain. Happiness is synonymous with thriving in human life, i.e. a kind of living that is active, inclusive of all that has intrinsic value, and therefore also of what I call 'the relational order of society'. It is a direct or indirect result of the practice of human virtues. Going beyond a restricted interpretation of Aristotle, who claims that pleasure is an *enérgeia* (act of being = intrinsic operation) of the human body and mind (*Nicomachean Ethics*, Book X, chapters 1–5), I will apply the concept of *enérgeia* to social relations as such. This means to talk about the 'act of being (the intrinsic operations) of social relations', which is proper to social reality to the extent that it is human.

Aristotle understood human happiness on two levels. On the individual level, as the satisfaction of the human being's natural needs (physical, psychological, and sociocultural), with the purpose of enhancing the more elevated human qualities, however one defines them (rationality, contemplation, *otium*, spiritual virtues). On the social level, life consists in enjoying interpersonal friendship and in conducting a commensurately active and peaceful life in the public sphere of the *polis*, with the intention of pursuing the common good. Aristotle did not examine in detail the relational nature of eudaimonia, limiting himself to making individual happiness dependent on the happiness of the political community, the latter having primacy over the former.

What I wish to recall is the fact that in classical thought and until the beginning of modernity, eudaimonia is related to two basic conditions: (i) it refers to the naturalness of human needs and thus *presupposes a human nature*, however this is defined, and (ii) it implies that the political community is capable of pursuing the common good by resolving social conflicts and giving citizens the security necessary to enable their human potentialities to flourish. These potentialities are generally understood as virtues.

In premodern thought, including Aristotle, virtue has a stable disposition called *habitus* as its prerequisite. *Habitus* is a fundamental means for achieving the good life in that it regenerates a social order conceived as an ideal that is stable and immutable in its principles. From this comes the idea that a happy society and a good life for its citizens is achieved by a strict correspondence between personal virtues and the social order, and that it is reproducible over time. The idea that individuals' happiness (as the realization of their virtues) projects itself onto the entire society prevails so that if individuals, as such, act for the good and are happy, the society will also be happy.

With modernity, this framework is progressively called into question. To the degree to which the individual is no longer incorporated (embedded) in a given community and becomes 'casual' (as Marx defines it in his *Manuscripts of 1844*), the distance between the individual and society grows increasingly greater. With the advance of the nation state and the spread of capitalism, the two assumptions of premodern thought fall: the notion of human nature and that of the common good are radically changed, altered, overturned, and, with them, the meaning of eudaimonia as well.

Once the great metaphysical-religious scaffoldings of the past have fallen away, the problem of how to sensibly conduct one's life (the Weberian *Lebensführung* or 'conduct of life') becomes an increasingly fraught problem. In a society in which the values that guide life are no longer 'founded' but simply subjectively chosen (Max Weber), eudaimonia presents itself as always problematic and somehow an unreachable goal. The fact is that all of modern culture, from its beginnings to the present day, is marked by the drama of defining 'what is human' (Archer 2000) and consequently what human happines is or can be.

With post-modernity, the process of change becomes ever faster and deeper. On the one hand, there are those who hold that the good life consists in the emancipation and liberation of individuals' subjectivity from any system of constraint (a new form of the hedonic ethos); on the other hand, there are those who believe that it consists in the possibility of building highly techno-functional impersonal social systems that can relieve individuals from their material needs (Arnold Gehlen's concept of *Entlastung*), which is a technocratic reformulation of the eudaimonic ethos.

In reality, Western modernization mixes both of the above tendencies: individualism and systemic functionalism intermingle with one another. They support and feed off each other. Once the possibilities of basing moral values in an objective reality are lost, social structures function as if the problem of living in a good society can be reduced to a question of individual preferences and tastes that are allowed or prohibited by the system. The happiness of individuals is relegated to the private sphere, where it is subjectified and becomes narcissistic (Lasch 1984), while public happiness (the well-being of social systems, as Jenks 2004 calls it) is entrusted to the chance of creating 'reflexive systems' (Beck et al. 2003). Modernity requires more and more reflexivity in order to pursue happiness (Archer 2012), but systems as such cannot be reflexive (they can only be 'reflective' in a mechanical way), whereas Beck, Bonss and Lau fail to make these distinctions. Here it seems clear that the problem of human happiness is being posed in radically new terms, for at least two major kinds of reasons.

(a) Social and cultural systems no longer presuppose the existence of a human nature. On the contrary, they tend to alter existing reality to enter into the realm of the 'post-human', the 'transhuman'; they create the cyborg. All prior forms of humanism become obsolete. If it is true that all the concepts of eudaimonia (happiness, *oikéiosis*, human flourishing, etc.) presuppose a human nature, the abandonment of any concept whatsoever of human nature (defined *ex ante* or *ex post*), the refusal to trace clear distinctions between the human and the non-human, and the project of rendering the human person continually modifiable put the concept of the good life into a state of fluctuation. In short, human happiness no longer consists in the realization of potentialities that are proper to human nature and only to it, but exists 'elsewhere', an 'elsewhere' that cannot be defined because it does not have either an identity or stable boundaries. It is said that society becomes liquid, and people must live on the edge of chaos.
(b) The processes of social differentiation erode the concept of the common good and, with it, the idea that eudaimonia can be guaranteed by a political community. The common good is identified sometimes with total goods, that is, with impersonal entities created by a simple aggregation of individual goods. The idea that public happiness can avail itself of private vices, indeed, that it is the product, even if an unintentional one, of private vices becomes a social norm. The logic of the production of the goods in which happiness consists is left to the neo-liberalism of the market regulated by the state (*lib/lab* arrangement).

As a consequence of all of the above, happiness becomes a mysterious object, a dream, a passion, a conduct of life without a symbolic and normative 'center'. It is no longer a project. It is abandoned to the intrinsic ambivalence of a Western morality that puts everything into doubt (Smart 1999) and is thought of as being purely 'liquid'. In reality, this society does not see that the liquid life and the risks that hinder the possibility of achieving the good life depend on precise social and cultural structures. We can ask: where can such a society, which appears to limit itself to being aware of its own inability to solve the problems that it generates, find happiness?

Certainly not in material welfare. Various scholars have evidenced the 'paradox of happiness', which states that, beyond a certain threshold of material welfare, increases in income and material goods do not, in fact, lead to increased happiness but generate its opposite, that is, unhappiness and a whole set of connected individual and social pathologies. Where is the 'good society'? The economists and psychologists of the so-called 'economics of happiness' are still far from giving a convincing answer. In my opinion, the reason for this shortfall lies in the fact of not having really understood the role that social relations play in fostering human flourishing. The human being is a *sui generis* potential that can be actualized only through their relationality with other human beings. It makes no sense to ask which is more important, the potential (inherent in the nature of the human individual) or the social relationship. The fact is that, without the potential, there is no proper relationality, and, without relationality, the potential (nature) is alienated and lost.

The central point becomes that of understanding how the logic of opportunities, which is supported by the morphogenetic society (Archer ed. 2013, 2014, 2015), puts social relations into a state of intensive change and what consequences this has for the good life.

The Modern Logics of Opportunities and the Morality of the Good Life

Three Moralities of the Good Life

In typically modern conceptions of the good life, goods are of an either individual or collective nature. The differences between the various moralities consist in the norms that regulate the ways of generating and using opportunities for individuals and the collectivity. In a nutshell, we can say that there exist two moralities of the good life that drive social changes, and a third morality that is generally considered auxiliary, complementary, but, in any case, residual compared to the other two.

The two driving moralities are those of the capitalist market and the state (or political system). The morality of the economic market extols the ideal virtues of honest and efficient competition in producing a never-ending supply of new goods that are supposed to improve the well-being of individuals and society. As a matter of fact, these virtues are not actually practiced. What is really at work is the idea that a good society should allow agents to engage in their free and private activities through which they are expected to enrich themselves and the social body (liberal morality). For this morality, opportunities are created by the capitalist market. Of course, there are other kinds of markets, with different moralities, based on different norms of exchange, but rampant capitalism marginalizes these different (civil) economies.

Collective morality, instead, extols the civic virtues of agents' participation in and responsibility toward the public good, which is identified in the total good of the redistributive state that guarantees the rights of citizenship and equality of material starting conditions (socialist morality). For this morality, opportunities are created by the state or the political-administrative systems existing at the different territorial levels.

The third morality, the most marginal one, is that of the social spheres in which the virtues are neither those of the market nor of political citizenship, but make reference to relations of trust, cooperation, and reciprocity in the lifeworlds. Opportunities are created in and by the primary and secondary social networks of civil society whose morality is based neither on profit, exchange nor on redistributive norms, but on criteria of reciprocity (peer-to-peer production, coproduction, open coordination, social partnership, etc.). The marginality of this third morality is attested to by the fact that its guiding-value (*fraternité* or solidarity) is not institutionalized in the cultural system as are the other two guiding-values (*liberté* and *égalité*).

These three moralities refer to different logics of opportunity, which are opportunities in liberal, socialist, and 'associational' terms. All three have their own specific conception of what we call 'life opportunity'. The opportunities offered by the market, those offered by the state, and those offered by the networks of everyday lifeworlds respond to different relational logics intrinsic to the three moralities above, respectively those of economic exchanges, political safeguards of citizenship, and associative relations. Each logic of opportunities reflects and fosters a different morality of social relations.

It then becomes a matter of analyzing *who* offers the opportunities, *how* the opportunities are selected and utilized, and what their *effects* on the good life are. I will argue that, while, within Western modernity, the market and the state have institutionalized the devices (*dispositif de médiation*) by means of which they can solve potential economic and political conflicts (respectively through the legal contract and the rules of democracy), the associational realm does not have any. The morphogenic society has to find such devices in a new relational logic of opportunities. This process becomes more urgent and necessary to the extent that the devices of the economic and political systems work less and less adequately.

Eudaimonia in the Crucible of Morphogenesis

The concept of *opportunities* is often defined in a generic way. It is a possibility assessed as being potentially positive for one or more subjects who can choose and exploit it. Defined in terms of logical relations (Archer 1988: 258), opportunity is a positive variation in the situational relation of 'contingent complementarity' between two or more elements. As I interpret it, two or more items come, are discovered, or are put into relation with one another in a contingent way and turn out to be complementary and to generate a new possibility. For example, inserting a computer chip into a human brain in order to produce an enhanced human body seems to constitute an opportunity. In any case, the concept of opportunity has to do with a circumstance (or combination of circumstances) that is favorable or advantageous to a subject, that is, useful for enriching his/her life, which requires a certain choice on the part of the subject.

I will argue that, vis-à-vis the shortcomings of 'modern logics', a new *situational logic* of opportunities emerges. This new *situational logic* of opportunities refers to the specific modalities with which combinations are created among the various elements brought about by over time. Such modalities favor or discourage, channel or somehow influence the conditions in which acting subjects make their choices for action, whether individual and/or collective, in the various social spheres (economic, political, cultural, etc.). Given that not everything can be combined, the logic of these combinations responds, in an explicit or implicit manner, to a morality.

It becomes a matter of analyzing the rules with which the combinatory modalities operate and, thus, the vision – whether normative, 'transnormative' (Fitzi 2012), or even involving 'anormative' regulation (Archer 2016) – to which they lead, with a view to achieving the 'good life' in late-modern society. To this end, I propose to use the morphogenetic framework (Archer 1995). Figure 7.1 describes the three phases of the morphogenetic process of morality, starting from the assumption that the current social and cultural structures of modernization still support a *lib/lab* logic of opportunities.

(a) *The starting structure.*

At time T^1, the question is: what is the morality of the good life promoted by current social and cultural structures? CTMN-1 represents the starting structure. [CTMN is the acronym that describes the relational structure of a morality in which: – C is the latent cultural value that the relational structure incorporates; – T is the concrete and situated target/goal of that relational structure; – M stands for the means used to reach the goal; – N represents the norms that relate C,T & M according to the internal logic of the relational structure (Donati 2014: 144–159)]. It includes the moral norms of the good life that regulate the actions and relations among agents/actors interacting with one another on the basis of a situational logic of opportunities. In *lib/lab* systems, opportunities are essentially offered and configured by the political system and the economic market according to their own logics, which are managed in terms of relations of contingent complementarity, depending on the situations.

The individual's and society's pursuit of happiness (eudaimonia) takes place by including in human flourishing certain specific opportunities that did not belong to them previously. These opportunities (called provisions) are produced by the market and are guaranteed by the state (as entitlements). In terms of the morphogenetic approach, eudaimonia is configured as a process of creating a variation/selection of an opportunity and stabilization of the possibility of acting and of receiving goods that are not given in nature. According to the *lib/lab* vision (Dahrendorf 1994), the good life consists in the possibility of increasing access to as many opportunities as possible for everybody. Such a view makes at least two fallacious assumptions. First, it assumes that all people want everything, which isn't true, because many people don't (some refuse to use certain therapies, others reject T.V. or cannabis or

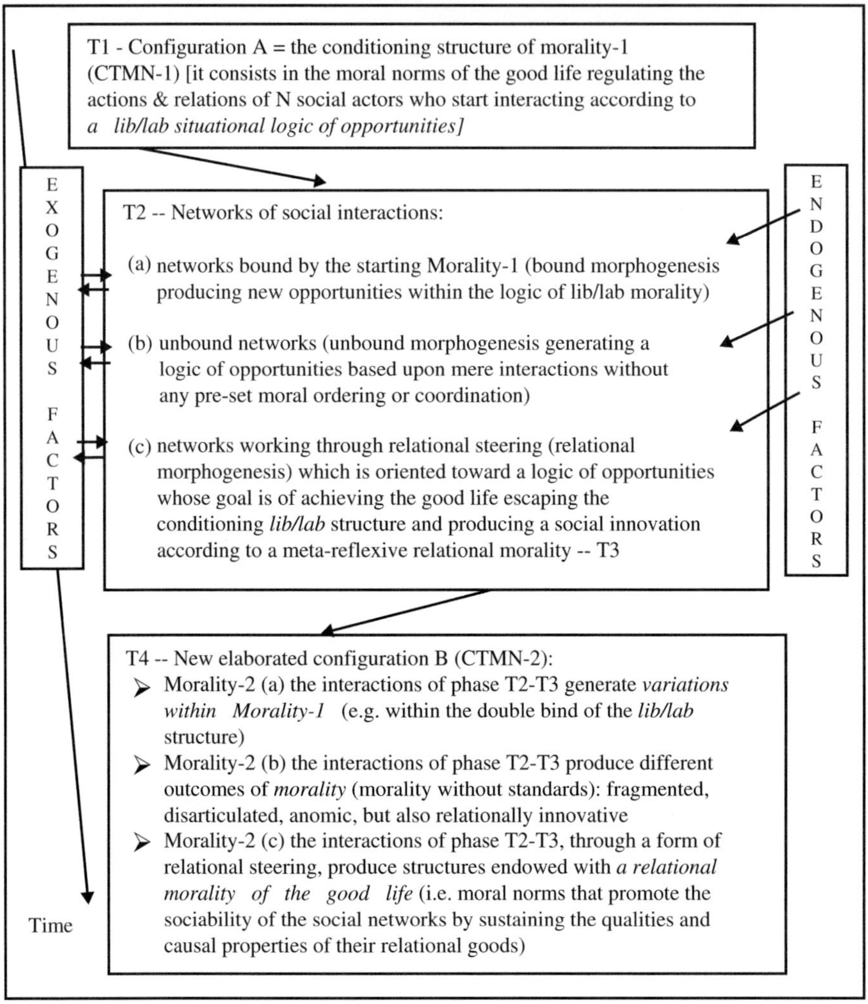

Fig. 7.1 *The different morphogenetic paths through which different moralities of the good life emerge in late modernity in a cycle T1-T4* (for more details on this scheme and CTMN, see Donati (2013: 216) and (2014: 144–159))

new tecnologies, etc.). Second, it assumes that the welfare state guarantees equality of opportunity to all individuals, through a minimal safety net on the basis of which everyone can enjoy the fruits of his/her own merits. But also this assumption is not true.

(b) *The phase of interactions.*

In the phase T^2-T^3, the agents/actors use the opportunities offered and interact with one another, creating new ones. This takes place through the networks of social interactions that are allowed or fostered by the starting structures, but which can be contested and modified by the acting subjects.

Simplifying, we can have three types of interactive configurations. We can analyze them on the basis of the following questions. Who offers the opportunities? How are they used? With what effects?

(I) Many of the interactive networks produce new opportunities within the *lib/lab* logic. The underlying morality remains unchanged. Here, morphogenesis is bound to, limited by, the existing structures (Morality-1). It is important to point out that these networks are not morphostatic, but generate new opportunities, but ones that do not however alter the *lib/lab* morality of the good life.

Obviously, the analysis of these networks is complex. A constant source of crisis derives from the fact that this logic always involves exclusions. These have to do with factors of exclusion from access and use of information, knowledge, and technologies that expand human capacities only for those who are able to take advantage of the opportunities.

(II) Due to the failures of *lib/lab* systems and their obsolescence, a growing number of interactive networks are adopting modalities that escape the logic of existing structures. Here, the morality of the good life must be untethered from existing structures. Basically, the offer of opportunities lies outside of the compromise between state and market. In this process of unbound morphogenesis, various types of networks emerge which, at least initially, adopt a situational logic of opportunity based on mere interactions without a pre-established moral order. This is a new 'globalized society' that mixes civil 'demands' (for new civil rights, more social justice, etc.) with amoral or uncivil behaviors (for instance, cheating on the internet). Eudaimonia becomes an extremely problematic concept and a challenge for most people. What emerges is a societal context in which, alongside anonymous communication networks, ever new social networks are created, which, over time and under certain conditions of transnormative interactions, generate communitarian or associational forms of life, work, civic participation, and volunteerism. I will consider these dynamics below.

(III) There is a third type of social networking in which the interactions are in some way managed ('guided') by a set of multi-stakeholders. I am thinking, in particular, about forms of relational steering that produce social practices leading to a *relational* morphogenesis (Donati 2013). There emerge, in other words, new social networks that are propelled by a logic that creates and uses opportunities in order to pursue a good life *outside* the conditionings of the initial *lib/lab* structure. They can operate though more or less 'chaotic states', but what is important is the fact that they, in the end, produce social innovations 'oriented' toward generating collective goods. Independent of their final achievements, they intentionally pursue the goal of a 'relational good life' by acting upon their own relational configuration as a common project. It remains to be seen what the eudaimonic conception of the innovations is and what type of reflexivity they contain (the answer lies in the following phase T^4 of the same Fig. 7.1). Generally speaking, this has to do with meta-reflexivity, and not purely communicative, or autonomous, or fractured reflexivity.[1]

---

[1] According to the modalities explained by Archer (2012).

(c) *The outcomes (elaborated structure) at time T^4.*

In phase T^4, different moralities of the good life emerge that are produced by the preceding phase. CTMN-2 is the elaborated structure of morality. In parallel to the three interactive dynamics, three different types of structural situations can emerge.

(I) In the case of a *lib/lab* morphogenesis, the elaborated structures represent a morality that offers a further expansion of opportunities which aim to satisfy individuals' welfare on the basis of an ethics of 'equal opportunities' pursued through combinations of market provisions and political regulations. Parsons' (1977) theory can be considered as emblematic of this arrangement. Parsons holds that the good society is structured as follows: the latent value model is given by the equality of all citizens in respect to fundamental rights (function L), social integration is given by conferring equality to people in the starting status (function I), the goal is to place the subjects in functional positions with different powers and responsibilities (function G), on the basis of the inequality of results that reflect the subjects' capacities (function A). Clearly, this scheme is encountering growing difficulties and failures for many reasons, which I have discussed elsewhere (Donati 1991: 294–299). As a matter of fact, the Parsonian theory has been reformulated by Luhmann (1995) in neo-functionalist terms of 'opportunistic adaptations' operated by systemic structures on the basis of an 'amoral morality', according to which all that is possible is also licit.

(II) In the case of unbound morphogenesis, it is difficult to say which structures come to be elaborated, given the variety of possibilities. Generally, however, structures support forms of morality of the good life that do not follow pre-established standards. The networks of interactions without a pre-set order can have very different outcomes, positive, negative or ambivalent. Negative outcomes include 'network failures', involution, contested collaboration, fragmentation, dis-articulation, anomie. Positive outcomes can take the shape of a collective movement in search of an ideal society; but we witness also the emergence of new structures embedding 'local moralities' that could, in a successive morphogenetic cycle T^1-T^4, generate social innovations able to stabilize practices of the good life among those endowed with an adequate reflexivity. In other cases the outcomes remain ambivalent (for example, the so-called 'Arab springs').

(III) In the case of social networks of '*relationally guided*' interactions, we can have various outcomes in terms of elaborated structures that can reflect the ends directly pursued or not. Most of the time the outcomes have a good deal of spontaneity within the ambit of common guidance. What is relevant is the fact that the interactions following some form of relational steering produce structures endowed with *a relational morality of the good life*. With this expression, I mean moral norms that promote the sociability of the social networks by supporting the properties and causal powers of their relational goods (Donati and Martignani eds. 2015).

A General Overview

A general overview of society in the process of globalization suggests a question: which logic of opportunities dominates the globalized world in the T^2-T^3 phase? At first glance, this logic is driven by an 'aesthetic energy' that makes individuals choose favorable opportunities on the basis of a type of contingent utility, with no constraining finalities corresponding to a long-term project. Without norms that potentially make the choices stable, individuals end up aggregating and disaggregating with a growing variability that no longer responds to any social order except that of expressing a market-driven behaviour.

These new situational logics of opportunity seem to correspond to an underlying impulse that Teubner (2011) calls '*collective addiction*', i.e. systemic pathological compulsions to a self-destructive restless growth that produces catastrophes (e.g. financial crises, global poverty, masses of those drug addicted, etc.) through information flows responding to the addictive imperatives of globalized capital, favored by the medium of an anonymous communication matrix. It is a logic of the search for happiness through an unchecked availability of all possible innovations. In effect, if we observe the major changes in Western society, we see that the T^2-T^3 phase of morphogenesis has many of the same features of what Teubner (2011: pr. 1, 2) calls the '*addictive society*'.

In this scenario, we can ask: is it possible that, passing through a phase of unbound morphogenesis, new conceptions and effective social practices can be generated in which agents/actors (new creative minorities) find a stable consensus among themselves and build alternative forms of good life?

In the following sections I would argue the following thesis. If we look at the interactions through the lens of the critical realist relational paradigm (Donati 2015), which is neither relational*ist* nor formalist,[2] we see acting subjects faced with the need to confer a normativity on social relations that is adequate to successfully achieving the promise of a good life. This need can only be met with an adequate reflexivity leading to an agonistic understanding of normativity (Maxwell 2012). In other words, so that interactions can produce alternative forms of good life, it is necessary for acting subjects to acquire the characteristics of '*contesting relational subjects*'.

People create an innovative morality of the good life to the extent that they act as subjects who reflect *on* social relations as emergents and, without necessarily sharing the same tastes and opinions, are nonetheless able to build a *we-relation*. This entails understanding the meaning and practical implications of how a relational subject is constituted, whether this is a single person or a set of people who act as a collective entity or as social network (Donati and Archer 2015).

[2]Relation*ism* differs from relational realism in these respects.

The Moral Trap That Characterizes Current Human Morphogenesis

The analysis of phase T^2-T^3 in morphogenetic processes reveals the existence of moral traps (on a micro, meso, and macro level) and the need for relational guidance so that the logic of opportunities (which, like it or not, necessarily involves social norms) does not create social pathologies, inequalities, relational evils, etc.

In particular, the morality of the *lib/lab* configuration of society is based on an injunction: 'you *must* be *free'* to seek any opportunity that can fulfill you. This injunction is a well-known 'double bind' that consists in one's being at the mercy of a paradoxical message: if you obey this injunction, you show that you are not free because you do it out of obligation; if you do not obey this injunction, then this means that you renounce being free. Apparently, there is no way to escape this paradox, which is notoriously at the origin of so many psychic and social pathologies and was elucidated as 'the trap of postmodernity' by Michel Foucault (1966).

This paradoxical message of late modernity is inscribed in the social and cultural structures that impose on individuals the norm of having to realize themselves by making themselves independent of every social bond. From this systemic injunction derives a clear deception that consists in attributing to lone individuals the responsibility for everything that happens to them in life. Theirs is the fault, theirs the shame. From this comes the repressive sense of human and social relations in present-day society, and a lot of moral traps that go with it. This social norm is not saying, as some think, that the human person has the moral obligation to fulfill his/her capacities: it commands individuals to transcend themselves, to go beyond their capacities and potential to take on properties and powers that the human does not have. This is the post-human, the hyper-human, the trans-human, the cyborg.

In the private sphere, interpersonal bonds are replaced by technologies: for example, procreative relations are replaced by reproductive technologies; primary relations are replaced by virtual communication on the internet; in the public sphere, collective bonds are replaced by systemic bureaucracies and mechanisms; in large organizations, the bonds between people are replaced by technological tools; in public debate, dialogue between face-to-face participants is replaced by mass media and new *apps*. In all of these cases, social bonds become increasingly virtual. What was considered the 'natural' quality of the bond between human beings loses its meaning, is rendered artificial, and, as a result, the bond can be constructed and altered at pleasure.

In reality, a different way out exists. But in order to see it, it is necessary to escape the paradoxes of modernity with a process of cultural breakthrough. This process consists in semantisizing the injunction, turning its meaning upside down, that is, by resorting to a *counter*-paradox. The injunction 'you must be free' is reversed into '*you must choose whom to depend on*' because freedom consists in having the possibility of choosing the relation to which to belong, i.e. the bond that, through your choice, is the foundation of your free identity.

The fact is that, when talking about eudaimonia, we have to reconsider what we mean by 'human nature' and, correspondingly, what the demands that social and cultural structures impose on people's action are, especially with respect to the social bond. We have to understand the complexity of the morphogenesis of the human in order to grasp the novelty of the human wherever it is regenerating rather than destroying itself. My argument is that *the regeneration of the human,* wherever it is not being lost but is instead flourishing, *emerges as the product of a qualified morphogenesis of the social bond.* I would like to explain this statement by analyzing the causes that make the transition from *lib/lab* morality to a *relational* morality necessary. This transition is confirmed by many empirical phenomena that I will discuss later.

The Displacement of the Morality of Opportunities From a *lib/lab* Logic to a *Relational* Logic

Two Logics of Opportunity

The diagram (Fig. 7.1) offers us an instrument for understanding in greater depth the differences between the logic of opportunity according to the *lib/lab* paradigm and according to the relational paradigm. At the same time, it allows us to explain if and how it could be possible to escape an anomic fluctuation of the morality of the good life through the interactive phase (T2-T3).

The sequence (a) → (b) → (c) in Fig. 7.1 describes the distancing from the system of opportunistic logics supported by the *lib/lab* arrangement. It indicates the opening of possibilities that the morphogenetic process can cause to emerge under certain conditions, with a view to a new social morality for human flourishing.

The sequence is the following:

(a) *creation of variations/variability*: there is an increase of opportunities within the *lib/lab* framework;
(b) *selection*: the opening of new contingent opportunities creates a space-time in which the selection of alternatives must take place; selections may abandon the rules of the *lib/lab* morality and follow other rules, which, may *refer to new relations that should be generated in order to achieve a different modus vivendi;*
(c) *stabilization*: if choices are enacted that, in a targeted way, guide the creation and use of opportunities according to an adequately reflexive relational logic, stable social innovations emerge in which the goal of humanizing these same social relations can prevail.

We can delineate the discontinuity between *lib/lab* ethics and relational ethics with respect to their creation and use of opportunities as follows.

In the *lib/lab* paradigm: (a) the ethics of eudaimonia is a private choice and becomes public only as an external constraint on action; (b) the social quality of objectives and outcomes is independent of inter-human relations because it refers to the achievement of the maximum of individual opportunities. The 'advantageous' new forms of 'variety' are necessarily appropriated by those who, even if they start from supposedly equal positions, have the capacities and means for appropriating them.

In the relational paradigm: (a) the ethics of eudaimonia pertains to the social relation in that it is a bond between humans, i.e. inter-human; (b) the social quality is that which derives from the respect for and fostering of values and norms that give priority to caring for the relations between the acting subjects. In this case, the appropriation of 'advantageous' new forms of 'variety' by some to the detriment of others is hindered or very limited because here the moral norm of reciprocity, understood as symbolic exchange, is in force.

What is reciprocity as symbolic exchange? It is a form of exchange that generates, maintains, and organizes social relations. The difference from other forms of exchange is that the exchange value does not lie in the objects exchanged, but in the relationship itself. Symbolic exchanges are not aimed at establishing equivalence (equal value) between two exchanged tokens, as in the exchange of money for goods or services. The aim of people involved in a symbolic exchange is to generate and regenerate a meaningful relationship with significant others. It can be a move to start a relationship of reciprocity, wherein reciprocity cannot be reduced to a mere utilitarian exchange (*do ut des*), since it means the readiness to return what has been received according to need. Its actual utilitarian value is superseded by the value of the relationship. The circle can be restricted to two persons or enlarged to include many people. In any case, the exchange is not calculated in monetary terms but is part of a series of acts that maintain and sustain a relationship. It is in the spheres of society where reciprocity is the foundational norm in which the new eudaimonia resides.

The original sin of the *lib/lab* arrangement lies in the fact that, by ignoring the value and intrinsic norms of social relations inspired by the symbolic exchange, it generates relational evils. The passage from a *lib/lab* arrangement to a societal arrangement in which morphogenesis is relationally steered requires the construction of a social context regulated by positive norms (e.g. caring for positive relations such as voluntary work for the social inclusion of marginalized people, concern for an integral ecology) and negative norms (e.g. opposing relations that favour prostitution or exploitative uses of labor). The complex of these norms should follow a logic of opportunities in which the common good is redefined as a relational good. The reason for this assertion is the fact that a common good without relationality between those who produce it and those who use it renders the ethics of the good life sterile and indifferent.

The relational vision of society reveals that social problems arise from specific contexts that generate relational evils and that the morality for combating these must be inspired by relational work on these networks.

Let us take the case of poverty. As very many studies demonstrate, poverty is not only the product of individual characteristics, but above all of differences in access to opportunities. Social networks are the factor that conditions access to goods and services that can be obtained in markets (Marques 2012). Social inequalities have often been analyzed from the point of view of characteristics of individuals or the workings of large opportunity structures such as the job market or the offer of direct income transference policies. In reality, the best solutions to poverty are those inspired by the paradigm of relational work. Note the following difference. In the U.S. relational work is taken to be assistance toward pursuing a life plan in which material help is given to poor or indigent people within a long-term relation in order to valorize the *individual* capacities of the poor and unemployed. This way of intervening has some value, but it does not alter the structures that generate social inequality, because it does not change the morality of the *lib/lab* social structures, even when welfare measures are performed by third sector agencies (Jindra and Jindra 2015). In Europe, on the contrary, relational work is theorized and practiced as an attempt to modify the social, cultural, and economic structures, at least at the local level, by building collective networks (see the contributions in Donati and Martignani eds. 2015). I would like to develop this topic in the following sections.

Assessing the Morality of Social Networks

Social networks can foster human flourishing or human deprivation. The question is: can we assess the morality of social networks, that is, whether and how a network produces moral values such as justice, solidarity, subsidiarity, etc. or, vice versa, injustice, oppression, marginalization, exploitation, etc.?

The answer can be affirmative, but a relational framework is necessary to understanding this because it involves giving an assessment about relations and the networks of relations, and it is not enough to consider only individuals' intentions (or their 'altruism'), or only the morality of the social structures that condition individuals.

In my view, the morality of a social relation (or network of relations) consists in the fact that it can produce relational goods or relational evils for those who take part in it, apart from agents' intentions.

For instance: (i) the freedom to dismiss an employee can be intentionally good in order to save a company or increase its competitiveness, but it can produce poverty or social inequities (not as a simple 'fact', but as a *relational* evil); (ii) redistributive state policies can have good intentions aimed at assisting the poor, but they can generate a 'poverty trap' or other social traps (relational evils). When, how, and why can we say that a social relation is good or bad?

In order to produce relational goods, a dyadic social relation (or the relationality of a network of social relations) should meet the following requisites: (1) a necessary requirement, but not a sufficient one, is that *the social relation be good in itself*, i.e. in its own structure or 'molecule' (and, therefore, in its own elements, which are its goal, means, guiding norm and value pattern), and not only in the feelings, aspirations, or intentions of the subjects/agents; (2) the social relation *should generate an emergent phenomenon that brings a good to each participant*; and (3) *the good enjoyed by each participant could not be obtained 'otherwise'*, i.e. in a way that is lacking the we-relation.

For instance, a 'mafia relation' does not meet the first requisite, since its structure is morally bad, although it can meet the other two requisites. On the contrary, a measure of redistribution pursued by public (state) policies can be morally good in itself, but generate relational evils because it does not meet the second and/or the third requisite.

The fact is that social networks are highly ambivalent. They offer opportunities and resources, but also constraints and obstacles to accessing and using opportunities. This can be seen in the research on structural holes and on the brokers that occupy positions of intermediation of information and exchanges between the nodes of the network. According to some authors, brokers play a positive role in offering opportunities (Burt 1992). It is argued that the wealth of a society's information depends on the informational potentialities of social circles (structural holes) that social entrepreneurs (bridges) are able to put into contact with one another. According to others, brokers play a decidedly ambivalent role; for instance, Ahuja (2000) claims that structural holes have both positive and negative influences on subsequent innovation. According to still others, they have different functions; for example, the results of the research done by Fleming et al. (2007) illustrate how collaborative brokerage can aid in the generation of an idea but then hamper its diffusion and use by others.

Certainly, social networks are 'assets' (Lazega 2007; Gulati 2007), but we must draw distinctions between the characteristics of each network because *the fact of producing relational goods or evils is correlated with – if not causally connected to – the morality of the good life that each network supports*. It is important to reiterate that relational goods are goods that consist of relations: they are not material entities, they are not performances, they are not ideas – they are none of these things. They are relations. Let us take two examples, one negative and the other positive.

The negative example is when relational goods are lacking. A very common case, whether in families or in universities and work places, is the presence of *structural holes* in the networks of relations among people who are managed by brokers who hinder rather than foster communication among all the nodes in the network. The brokers are mediators who prevent people from being able to relate to one another and thus hinder the creation of a relational good. Recent investigations demonstrate how important the attributes of nodes are in configuring the characteristics of social networks (Wang et al. 2015).

The positive example is friendship. Friendship is a social relation that goes beyond individual dispositions. Certainly, friendship flows from people, and only people can be friends and create friendship, which is a virtue for them as persons. But it cannot be an individual undertaking. Ego and Alter are not friends as individuals. Friendship is the acknowledgement of something that does not belong to either of the two, although it is generated by both of them. This is the relational good (Donati and Solci 2011). It is the good that exists in common between people; only they can create it, but it does not belong to either of the two people, even if it is their joint product. Likewise, friendship cannot be the product of a social structure;

it cannot become an institution, a structure to which people must conform. To be friends, there have to be at least two people who must share and exchange something on an interpersonal level. As Lazega and Pattison (2001) have shown, friendship mitigates competition in social networks and fosters the creation of social capital. It is the sharing, that is, the reciprocal action that generates the we-relation, the relation as the reciprocal action of We, which gives sense and form and content to friendship. Sharing cannot be a fact explicable in individual terms, even if it is not a collective reality: it is not imposed by anyone, it cannot be dictated by any authority, and no one can experience it as something constrictive or external. To understand this, it is necessary to move beyond both methodological individualism and methodological holism, which are the two great currents of thought that still dominate the social sciences today. They do not seem to have understood the new realities that are emerging in the worlds of the economy, as well as in those of the production and consumption of goods and services, including the worlds of welfare and the internet.

In these worlds we see the spread of productive practices that operate on the basis of a 'relational logic' so that the value of goods and services refer to (depend on) the quality of the social relations they convey, and not other parameters (such as the quantity of the time taken by the work that was employed in producing them). In this way, the validity of all the classical economic theories, which computed the value of a good or service in terms of the time necessary to produce it or other parameters, as *lib/lab* logic still does to a great extent, is overturned. This new 'relational logic' is intrinsically a form of social morality because it involves the fact that a criterion of value is introduced (the quality of the relation) in place of ethically neutral quantitative parameters.

An ethical economy rests upon 'ethical labour', i.e. an economy in which the social relation is a 'value' because what matters in every exchange or financial transaction is neither the thing exchanged or transacted in itself or its monetary equivalent but the morality of the relationship. It is the relationship that determines the 'good exchange' or transaction, not the money or material advantages obrained by the parties. An ethical society depends upon an ethical economy in which, behind the financial transactions and the sheer money, people can see and be fair to the relationships that underpin them.

A New Relational Logic

The information society brings with it an important structural transformation: the growth of a number of strategically central, though still quantitatively marginal productive practices, all working according to this *relational logic*. This 'logic' is intrinsically a form of social morality that comes to define a new civil economy. What kinds of eudaimonic morality emerge through these phenomena?

The idea of happiness, the good life of individuals as well as of society, come to depend on the creation of relational contexts able to produce common goods. In a complex and globalized society, common goods must be interpreted as relational goods within particular networks that have positive externalities for the surrounding community.

In this regard, it is necessary to consider how the new communication media (ICTs) are revolutionizing 'real' (interpersonal and structural) social relations through virtual relations. Clearly, we must distinguish between the different types of media, the different ways of using them, and their specific outcomes. There are media that allow for the production of relational goods and others that generate relational evils. This is what the morphogenetic approach proposes to explain concerning the morphogenesis of the human person (agency), as well as social and cultural structures, in relation to a possible 'good life'.

If and when people become aware of all of this, social change begins. New processes emerge that are aimed at reassessing relations with others. Most people discover that working as a team, i.e. cooperating with others rather than acting individually, is more effective and satisfying, on condition, obviously, that the task has not been imposed and that teamwork is not a tool used by those in charge to make higher profits. Family bonds are rediscovered as relations that, while being constraints, give a meaning to one's life that other relations cannot give. A growing number of people realize that they can achieve their goals only through new forms of association and new social movements. New demands for justice and social solidarity arise requiring a vision capable of putting the needs and rights of all of a community's members into relation with one another. Indeed, many discover that we are all deeply connected to one another. Each person's decisions, choices, and actions are not purely individual matters, but are enacted in relation to others. It is irrational to think of them as simple expressions of the autonomous Self. One comes to realize that, in reality, each person lives in dependence on and interdependence with so many others, without whom one could not be the person one is, and could not become the person one desires to be.

It becomes apparent that each individual's history resides in relations with significant others. The human person is not a self-sufficient entity: he/she is an '*individual-in-relation'*, where the relation is *constitutive* of the person.[3] We are all in the same boat, in the sense that we depend on one another. And so the question becomes: what kind of boat is this? I think that we can call it: the 'We-relation'. But what kind of relation is that? In other words: how should the relationality between us be such that individuals fulfill their own humanity and do not become alienated from themselves to become someone or something else?

Traditional mass movements no longer offer adequate answers in that the identity they confer is of an aggregate type and is not relational. The identity acquired by the individual from the fact of belonging to a collective movement based on identification with a symbol (for example, ecological, anti-global, civil rights etc. movements) can become significant only on two conditions: (a) if it is mediated by an adequate

[3] Although parts of natural reality other than the social (relations with Nature and Material Culture) also play a part in this constitution (Donati and Archer 2015: 53).

inner (personal) reflexivity and (b) if the personal reflexivity is capable of realizing a relational (social) reflexivity with others. Both of these conditions are hardly ever met by collective movements if they are purely aggregative. They can be present, instead, in collective movements in which people have real relations, and not only virtual ones, with one another, and these relations cause a social form (instituted form) to emerge that is capable of stability and its own action. Social networks (ICTs) can do this on the condition – which is by no means a given – that the virtual relations are only a tool, and not a replacement, for inter-subjective relations.

The Logic of Opportunities Differentiates the Ways of 'Making the Social Fabric': The 'Society of the Human' and Other Societies

What does 'society building' mean according to a virtuous logic of opportunities?

I stated above that a certain logic of opportunities always implies and at the same time fosters a certain morality of the good life. Any morality has to do with the norms with which elements, used in a complementary way, are combined. Their combination is not a mere logical relation, but is the activation of a reciprocal action that creates a *sui generis* social bond and not a different one.

Many and diverse situational logics exist to manage opportunities, which obviously have different consequences in terms of the social bonds they create.

Here, I limit myself to examining the criterion that, in my opinion, is the most sociologically meaningful and relevant for explaining and assessing the greater or lesser goodness related to new opportunities. This criterion makes reference to the quality and causal properties of the social bonds the new opportunities made possible in 'making (a certain type of) social fabric'.

I propose to address the morphogenetic differentiation of society, of any society, from the smallest (single families or small companies) to the largest (global society), in light of the fact that 'doing society' today means building *networks of relations in which the situational logic of opportunities can commodify or decommodify well-being* and more generally human flourishing through the generation and transformation of social bonds. Social networks always entail the presence of social bonds, which are continually created, altered, or destroyed.

The dynamics of creation and destruction of social bonds characterizes the morality of a social networks. It is interesting to observe that, by continually adding new nodes to a network, the number of social relations of the first, second and third order increases with incredible progression according to the following formula (this algorithm is proposed here for the first time):

$$\sum_{1}^{k} F_k\,(n_k)$$

where: F_k is the number of relations of k order; n=number of initial nodes ≥ 2; $n_k = F_{k-1}(n_{k-1})$; $F_1(n_1) = n(n-1)/2$.

For n = 3 and k = 3, the total number of relations is equal to 9. For n = 4 and k = 3, the total is 126. The increase of the nodes brings with it a higher complexity of the network and therefore raises issues of social and cultural integration (with the formation of sub-networks diverging between them). This complexity leads to the emergence of conflicts that modify the bonds and the nodes themselves. In short, the morality of the social networks becomes increasingly critical the greater is the number of nodes. If the nodes are seen as opportunities for potential exchanges, or at least symbolic references, the rationale of the argument is clear: for the creation of stable and morally good bonds, it is necessary that people are able to manage the relations (whatever their order) as relational goods.

An empirical test is represented by what happened to the so-called ‘Arab Springs’ (2010–2012). These movements were supported by many social networks on the internet and were successful due to a rapid increase in the number of nodes. How did the morality of these ‘democratic’ networks work? Although some scholars have theorized that these networks worked on the grounds of morally good relations (i.e. the relational goods defined as individual rational choices made by many people together, according to the interpretion of Uhlaner 2014), these networks revealed a highly tribal character, and in the end produced a lot of relational evils, e.g. widespread regional, national and international conflicts, the fragmentation of some nation-states, the inability to build a democracy, the birth of Daesh. The explanation of these outcomes lies in the fact that the morality involved in these networks was aggregative and non relational. In other words, to get a good society we need networks able to produce truly relational goods, and not an aggregation of large numbers of individual nodes.

How should we assess these networks from the perspective of the good life? To grasporseize their diversity and vicissitudes, we need a certain understanding and explanation of what a social bond is ontologically and what it means epistemologically.

The expression ‘social bond’ is polysemic because it designates at least three different entities: (a) the history of reiterated reciprocal actions that generated a social ‘relationship’, (b) a structural bond inherent in this ‘relationship’, and (c) the nature of social agents’ reciprocal subjective expectations.

The bond is not just any relation: it is the structurating of a relation that gives life to a specific ‘social molecule’ (Donati 2014). For example: is the couple relationship a system of interactions that can take on the form of a ‘pure relationship’, which is continued only in so far as it is thought by both parties to deliver enough satisfaction for each individual to stay within it or, on the contrary, should it be configured as a stable bond to which the realization of a project is entrusted?

The history of the relation and its structuring in a bond (understood as an emergent system of expectations, that is, a set of rights and reciprocal obligations) can be seen as a dynamic process (*emerging* bond) or as instituted reality (*instituted* bond). For example, a bond is of an associative type (I am referring to the associations of civil society) when subjects associate with one another (association as process) or is an elaborated reality (the association as a structured autonomous institution). As such, the bond, whether in the *generating* phase or in its reality as *generated*, reveals its own dynamic, that is, its own causal powers and properties. This autonomous 'order of reality' (the order of reality of the social relation) not only entails the fact that the subjects involved in the bond have rights and obligations toward one another as individuals, but they have a complex of rights and obligations toward the bond itself, the bond *qua talis*.

In what I call 'the society of the human', well-being is constituted by the good of the social relation as the path towards obtaining individual goods. The relational good consists in all those relations that can be generated and enjoyed together with others and on which individuals must rely in order to obtain everything that they could not have without such a relation. Examples are all of those immaterial, yet real, goods such as trust among the members of an association or community, cooperation, friendship, recognition, solidarity, mutual help, a positive climate in a classroom or workplace, social innovations like a social street or a commons on the internet, and so on, which meet most daily human needs (Donati and Solci 2011).

Let me give an example: the *social streets* (http://www.socialstreet.it). In my town (Bologna), in a street close to that in which I live (its name is via Fondazza), one Sunday in 2014 it happened that a father, seeing his 6 year old son playing alone and in silence at home, while other children were shouting in joy playing together nextdoor, thought to create a profile on facebook so as to connect his family to the others around, and in general to link the people who lived in that street in order to get acquainted and exchange company and mutual aid in ordinary life. In a few days, many people had joined the initiative. The profile was called the '*social street of via Fondazza*'. After few months, the members of this social network numbered more than 1500. The social street network developed quickly as a way to facilitate the reciprocal knowledge of the residents of the street. They began to greet when they met on the street, and started to organize meetings and parties, take care of the public garden, clean the walls of the buildings that face the street, arrange common facilities and, more generally, create relational goods. Following this experience, many other social streets were set up in Bologna and in other cities in Italy. Now the 'social streets' are spreading in other countries, in Europe and other continents (now numbering several hundreds). They do not follow the same pattern. Some of them are wholly independent and do not want to be influenced by political parties wishing to use the social street as a constituency or be colonized by multinational companies for purposes of consumption. They conceive of themselves as an expression of a 'pure' civil society. Other social streets make agreements with the local authorities or other partners (e.g. companies) in order to get facilities and aid of various kinds. In a way, this is an example of 'agonistic solidarity': different patterns of social streets are developing depending on their different needs, contexts, agents, with the idea of competing in the quest for new ways to organize the social network so to be able to produce relational goods for the people involved, ways that can also be attractive for other social streets.

With reference to my Fig. 7.1, the process can be described as follows. At time T^1 the starting social structure was that of a town where individual people and their facilities were administered by the local authorities (the impersonal administration of the public institutions) in a *lib/lab* configuration. Common goods were lacking. People living next door did not relate to each other. On the initiative of a person and the group that this person succeeded in mobilizing, a process of local social interactions began through which a new social network was constituted (phase T^2-T^3) linking the people living in the same street. In this phase, the social system based upon the confrontation between single individuals (micro level) and the public bureaucracy of the Municipality (macro level) has been changed through the formation of a meso level collegial movement that, at time T^4, has generated a new social institution, the social street, which is now a meso level social structure taking care of the relational goods produced by the local community. Of course, if we look at Fig. 7.1, other possibilities were (and still are) open. The *lib/lab* structure could neutralize the social street by reabsorbing it somehow (alternative *a* in Fig. 7.1); the social network of the social street could face a process of unbound morphogenesis induced by internal and/or external interests that conflict with the creation of relational goods between the inhabitants (alternative *b* in Fig. 7.1).

The point that I want to emphasize is that, in my relational paradigm, the shared good is not "a state of affairs that is, as far as possible, good for us all", but is a moral relationship. The relational character of the moral good *is defined by what we include in it and by what we exclude from it through specific relations, which are activity-dependent and context dependent.*

Conclusions: The Good Life According to Relational Realism

Relational analysis leads one to conclude that postmodern morality erodes the common good because it erodes social relations. There are obviously good reasons for assessing social relations negatively when they are used to exploit people (such as in human trafficking or forced prostitution), to organize social groups for the purposes of common criminality or corruption, or for other morally negative ends (mafia & Co.). On this basis, however, the postmodern morphogenetic society has elaborated a social morality according to which the good life consists in an indefinite increase in life opportunities, on the assumption that human identity can continuously change, endlessly altering its social relations. Today's moral norm dictates the celebration of 'relationalism' as the path toward the individualization of the individual. In the postmodern cultural system, it is assumed that happiness consists in this process.

Reality ends up debunking this morality. The idea that in order to achieve a good life the logic of opportunities must be detached from the value and norms of social relations leads to continual failures. Happiness is sought in the *creation of ever new social relations; it becomes possible to enjoy all possible opportunities only on condition of immunizing oneself from the relations themselves*, that is, on condition of not rendering any particular relation (any opportunity) necessary: thus, on condition of not binding oneself to anything or anyone, if not for the opportunities of the moment (this is the 'pure relation' theorized by Giddens).

The moral norm celebrated by the radically unbound morphogenesis emerging from the crisis of the *lib/lab* system leads late modern society to the imperative of maximum contingency and relational*ism, not relationality*.[4] This society celebrates relationality while negating it at the same time. But negating the identity of the relation (its emergent character, or its 'act of being') means also negating the identity of the subject, since the subject is relationally constituted (though not only by the social order). Hence, the impossibility for the individual of achieving authenticity in his/her identity. Such is the paradoxical outcome of this conception of the good life, that is living in relations without tying oneself to them. In this way, the individual can increase his/her life opportunities always on condition of not privileging any one social relation over others. Choosing one relation instead of another would involve self-imposed limitations and discriminations. It is a morality of non-distinction because the moral norm dictates that one has not to distinguish, because every distinction is a discrimination. But in this way, a 'reverse discrimination' operates because one chooses to not choose (one decides not to distinguish). This is a moral norm that leads to form of eudaimonia in which we observe a cultural and moral regression because human civilization requires the continuously renewed and creative use of distinctions.

Considering every thing and every human action within the relation in which we find it and looking at it from this point of view is essential to giving meaning to things and actions. Human life in pursuit of happiness – in a couple, in a working relation, or in the search for a job that isn't there – does not mean alienating people within the limits of the relational situation in which they find themselves, but the complete opposite. It means giving them a perspective for managing their human condition in a horizon of openness to meaning – that is openness to other relational contexts.

The logic of opportunities necessarily requires a morality of action because when opportunities are not infinite, but limited, competition arises. However, competition can be of various types. There is the 'excluding competition' that allows only some to obtain resources and benefits, excluding others, and there is the 'inclusive competition', that is, 'agonistic sociability', which consists in competing with others to create new opportunities under the condition that, subsequently, these will be shared with others in a circuit of reciproccity. In other words, agonistic sociability is a mechanism that creates opportunities for everyone without generating unwarranted structural inequalities. Competing, not in order to appropriate a good for oneself, but to achieve better solutions to share with others who will do the same thing according to the reciprocity rule (this is the meaning of the Latin word *cum-petere*, i.e. to 'strive together' for something that will benefit all, a *win-win* solution, without winners and losers).

[4]Donati and Archer (2015: 176–179, 271).

In conclusion, we must acknowledge that today we still lack a proper reflexivity on the relational nature of the good life, if we understand this expression in the sense that the good is constituted by certain social relations *sui generis* instead of others. The challenge that social morphogenesis has to face is how to distinguish and foster the relational goods that bring true human happiness beyond material welfare instead of fueling relational evils.

References

Ahuja, G. (2000). Collaboration networks, structural holes, and innovation: A longitudinal study. *Administrative Science Quarterly, 45*(3), 425–455.

Archer, M. S. (1988). *Culture and agency*. Cambridge: Cambridge University Press.

Archer, M. S. (1995). *Realist social theory: The morphogenetic approach*. Cambridge: Cambridge University Press.

Archer, M. S. (2000). *Being human. The problem of agency*. Cambridge: Cambridge University Press.

Archer, M. S. (2012). *The reflexive imperative in late modernity*. Cambridge: Cambridge University Press.

Archer, M. S. (Ed.). (2013). *Social morphogenesis*. Dordrect: Springer.

Archer, M. S. (Ed.). (2014). *Late Modernity. Trajectories towards morphogenic society*. Dordrecht: Springer.

Archer, M. S. (Ed.). (2015). *Generative mechanisms transforming the social order*. Dordrecht: Springer.

Archer, M. S. (2016). Anormative social regulation: An attempt to cope with social morphogenesis. In M. S. Archer (Ed.), *Morphogenesis and the crisis of normativity: Normogenetic processes*. Dordrecht: Springer.

Beck, U., Bonss, W., & Lau, C. (2003). The theory of reflexive modernization. Problematic, hypotheses and research program. *Theory, Culture & Society, 20*(2), 1–33.

Burt, R. S. (1992). *Structural holes: The social structure of competition*. Cambridge, MA: Harvard University Press.

Dahrendorf, R. (1994). The changing quality of citizenship. In B. van Steenberger (Ed.), *The condition of citizenship* (pp. 10–19). London: Sage.

Deveaux, M. (1999). Agonism and pluralism. *Philosophy and Social Criticism, 25*(4), 1–22.

Donati, P. (1991). *Teoria relazionale della società*. Milano: FrancoAngeli.

Donati, P. (2009). *La società dell'umano*. Genova-Milano: Marietti.

Donati, P. (2013). Morphogenesis and social networks: Relational steering not mechanical feedback. In M. S. Archer (Ed.), *Social morphogenesis* (pp. 205–231). Dordrecht: Springer.

Donati, P. (2014). Morphogenic society and the structure of social relations. In M. S. Archer (Ed.), *Late modernity. Trajectories towards morphogenic society* (pp. 143–172). Dordrecht: Springer.

Donati, P. (2015). Manifesto for a critical realist relational sociology. *International Review of Sociology, 25*(1), 86–109.

Donati, P., & Archer, M. S. (2015). *The relational subject*. Cambridge: CUP.

Donati, P., & Martignani, L. (Eds.). (2015). *Towards a new local welfare. Best practices and networks of social inclusion*. Bologna: Bononia University Press.

Donati, P., & Solci, R. (2011). *I beni relazionali. Che cosa sono e quali effetti producono*. Turin: Bollati Boringhieri.

Etzioni, A. (2014). *The new normal: Finding a balance between individual rights and the common good*. New Brunswick/London: Transaction Publishers.

Fitzi, G. (2012). A 'transnormative' view of society building: Simmel's sociological epistemology and philosophical anthropology of complex societies. *Theory, Culture & Society, 29*(7/8), 177–196.

Fleming, L., Mingo, S., & Chen, D. (2007). Collaborative brokerage, generative creativity, and creative success. *Administrative Science Quarterly, 52*(3), 443–475.

Foucault, M. (1966). *Les mots et les choses*. Paris: Gallimard.

Gulati, R. (2007). *Managing network resources: Alliances, affiliation, and other relational assets.* New York: Oxford University Press.

Jenks, C. L. (2004). The well-being of social systems. *Systems Research and Behavioral Science, 21*(3), 209–217.

Jindra, M., & Jindra, I. W. (2015). *A revolutionary change: Relational work in the new safety net.* Notre Dame: Dept. of Anthropology University of Notre Dame.

Korsgaard, C. (2013). The relational nature of the good. In R. Shafer-Landau (Ed.), *Oxford studies on metaethics* (Vol. 8). Oxford: Oxford University Press.

Lasch, C. (1984). *The minimal self: Psychic survival in troubled times*. New York: Norton.

Lazega, E. (2007). *Réseaux sociaux et structures relationnelles*. Paris: Puf.

Lazega, E., & Pattison, P. E. (2001). Social capital as social mechanisms and collective assets: The example of status auctions among colleagues. In N. Lin, K. Cook, R. S. Burt (Eds.). *Social capital: Theory and research.* New York: Aldine de Gruyter, ch. 8.

Luhmann, N. (1995). *Social systems*. Palo Alto: Stanford University Press.

Marques, E. (2012). Social networks matter in gaining access to goods and services obtained from outside markets. *International Journal of Sociology, 41*, 10–27.

Maxwell, L. (2012). Toward an agonistic understanding of law: Law and politics in Hannah Arendt's Eichmann in Jerusalem. *Contemporary Political Theory, 11*(1), 88–108.

Parsons, T. (1977). *The evolution of societies*. Englewood Cliffs: Prentice-Hall.

Smart, B. (1999). *Facing modernity. Ambivalence, reflexivity and morality*. London: Sage.

Teubner, G. (2011). A constitutional moment. The logics of 'hitting the bottom'. In P. Kjaer, G. Teubner, & A. Febbrajo (Eds.), *The financial crisis in constitutional perspective: The dark side of functional differentiation* (pp. 3–42). Hart: Oxford/Portland.

Uhlaner, C. J. (2014). Relational goods and resolving the paradox of political participation. *Recerca. Journal of Thought and Analysis, 14*, 47–72.

Wang, P., Robins, G., Pattison, P., & Lazega, E. (2015). Social selection models for multilevel networks. *Social Networks, 44*, 346–362. doi:10.1016/j.socnet.2014.12.003.

Chapter 8
Flourishing or Fragmenting Amidst Variety: And the Digitalization of the Archive

Mark Carrigan

Introduction

What should I do? Who should I be? How should I live my life? Theorists of late modernity have understood these questions as constitutive of the existential horizons of contemporary social life. Collective bases of identity are seen to melt away, normative conceptions of the life course disintegrate and life becomes a do-it-yourself project (Giddens 1991; Beck and Beck-Gernsheim 2002; Bauman 2000). The empirical inaccuracies of this body of work are pronounced (Smart 2007). So too are the methodological deficiencies and conceptual difficulties (Thomson et al. 2002; Carrigan 2014). But it's a useful starting point for the present chapter because it reintroduced existential concerns into the mainstream of British Sociology of the sort that will be addressed in this chapter. These may seem parochial disciplinary concerns but they have profoundly shaped the intellectual context within which the present project has been pursued, as the speculative notion of 'morphogenic society' and the increasingly sophisticated account of 'social morphogenesis' as a process have been orientated towards a move away from talk of *risk society*, *liquid modernity* and the *runaway* world (Beck 1992, Bauman 2000; Giddens 2011). Another target has been Rosa's (2013) account of *social acceleration* which, though rightfully subject to critique, surely represents an intellectual trend distinct from the aforementioned literature.

M. Carrigan (✉)
Centre for Social Ontology, University of Warwick, Coventry, UK
e-mail: mark@markcarrigan.net

M.S. Archer (ed.), *Morphogenesis and Human Flourishing*, Social Morphogenesis,
DOI 10.1007/978-3-319-49469-2_8

Personal Change and Social Change

Over the last 2 years my own developing inclination has been to consider the project as offering an alternative framework through which to think about social change, as opposed to being an account of what comes *after* late modernity or an alternative theory *of* it. Over the course of Carrigan (2014) I used an empirical case study to explore the deficiencies of the prevailing body of work on late modernity and to elucidate the conspicuously absent issue of *personal change* underlying it. Without a conception of personal reflexivity and personal change, the theorists of late modernity are unable to take the existential questions they raise seriously: nothing rests on their answers to these because such theorists all fail to conceive of relations of concern by virtue of which the outcomes matter to the subjects concerned (Sayer 2011).

Elliott and Lemert (2008) actually embrace this stance, arguing that "in current social circumstances – in which our lives are reshaped by technology-induced globalization and the transformation of capitalism – it is not the particular individuality of an individual that is most important" but rather "how individuals create identities, the cultural forms through which people symbolize individual expressions and desire, and perhaps above all the speed with which identities can be reinvented and instantly transformed" (Elliott and Lemert 2008: 53). In other words, it's the form taken by serial reinvention which matters, as well as what that can tell us about 'globalisation', rather than any consequences this might hold for individual or collective reproduction or transformation of the social system. The paradox here is a fascinating one: the theorists of individualization are oddly incapable of taking individuality seriously. We see a comparable problem in Bauman's work, which presents us with a world in which subjects passively reproduce systemic commodification, shaped and reshaped by the 'liquefying' forces of an economy that operates deterministically. As Rattansi (2014: 909) insightfully observes, "it is archetypes such as 'strangers', 'nomads' and 'vagabonds' who populate Bauman's world" rather than "concrete individuals". Bauman offers us a morality play, ceaselessly reiterated in books published at a rate which has demonstrably involved self-plagiarism on a massive scale: up to 15,000 words reproduced verbatim or non-verbatim without acknowledgement in the most serious cases (Walsh and Lehmann 2015). We can see more substance in Giddensian people but they are strangely divided creatures, either exercising autonomous reflexivity to 'colonize the future' or gripped by mindless compulsion. As Adam (2004: 393) describes it, Giddens paints a "peculiarly arid picture of the processes we utilize to make sense of the world and of ourselves", in which we are understood either to "reflexively control our activities, or else fatalistically resign the outcome of events to chance". The Giddensian subject is normatively rudderless because lacking any second-order personal emergent properties: in thrall to the affective dynamics which characterize the 'intimacies of the self' while rationally assessing the risks emergent from 'distant happenings', without the emerging constellation of concerns by virtue of which the expected outcomes of potential courses of action would actually *matter* to the subjects concerned (Archer 2000; Maccarini 2012: 109; Sayer 2011).

All the accounts criticized above share an underlying assumption of a zero-sum relationship between traditionalism and reflexivity. But they lack any account of the *variability of reflexivity* or *relations of concern* to more or less enduring features of the environment. Thus, the choice opened up by this extension of reflexivity becomes vacuous because the choosing is necessarily arbitrary and capricious. As Archer (2007: 37) notes of Beck, "[t]he decisions taken, and what reflexively went into their making, becoming uninteresting because they are *given* all the interest of people playing the lottery".

The theorists of late modernity open up a space for questions which they prove themselves to be systematically unable to answer. This is not just a matter of changes in how reflexivity is exercised throughout the population, as important as these are to understanding the trajectory of social transformation. I share Maccarini's (2012) conviction that we may be seeing the emergence of types of reflexivity that escape the concern-orientated model. Archer's (2012) account of expressive reflexivity represents one such possibility and in the previous volume I sought to build upon this by considering how many factors productive of expressivity may also be tipping practitioners of others modes into a more circumscribed exercise of this personal power (Carrigan 2016b).

In the present chapter, I intend to develop this contribution further by exploring how this new socio-technical environment influences the *future* orientation of subjects: how the present 'I', always conditioned by the past 'me', relates to the 'future' you. As Wiley (2006: 9) puts it, "if we attempt to foresee the various paths along which we might go, we can clearly see what is right for us". How does digitalization influence this activity? What changes can be found in how subjects orientate themselves towards their future selves in an environment transformed by what Rainie and Wellman (2012) call the 'triple revolution' of social networks, the internet and mobile computing? How does this influence the process of *shaping a life*? Giddens (1991: 84) gestured towards these questions in his discussion of the globalisation of media, suggesting that it renders "a multifarious number of milieux ... visible to anyone who cares to glean the relevant investigation" and that the "collage effect of television and newspapers gives specific form to the juxtaposition of settings and potential lifestyle choices". But he was unable to offer traction upon the conditions under which some outcomes are more likely than others. Archer (2014) and Maccarini (2012) observe a similar problem in Rosa's (2013) acceleration theory and its claim that the *good life* has come to be conceived as the *full life*: doing as many things, with as many people, in as many places as we can. As Maccarini (2012: 64) notes, the steps leading from a change at the level of temporal structures to the embrace of this ethos are far from automatic and call for a theory of culture, personal reflexivity and human fulfilment which is lacking in Rosa's work. As a corollary to this, Maccarini makes a crucially important observation that because "the cultural system is never fully integrated, people can tap into these *or other* resources" (Maccarini 2012: 63). Affirming this contingency is crucial but explaining it necessitates that we account for how the cultural system is mediated socio-culturally. The aforementioned 'triple revolution' has profound implications for this question and crucially they are ones which operate at the level of the person. With a personalised web, accessible from any device, there is no such thing as 'offline': we increasingly carry the archive with us as we make our way through the world.

An example from a film nicely illustrates the point here. *Six Degrees of Separation* was a popular comedy from 1993 in which a con artist appears at the door of a wealthy New York couple one night claiming to be a university friend of their children. Charming and loquacious, as well as apparently injured, he soon insinuates himself into their lives and becomes the beneficiary of their financial and emotional generosity. His scam is revealed when they eventually become suspicious of his claim to be the son of Sidney Poitier. Their capacity to verify this claim rests on going to a book shop in order to consult a biography of the famous actor. The whole narrative arc rests on the necessity of identifying and consulting physical records in order to verify a claim made about a relation to a famous figure. To remake the film for 2016 would be difficult, as the same scene would almost certainly[1] lead those involved to remove an iPhone from their pocket, consult Wikipedia and immediately conclude the figure at the door is an imposter because Sidney Poitier has six daughters but no sons.

What I will analyze in this chapter as the *digitalization of the archive* has profound consequences for the entirety of social life. Theorizing this process of transformation is an extensive project far beyond the confines of a single paper. Instead, my focus will be on a single aspect of it: how does the digitalization of the archive influence how subjects represent their future selves and orientate their present actions in terms of the people they seek to become or to avoid becoming? In asking this question, I understand the archive as the store of *cultural variety* within a social order and by 'cultural variety' I mean ideational content susceptible to *thinking with* and *thinking through* by subjects: propositions, categories, labels, metaphors and analogies. The question of how specific cultural items (books, websites, articles, films, plays etc) are composed of such elements, as well as processes of decomposition through which they can enter into mental life is beyond the scope of this paper. So too are different forms which such cultural variety can take: for instance the *resources of the self*, discussed by Porpora (2003). Cultural variety is drawn upon internally in "modeling our options, internally, so we can visualize the choices that lie before us" (Wiley 2006: 14), but this may be done in a range of different ways.

We always have an orientation towards a future 'you': the possible self, or field of possible selves, which define the horizon of our present actions.[2] In the absence of a substantive representation, we have a vacuum which itself reflects an uncertain relation between present action and future consequences. These representations are not constructed *ex nihilo* in a private language, but rather are cobbled together,

---

[1]Intended as a tendential claim about the diffusion of smart phones within a socio-demographic group rather than an assumption of their universality.

[2]See Carrigan (2014) for an extensive discussion of this, building upon the work of Archer (2000, 2003, 2007). See also Stevenson and Clegg (2011).

sometimes deliberately and often not, from the cultural raw materials available to us. The present chapter is an inquiry into the source of these cultural raw materials, what from this point onwards I will simply refer to as the *archive*, as well as how fundamental transformations of it are giving rise to profound changes in how we are orientated towards the people we might become. My argument will be that the digitalisation of the archive has important consequences for how we seek to make our way through the world under conditions of intensifying social morphogenesis. In offering an account of the digitalisation of the archive and its epochal significance, I will explore the structuring of the archive which is so overlooked in the aforementioned accounts of radical social and cultural change. In doing so, I hope to gain traction upon why some subjects flourish while others fracture in the face of the opportunity and choice opened up by social and cultural change, as well as how these contrasting fortunes manifest themselves as individual and collective contributions to further transformation.

The Digitalization of the Archive

To talk of the digitalisation of the archive implies a historical process, involving the transition from an *analogue* archive to one which is *digital*. While it was certainly the case that the archive was once exhaustively analogue, encompassing the contents of books and other media through which information was encoded in a physical form, the historical picture is more complicated than the opposition of an analogue archive to digital one would suggest. My focus here is not to tell the story of this transition, which is necessarily multifaceted and unfolded contingently across a range of contexts, but rather to focus on digitalisation as a process. This does not imply it is a *unitary* process, for the historiographical reasons offered above, but instead proceeds on the understanding that we have moved through a 'tipping point': one which can be tracked, through empirical indicators, as Porpora (2013) notes. This justifies our considering whether the *digitalisation of the archive* has led to a qualitative change in the cultural conditions of human life. Past tipping points can be seen in the emergence of language itself, as well as the origins of the archive in the earliest instances of information storage outside the brain, expressed in the cave art and bodily adornment that proliferated in Europe 35,000–45,000 years ago (Bentley and O'Brien 2012). Seen on such a time scale, the 'messy' history of digitalisation that too easily gets reduced to a simple narrative about the internet or globalisation and comes to seem more manageable. Or at least sufficiently so to license attention to the cumulative results of the process at a certain level of abstraction.

With these considerations in mind, I wish to proceed by looking at a specific case study: the relationship between the archive and memory. This might seem superficially counterintuitive. But the memorialising use of the archive is an interesting reflection on the primary consideration of this chapter. Looking at how people use the archive to construct a sense of the *past* will hopefully prove to be a useful route in to considering how the same facilities can be drawn upon to construct a sense of their *future*. In her study of what she terms 'mediated memories', Van Djick (2007) describes the digitalisation of the archive in terms of a transition from 'memory objects'[3] being predominately analogue to one in which digital objects are the norm. This is not a matter of the former being exhaustively replaced by the latter. Such a claim would be both empirically implausible and serve to occlude the second order effects through which analogue technologies come to be valued in a renewed way driven by their relative decline.[4] But such cases illustrate how analogue memory objects are becoming exceptional, something utilised as a deliberate choice rather than a quasi-automatic response to a restricted repertoire of possibilities. As Hoskins (2009) observes, digitalisation transforms the *potential* circulation of memory objects in ways which feed back into the culture of memorialisation underlying their production. Much activity which would have once been predominantly or entirely private becomes something at least implicitly orientated towards public self-presentation. Personal experiences can become publically available memories with an unprecedented degree of rapidity (Reading 2009).

Digitisation reshapes our remembrance of things past and our imagination of things yet to come, as two aspects of the same underlying process (Garde-Hansen et al. 2009). To use boyd's (2014) useful framework, the mediation afforded by digital technologies is characterised by *persistence, visibility, spreadability* and *searchability*. Each of these affordances has implications for (past) memory and (future) imagination but also for the relation between them, for instance as the persistence of records of past action makes it much harder to reinvent ourselves in the present, leading to what some have called the 'end of forgetting' (Mayer-Schönberger 2011). The tendency of digitialised memories to *spread* through digital channels or their susceptibly to being found through *search* radically expands the possibilities for the memories of others to influence our present selves. An experience once limited to those with whom we were close, in which the recorded memories of others cause us to look differently (however minutely) at the person we are and which we might become, now becomes a recurrent feature of digitalised social life: it might be far from universal but the intensely personalised social environment engendered by the ubiquity of social media is one in which the memories and imagined futures of others have an unprecedented capacity to impinge on our own lives. We might evade, ignore or obscure them. But such agential responses themselves speak of the biographical ramifications of this new environment. Nonetheless, this is not simply a matter of memory, but one of *mediation* more broadly. Van Djick (2007: 24) observes,

> *Since the 1950s, we no longer need to derive our personal tastes or cultural preferences mainly from social circles close to us, because media have expanded the potential reservoir for cultural exchange to much larger, even global, proportions.*

---

[3]Objects which serve to scaffold remembering through their association with, ascription to and/or use in recounting particular events.

[4]Consider for instance the 'vinyl revival', the thriving trade for old instant cameras, 'retro gaming' cultures or the fashion for luxury stationary. See Parikka (2012).

What Thompson (2013: 233) describes in a similar vein as "new opportunities, new options, new arenas for self-experimentation" was analysed in my contribution to the previous volume as the *problem of cultural abundance* (Carrigan 2016a). There is so much to read, to watch and to hear. We are overwhelmed by what are, at least in potentia, *cultural resources*: representations of things we could become or perhaps should avoid becoming. What can be celebrated as a freeing of the self from situational constraint through 'disembedding mechanisms' can equally be presented as a terrifying vertigo into which people find themselves spiralling (Giddens 1991; Young 2007). My objective in this chapter is to move beyond these parallel framings, which reflect a broader style of theorising social change addressed in the opening section, instead using an analysis of the digitalisation of the archive to consider the challenges for shaping a life to which the intensification of social morphogenesis gives rise.

The Problem of Abundance

It has become a commonplace to remark upon the explosion of cultural production facilitated by digital technology. Cyber-utopians like Shirky (2008, 2010) have lauded the 'mass amateurization' liable to result from these innovations. Less utopian but nonetheless optimistic figures such as Gauntlett (2013) point to a long history of 'amateur craft' being disregarded, seeing contemporary critiques of the 'cult of the amateur' as being another instance of experts and elites 'policing the borders of their practice'. This much invoked blurring of boundaries between the role of *consumer* and *producer* has been conceptualized in terms of the so-called 'prosumer' creating content while also responding to it. Either reflecting upon it as an extrinsic object or through its recombination or remixing to produce something new from the component parts. For instance, many of the nearly 3,372,000,000 videos viewed on YouTube today will be such 'remixes' or 'mashups' (Internet Live Stats 2015). Their production necessitates a remarkable degree of media consumption: to splice together a whole sequence of existing video clips into a whole that is intended to be more than the sum of its parts, as well the consumption necessary to engender the background literacy which facilitates selection of these components.

We can see comparable *escalations* across the field of cultural production. If we point to the 77 billion e-mails, 1.5 million blog posts, 215 million tweets, 30 million Instagram photos and 43 million Tumblr posts[5] that have been produced today at the time of writing. Not all of these have clear pre-digital precursors but what's notable is the *additive* rather than *substitutive* dynamic driving this discursive explosion: the emergence of one platform through which this activity is enacted does not entail the

[5]A popular micro-blogging service representing an intermediate point between Twitter and a traditional blog.

decline of a previous one (Carrigan 2016a). With almost 1.6 billion active Facebook users, 417 million active Google+ users and 326 million active Twitter users, the scale of the escalation is perhaps unsurprising but it's important to recognise the interests served by it (Internet Live Stats 2015). As van Djick (2013: loc 3290) notes, "the majority of large, mainstream platforms gauge content in terms of quantity, often measured by its potential to draw massive numbers of users": the whole attentional economy rests on sustaining this process of escalation, with specific platforms exhibiting a deliberate bias in their architecture towards creating a cadre of social media stars. The resulting tendency to "publicize successful outliers to propagate the illusion",[6] as Nichols (2015) puts it, has some profound implications for human flourishing which are returned to in the conclusion.

However this change must be addressed in terms of *quality* as well as *quantity*. If we understand *cultural variety* as ideational content susceptible to thinking with and thinking through by subjects, what's striking is how much contemporary cultural production doesn't meet this criterion. A quantitative increase in *output* does not entail an increase in variety. For instance, as Birnbaum (2015) observes, the vast majority of 'selfies', representing a nascent institution which is the key driver in the proliferation of online images, encompass a very limited range of poses and stances. Filtering existing material without expanding upon it has been central to the development of the blogosphere (Rosenberg 2009) and is arguably even more so on micro-blogging platforms like Twitter and Tumblr. Recognizing the empirical scale of cultural production is important because it invites us to inquire into the *escalatory* processes underlying a remarkable increase. Nevertheless, the fact of this escalation does not translate straight forwardly into an increase in cultural variety: the digitalization of the archive sometimes produces a homogenizing dynamic, as well as the more commonly recognized heterogenizing one. Thompson's (2013: 233) "new opportunities, new options, new arenas for self-experimentation" do not emerge in a linear way, as is so often assumed in the literature on the opportunities offered by late, liquid or post modernity (whether or not these opportunities are coded positively or negatively).

Furthermore, commercial incentives drive significant portions of this increase in output while simultaneously exercising a deleterious effect over the quality of the communication. We can see this in 'content farms' in which poorly paid international freelancers, incentivized to work at a pace which precludes meaningful reflection, churn out 'content' commissioned on the basis of algorithmic insight. But we can also see it in the slide towards banality which the competitive dynamics of online attention incentivize. In a prescient early analysis, Shenk (1997) warned of the 'data smog' clouding our capacity for evaluation and judgment. Escalatory dynamics are most pronounced with commercial communication, as tactics which

[6]A description used in a slightly different way, characterizing the unrealistic presentation of careers in coding by those with vested interests in the expansion of coding academies, but it's a remarkably apt one to describe the *cultural construction* of all manner of career hierarchies which are undergoing radical *structural constriction* under digital capitalism.

exhibit an increased capacity to win the attention of an audience (e.g. by differentiating themselves within an overcrowded inbox) are immediately liable to be copied by competitors, thus negating the competitive advantage and encouraging a new tactic, itself liable to be immediately copied in the event of success. Techniques which are rational for one actor generate problems at the level of the field as a whole, as both qualitative and quantitative escalations lead to further attentional fragmentation and provoke agential backlashes on the part of the audience that necessitate strategic negotiation. In one fascinating case, a concern for the consequences this has for social and political life has led one self-defined professional 'media manipulator' to call for an end to these techniques (Holiday 2012).

Finally, the conjuncture of computational innovation and marketing imperatives have led to a proliferation of what tends to be called 'spam', though this increasingly everyday term risks obscuring a complex phenomenon intimately entwined with the history of the internet (Brunton 2013). Its most familiar manifestations are 'constantly repeating messages of crushing banality' disseminated on a scale of production unlike anything in previous human history, leveraging thousands of computers to produce hundreds of millions of messages at near zero cost (Brunton 2013: loc 120). But automated spam bots also increasingly threaten to overwhelm popular social media sites, prompting an arms race in which these platforms incentivize technological innovation by in turn automating the process of identifying and banning spam bots. This torrential undercurrent of automated advertising perpetually risks pulling us away from the task at hand, amplifying the existing effects of social media and the background noise it injects into daily life (Losse 2012: loc 184). Could this second-order effect of the digitalization of the archive ultimately prove fatally self-destructive? The scale and scope of this accelerating process certainly risks feeding back into the relation between subjects and the archive in complex and confusing ways.

The Curatorial Bubble and the Filter Bubble

Under the circumstances resulting from this qualitative and quantitative escalation of cultural production, intermediaries become crucial, providing a necessary mechanism for filtering the extent of cultural variety. As discussed earlier in the chapter, cultural variety in the sense used here is not co-extensive with cultural production: the mere fact of a new cultural *output* does not entail any necessary addition to the total stock of cultural *variety*. But it does add to the stock of items of which subjects are *potentially* aware. Assessing salience becomes increasingly complex under these conditions, a problem intensified by the aforementioned tendency for online marketing deliberately to contravene the boundaries of relevance in a way intended to win the attention of a subject (Brunton 2013). Most, if not all subjects, require some form of assistance in 'bounding' the information available online if using digital technology is liable to prove consistently useful. Otherwise there is just too much *stuff.* But the question of what form this takes has been crucial to the develop of our present socio-technical environment, with the balance between two competing tendencies exercising an important influence over particular subjects.

These intermediaries take two broad forms: *curatorial* and *algorithmic.*[7] If we look to particular cases studies, such as Amazon and Google, we can recognize the tension between them as well as how the demands of scale which characterize the competitive environment in which tech corporations operate led the former gradually to lose out to the latter. For instance in the case of Google, internal conflicts about the limitations of algorithmic search led some to advocate editorial intervention but this strategy was ultimately subordinated, given the difficulties in scaling it, apart from boundary cases in which search results are deemed troublesome or potentially illegal (Vaidhyanathan 2012: 62). Another example can be seen in the eclipse of Amazon's editorial team, eventually replaced by the *Amabot* that inserted automatically generated recommendations in a standardized format where the outputs of the editorial team used to be presented (Stone 2013: 134). This scaling problem has led major platforms to, for the most part, turn away from human intervention in favour of algorithmic alternatives. In the early days of the web, the seeds of multi-billion dollar businesses were generated through the simple act of collating and categorizing links in order to present them to an audience. But the search for business models, in the case of those portals that had captured a significant audience ripe to be monetized, inevitably led to algorithmic considerations: the digital data produced by audience engagement with the portal allowed the 'click-finding' through which the audience was modelled and segmented, facilitating increasingly sophisticated understandings of the information seeking activity of the audience (Carlson 2015: 37–38). This paved the way for the algorithmic filtering which is built into major platforms, resulting in what Pariser (2011) calls the 'filter bubble': the personalization of our experience, generated through accumulated user data, shackles subjects into a digital environment that has been pre-structured for them on the basis of fundamentally opaque criteria.

Nonetheless, this didn't entail the death of curatorial intermediaries, only their exclusion from the architecture of major platforms. Indeed, as I discussed in the previous volume, a plethora of 'curation tools' seek to democratize curatorial activity by encouraging everyone to engage in the selection, organization and presentation of material they find online. The popularity of these varies but at the most visible end of the spectrum, the visually focused curation service Pinterest has 100 million monthly active users as of September 2015 (Hwang 2015). The uses to which these are put varies but the common feature they share is that judgments of salience are increasingly made on the part of these curators, as opposed to the

[7] *Curatorial* is a matter of deliberate human evaluation, whereas *algorithmic* entails pre-defined instructions performed in sequence by software of whatever sort. Both *ultimately* have their origins in human evaluation.

creators of the material that is itself being shared. We can see a similar trend in the evolution of blogging and micro-blogging, as the tendency of the former to reward curatorial 'filter blogs' with audiences has become a defining practice of the latter (Rosenberg 2009; Carrigan 2016a). In both cases, popularity varies immensely and many curators exercise little significant influence, but the aggregate trend is nonetheless significant. At the most prominent end of the spectrum, it means people are "in the business of locating and connecting interesting things", as co-editor of the popular *Boing Boing* describes himself (Doctorow 2002). But more diffusely, it represents an incorporation of curation into the fabric of everyday use of media, with important implications for the awareness subjects have of cultural variety. Any one example of this may seem trivial, but 'social traffic' has begun to outstrip traffic for search engines on many websites, suggesting the newly dominant place of curators (self-regarded or otherwise) in shaping the economics of online attention.

As I argued in the previous volume, responses to this increasingly personalized 'filter bubble' seem likely to vary in terms of mode of reflexivity (Pariser 2011). It is perfectly possible to escape the filter bubble but there are cognitive costs entailed by doing so. Presuming sufficient technical expertise, how much time and energy is a subject willing to expend upon escaping personalization? What are the opportunity costs? Particularly given the time gains that can be accrued through personalization, is it deemed worth it by any particular subject (who enjoys sufficient awareness of the socio-technical environment to be capable of posting the question).

Similar questions can be asked of the 'curatorial bubble' within which subjects now find themselves when using social media.[8] To what extent do they evaluate who they connect to on social media in terms of the quality or quantity of the 'content' they share? Do they choose people to follow based on a desire to acquaint themselves with the potential cultural variety they represent? Does contact with unfamiliar views make them uncomfortable and do they seek to prevent this? Considerations such as these preclude concrete forecasts concerning how different categories of subject will respond to these constraints and enablements characterizing their information environment.[9] Nonetheless, it may prove fruitful to consider speculatively how different dominant modes of reflexivity might entail divergent orientations to this environment. More importantly, this analysis opens up a space of mediation between the macro- and meso-social factors shaping the digitalisation of the archive, the micro-social dynamics this gives rise to, as well as how these feed back into the broader social and cultural arena.

[8]The use of algorithmic filtering of feeds on a service like Facebook illustrates how the two are in practice intertwined.

[9]Embodying as they do the irreducibility of personal reflexivity and the intrinsic character of open systems.

Bounding Variety and Shaping a Life

In the previous sections, I have offered an analysis of the archive in terms of the generation of cultural variety, emerging from concurrent heterogenising and homogenising processes. In doing so, I have tried to escape from the dominant view of the linear growth of variety, construed either positively or negatively, which dominates the literature on late, liquid and post modernity. Variety accumulates unevenly. Furthermore, the problem of abundance this creates gives rise to parallel *curatorial* and *algorithmic* strategies for facilitating access to it via the archive. Variety grows unevenly while these second-order effects generate what is in turn uneven access to it.

This multiple layering of contingencies is further complicated by the question of reflexivity: what do subjects do with this variety? Archer (2012) describes this in terms of 'bounding' variety: filtering the available opportunities in order to reach a point at which these existential (and practical) questions come to be experienced as manageable. *Communicative reflexives* rely on their interlocutors, with the difficulties facing this discussed below. *Autonomous reflexives* rely on the formulation of projects and goals, but these in turn become more difficult given the diffuse awareness of all the things which one could aim for. *Meta-reflexives* look to their concerns, but these provide no straight forward guides to action and exploring the cultural system in order to formulate projects but likely only complicate things further. *Fractured reflexives* struggle to bound variety and thus act purposively in relation to their future. Such considerations open up valuable questions concerning how personal reflexivity will reinforce or resist the *curatorial bubble* and the *filter bubble* which are the dominant mechanisms conditioning access to the digitalized archive.

My overarching point has been that the *curatorial bubble* and the *filter bubble* both exhibit independent dynamics which jointly influence the awareness subjects have of cultural variety. Algorithmic mediation infers *present* interests on the basis of *past* behavior, potentially eliminating serendipity and foreclosing cultural exploration by "freezing into place a future that rigidly reenacts the past" (Pasquale 2015). Curatorial mediation subordinates *cultural system mediation* to *socio-cultural choices*, potentially leaving us locked with inward looking and homogenous groups (Sunstein 2009). In both cases the effect is a potential one because subjects inevitably respond to these environments, even if they do so in ways which reproduce their underlying characteristics.

As suggested, I wish to draw speculative conclusions about possible tendencies on the basis of these considerations, considering the aforementioned orientations of different modes to 'bounding variety' in terms of the distinctive characteristics which constitute the digitalized archive. My contention is that *communicative reflexives* and *fractured reflexives* will tend towards passivity in the face of the 'filter bubble' and homophily in the face of the 'curatorial bubble': allowing their online activity to be structured through algorithmic mediation while seeking to connect with similar others – in many cases *already known* others – who reflect their own views back to them in a subjectively comfortable way. In contrast, autonomous reflexives are likely to exercise agency over the constitution of both the 'filter bubble' and the 'curatorial bubble', seeking and applying practical techniques to design an information environment[10] which they *believe* is likely to bound cultural variety in a way amenable to their *existing* goals. In contrast, meta-reflexives are likely to exercise agency over both but in a way mediated by *concerns* rather than *goals*, such that the defining factor becomes 'is this interesting?' rather than 'is this useful?'. This generates three distinct orientations towards cultural variety: *avoiding variety, applying variety and exploring variety*. In this sense, I want to argue that our new socio-technical environment leads to the stabilization of communicative reflexivity (through the provision of dispersed niches to support geo-local ones), does not exercise an influence upon the preponderance of autonomous reflexivity and leads to the *amplification* of meta-reflexivity through increasing the likelihood that meta-reflexives will engage with ever increasing swathes of cultural variety which is, under conditions of contextual incongruity, generative of meta-reflexivity itself.

However one could still object to the assumption that 'bounding' this variety is necessary. This takes us back to Maccarini's suggestion of non-concern based models of reflexivity which may be emerging in an environment characterized by intensified social morphogenesis. Could it not be possible to live in the stream? The metaphors which suffused the early popular reception of the internet certainly hinted at this possibility, preoccupied as they were with 'surfing the net' or exploring the 'information superhighway'. As Lupton (2014: 107) observes, the former metaphor has the connotation of "moving from website to website easily and playfully, riding over the top of digital information and stopping when we feel like". Instead, we're now more likely to encounter talk of the 'fire hose' of data, the 'data deluge' or the 'data tsunami' which threaten to 'swamp' or 'drown' us (Lupton 2014: 107). The possible pleasures to be found through immersion, indeed the possible transformation into something *more* through the willing embrace of digital capitalism's disorientating acceleration (Noys 2014), come to be replaced by a pervasive awareness of the potential threats. In my contribution to the previous volume, I argued that the many manifestations of productivity culture should be seen as responses to the demands this new socio-technical environment places upon personal reflexivity (Carrigan 2016a). Practices like the 'information diet', 'lifestyle minimalism', 'life hacking' and 'getting things done' are more or less systematic attempts to reorientate the subject towards *what really matters* amidst accumulating demands upon their attention (Johnson 2015; Allen 2015). The perils of distraction are a thread which runs through the products of this 'discursive

[10]The actual activities involved in doing this are much more mundane than these descriptions make them sound e.g. identifying particular useful instances of personalisation to attend to, identifying particular classes of people deliberately to connect with on social media networks.

explosion'[11] but it is sometimes unclear exactly what this distraction is taken to be. In a psychoanalytically orientated account, the political theorist Jodi Dean (2010) analyses what we might describe as a 'stuckness' that proliferates online: we get "stuck doing the same thing over and over again because this doing produces enjoyment. Post. Post. Post. Click. Click. Click." The popular comedy Portlandia describe this as a 'technology loop': the trap of frenzied overstimulation in which the cultural riches of online experience can leave one ensnared (Krisel 2011). The phenomenological accuracy of this perhaps goes some way to explaining the growing prominence of 'internet addiction' as both a lay and expert category. While it has yet to be officially recognised by the American Psychiatric Association, publishers of the globally influential Diagnostic and Statistical Manual of Mental Disorders, there are web addiction clinics operating in the US, the UK, the Netherlands, China and South Korea (Krotoski 2012: 40).

This proliferation of addiction clinics and the vested interests of those who work within them, fosters an often panic stricken discourse of social media addiction[12] and the pervasiveness with which people experience a lack of control *at times* in their relation to the internet jointly contribute to the institutionalisation of 'internet addiction'. But the prevailing psychiatric conception of addiction distinguishes between *substance disorders* (chemical dependence) and *impulse-control disorders* (behavioural compulsion) (boyd 2014: loc 1349). While some have claimed the internet is re-wiring our brains, see for instance Carr (2011), claiming that internet addiction is a matter of chemical dependence seems obviously untenable. But the causality at work in the latter is open to question, as the operational basis for identifying a disorder rests on the putative condition interfering with the subject's capacity to lead an active life (boyd 2014: loc 1349). The concept of 'internet addiction' risks treating it as axiomatic that 'excessive'[13] internet use is the *cause* rather than *consequence* of the putative dysfunction, when this is obviously an empirical matter. My suggestion is that we can more usefully analyse this in

[11]The more reflexive practitioners of 'productivity systems' can be seen to note the risks to productivity posed by reading about new approaches, discussing their virtues and experimenting with them in one's own life.

[12]One which focuses particularly on young people, reflecting a much longer standing concern with the purported ills of youth cultures, as boyd (2014: loc 1349–1368) insightfully diagnoses. This sits uneasily with the popular image of young people as 'digital natives', for whom the internet is second nature. These contrasting dystopian and utopian images of generational characteristics illustrate how a significant process has yet to find clarity in the popular imagination.

[13]The notion of 'excessive' use is itself problematic. Excessive in relation to *what*? If it is a matter of the population at large, we can always identify those who use the internet to a degree that would be deemed excessive on a *quantitative* basis but is licensed on a *qualitative* basis by this being intrinsic to an occupational role. The assumed standard of 'excessive' use is more nebulous than would appear to be the case prima facie, enfolding a network of assumptions which are rarely stated explicitly.

terms of a failure of second-order volition.[14] Frankfurt (1988: 19) distinguishes between two senses in which such a failure can occur: the 'unwilling addict', for whom a first-order inclination conflicts with a desire to refrain from acting upon it, and the 'wanton' for whom there is no such conflict between first-order desires. The former figure is mired in internal conflict, locked in a competition between competing inclinations, while the latter is simply mired in first-order desires. If the unwilling addict succeeds in the "formation of a second-order volition, with one rather than with the other of his conflicting first-order desires" then "[h]e makes one of them more truly his own and, in so doing, he withdraws himself from the other". In contrast, the 'wanton' exhibits a "mindless indifference to the enterprise of evaluating his own desires and motives", such that "it makes no difference *to him* whether his craving or the aversion gets the upper hand". The 'wanton' may sometimes experience an aversion to the object of addiction but these are *contrasting* first-order desires, rather than *conflicting* first-order desires that might prove generative of a second-order desire. To return to the case of the 'internet addiction' category: it is the difference between someone experiencing themselves as locked in Dean's (2010) loop of "Post. Post. Post. Click. Click. Click" while seeking to be free of this compulsion and mindless immersion in a technology-loop coupled with other urges that *may* include an inclination towards things other than being stuck in such a loop.

Digital Wantons are the specter haunting the discourse of 'internet addiction': digital zombies, something less than human, decreasingly able to function in the world. However the young people we meet in boyd's (2014) study represent 'conflicted addicts', as with the case of Andrew who eventually quit Facebook having reached the conclusion that "This is stupid and it's having control of my life and I don't want anything to do with it" (boyd 2014: 1279). She suggests that while "teens complain about how time drags when they must do things that they do not find enjoyable, time seems to slip away when in mediated environments with their peers" and that this experience, which can be "disorientating and a source of guilt", stands as the "root of anxiety about social media addiction" (boyd 2014: 1312). The point holds beyond the young people who are boyd's concern. If the experience of 'internet addiction' represents the extreme end of the behavioural spectrum, its quotidian correlate is *distraction* (Carrigan 2016a). But as Gitlin (2007: 32) points out, "[d]istraction is one of those terms – like freedom, responsibility, and alienation – that requires an object to make sense". But what is this object? The argument I develop in this chapter is that *digital distraction* and *internet addiction* are failures of second-order volition[15]: the cultural abundance which characterizes the socio-technical environment of digital capital transforms our experience of

[14]Second-order desires are *desires about desires*. For instance I may at this moment want another coffee (1st order) but I want to suppress this urge because I'm trying to limit the amount of coffee I drink while working at home (2nd order).

[15]Representing a spectrum, from occasional 'distraction' to debilitating 'addiction', defined by the extent of the tracts of everyday life within which this is experienced.

cultural variety. The anxieties and guilt which find expression in this cultural panic about internet addiction (our own or that of others) focus around a 'stuckness' concerning existing commitments or formulating new ones. My argument is that this can be understood in terms of a digitally induced crisis of 'bounding variety' and, so to speak, keeping it bound if this has been achieved in the past. Being 'stuck in the stream' or caught in a 'technology loops' represents an increasingly pervasive experience of *all the things there are to see, do or say* impeding meaningful action in relation to *projects which matter to us* or actually formulating such projects if we haven't already.

This might be construed in terms of expressive reflexivity in Archer's (2012) sense. But we might also, further exploring Maccarini's suggestion, consider the variability with which a subject experiences such a crisis of 'bounding variety': if expressivity is one end of the spectrum, are there more functional manifestations of this predicament we can identity? In a popular article on the Guardian website, the journalist Sophie Heawood (2013) attached the label *everythingist* to her experience of being unable to commit to courses of action, no matter how mundane, "unable to quite go with a plan or be in the moment because of all the other plans and moments where you might be, cheating on yourself with all your other selves". The comments on the discussion make for fascinating reading, as 261 people largely identified profoundly with her description ("You are me. You have just summed up my internal dialogue to a T") or sought to comfort her in a way oddly revealing about their own orientation to a shared predicament ("Don't try and be an alpha type: it's just one upmanship bollocks that leads to inner stress and mass pissing off of other people"). The problem recounted here is *committing to a course of action* without having other potential courses of action impinge upon consciousness during the ensuing activity. Not only is there always something else we could be doing, for *everythingists* it's seemingly impossible to expunge that awareness from their internal conversation when trying to do something. Under these conditions, life doesn't take *shape*. There's no unity to life. There are events, with resonances and rhythms, fleeting but intense meanings which lack coherence over time. But this is true of expressive and fractured reflexivity more generally. What makes *everythingists* distinctive is they crave this unity but find themselves systematically unable to achieve it. Every concern might represent a challenge to make a commitment, as Archer (2012: 105) claims, but for *everythingists* the commitment never comes because the endless possibilities are so bewildering, with each one pointing out to many others.

For Kenneth Gergen (2000: xviii) the problem here is the goal of unity. Describing his 'struggle' against "my modernist training for constant improvement, development and accumulation", he claims there are 'substantial rewards' "if one avoids looking back to locate a true and enduring self, and simply acts to fulfil potential in the moment at hand". Reflecting on this orientation, Rosa (2013: 297) suggests that "the absence of an integration of experiences into an identity-constituting whole can be affirmed as pleasurable and satisfying just insofar as it is possible to develop an ironic, playful relation to the uncontrollable vicissitudes of life". Obviously, it is probably easier to embrace Gergen's life philosophy when you're an internationally renowned tenured professor at a private liberal arts college.

Even if it is naïve, at best, concerning the accumulated material consequences of a failure to try and give shape to a life, what he advocates is not passivity, but rather that one “simply acts to fulfil potential in the moment at hand”. This is what *everythingists* fail to do and Gergen offers a therapeutic philosophy for them: commit to what you are doing, don’t worry about the opportunity costs and immerse yourself ever more deeply in the reality of your own (situational) existence.

Both Gergen and Rosa take it as a given that the ‘integration of experience into an identity-constituting whole’ can no longer be satisfactorily achieved, if indeed it ever could. My argument in this paper thus far entails that they have *underemphasized* the cultural dimension of this existential challenge: the difficulty some face in commitment does not come from ‘our modernist training’ but from our relationship towards cultural variety, reflecting what is for some a radically expanded awareness of potential opportunities and a concomitant difficulty in selecting from them, rather than a compulsion derived from character education. Conversely, they have *overemphasized* the structural dimension of this existential challenge: the social world has not become liquid, there is continuity and change between situations, hence the process of shaping a life is not impossible but merely unreliable. Certainly, unpredictability and instability – which we must distinguish – make instrumental rationality much more error-prone. We might respond to this by building contingencies into our life plans and returning to them with much greater frequency. These changing circumstances therefore encourage an intensification of reflexivity, an expansion of *life tactics* to ensure the endurance of our *life strategy*. This will work most effectively when our ends remain stable (e.g. becoming established and recognised within a given profession that remains securely existent) and only the means are subject to change (e.g. changing expectations attached to this professional role, changing practical activity necessary to establish oneself within the field).

An alternative strategy is to temporise, reducing the window of time within which we seek to enact a plan in order to preserve the efficacy of our planning, as can be seen in the example of Spotify’s 31 year old CEO who formulates 5-year ‘missions’ for himself, a period of time in which he could “achieve something meaningful but short enough so that I can change my mind every few years” (Seabrook 2014). But his ambitions seem anemic compared to those of Elon Musk, with his ground-breaking interventions in the commercialization of space flight and electrification of cars, as well as his long-term commitment to creating habitats on the moon (Vance 2015). Mark Zuckerberg seeks to transform global communication and create a world “in which we all become cells in a single organism, where we can communicate automatically and can all work together seamlessly” (Losse 2012: 201). Their ambitions are not confined to the locus of corporate life, with philanthropic capitalists seeking to leverage their wealth to remake the world in their own image, sometimes addressing social ills which have been produced in part through their own corporate activity. The billionaire financier George Soros once remarked that “sometimes I felt like a giant digestive tract, taking in money at one end and pushing it out at the other.” (Wilson 2015). It’s possible an awareness of this tension may go some way to explaining the scope of the ambitions displayed by the philanthrocapitalists, though of course we can see similar behaviour on the part of the super-rich through history (Armstrong 2010; Kampfner 2014). For these digital elites, giving shape to a life seems far from impossible. But their examples suggest how vast resources can mitigate against the cultural challenge discussed in this paper: it's easy to commit to a vision for your life if you have utter faith that you will possess the resources to carry out your most expansive dreams. For the rest of us, it is more challenging.

Conclusion

Contributing to this final volume left me reflecting on the meta-theoretical status accorded to the concept of *morphogenic society*. Is it a speculative provocation, entertained as a sensitizing device to orientate collective intellectual work? Is it a gradually emerging account of what comes *after* late modernity? Is it an alternative account *of* late modernity, accepting the underlying problematic of high modernity giving way to late modernity, but rejecting both the substance and method of Beck, Bauman, Giddens et al.? My own inclination is to treat it as a provocation which has anchored a framework for the analysis of social change: two elements which can in principle be detached and which I believe should be, at least now the initial work has been completed.

This chapter began with the theme of *flourishing* or *fracturing* amidst variety and ended with a consideration of life strategies and life experiences which one might conclude indicate a *need* for such a strategy. This descent into particularism might seem to constitute a retreat from the stated ambitions of the chapter but I would argue it indicates the strength of the approach that has been developed through this project, at least as I understand it. Utilized as a framework through which to address social change, it avoids the parallel pitfalls of epochal theorizing and empiricist generalization: grounding substantive statements about change in specific claims at the micro, meso and macro levels. It is an approach to inquiry which is intensely generative of new questions: ones which, in my case, emerged through my contributions in the later stages of this project and which I am now addressing through a book project. I remain disappointingly (and disappointedly) agnostic about the prospects of a morphogenic society and its potentially eudaimonistic character. However, I have nonetheless developed a deep commitment to 'social morphogenesis' as a meta-theoretical framework through which we can pose such questions, even if my substantive theorizing about the likely trajectories of social transformation lead me to rather gloomy conclusions that run contrary to the concrete utopia implied by the prospect of a 'win-win' social-formation.

References

Adams, M. (2004). Whatever will be, will be: Trust, fate and the reflexive self. *Culture & Psychology, 10*(4), 387–408.

Allen, D. (2015). *Getting things done: The art of stress-free productivity*. London: Hachette UK.

Archer, M. S. (2000). *Being human: The problem of agency*. Cambridge: Cambridge University Press.

Archer, M. S. (2007). *Making our way through the world: Human reflexivity and social mobility*. Cambridge: Cambridge University Press.

Archer, M. S. (2012). *The reflexive imperative in late modernity*. Cambridge: Cambridge University Press.

Archer, M. S. (2014). The generative mechanism re-configuring late modernity. In *Late modernity* (pp. 93–117). Dordrecht: Springer International Publishing.

Armstrong, S. (2010). *The Super-Rich shall inherit the earth: The new global oligarachs and how they're taking over our world*. London: Hachette.

Bauman, Z. (2000). *Liquid Modernity*. Cambridge: Polity Press.

Beck, U. (1992). *Risk society: Towards a new modernity*. London: Sage.

Beck, U. & Beck-Gernsheim, E. (2002). *Individualization: Institutionalized individualism and its social and political consequences*. London: Sage.

Bentley, R. A., & O'Brien, M. J. (2012). Cultural evolutionary tipping points in the storage and transmission of information. *Frontiers in Psychology, 3*.

Birnbaum, L. (2015). Presentation at crazy futures: Data crazy.

Boyd, D. (2014). *It's complicated: The social lives of networked teens*. [Kindle DX version]. Retrieved from Amazon.com

Brunton, F. (2013). *Spam: A shadow history of the internet*. [Kindle DX version]. Retrieved from Amazon.com

Carlson, N. (2015). *Marissa Mayer and the fight to save yahoo!*. [Kindle DX version]. Retrieved from Amazon.com

Carr, N. (2011). *The shallows: What the internet is doing to our brains*. [Kindle DX version]. Retrieved from Amazon.com

Carrigan, M. (2014). *Becoming who we are: Personal morphogenesis and social change*. Doctoral dissertation, University of Warwick.

Carrigan, M. (2016a). *Social media for academics*. London: SAGE.

Carrigan, M. (2016b). The fragile movements of late modernity. In *Morphogenesis and the crisis of normativity* (pp. 191–215). Springer International Publishing.

Dean, J. (2010). *Blog theory: Feedback and capture in the circuits of drive*. Cambridge: Polity.

Doctorow, C. (2002). *Essential blogging: Selecting and using weblog tools*. Beijing: O'Reilly Media, Inc..

Elliott, A., & Lemert, C. (2008). *The new individualism: The emotional costs of globalization*. New York: Routledge.

Frankfurt, H. G. (1988). *The importance of what we care about: Philosophical essays*. Cambridge: Cambridge University Press.

Gauntlett, D. (2013). *Making is connecting*. Cambridge: Polity.

Garde-Hansen, J., Hoskins, A., & Reading, A. (2009). *Save as… digital memories*. Palgrave Macmillan.

Gergen, K. (2000). *The saturated self: Dilemmas of identity in contemporary life*. New York: Basic books.

Giddens, A. (1991). *Modernity and self-identity: Self and society in the late modern age*. Cambridge: Polity.

Giddens, A. (2011). *Runaway world*. London: Profile books.

Gitlin, T. (2007). *Media unlimited. How the torrent of sounds and images overwhelms our lives*. New York: Metropolitan Books.

Heawood, S. (2013). *I'm an everythingist*. Guardian family. Available at http://www.theguardian.com/commentisfree/2013/jun/11/everythingist-craving-new-experiences. Accessed 17 Jan 2017.
Holiday, R. (2012). *Trust me, I'm lying: Confessions of a media manipulator*. [Kindle DX version]. Retrieved from Amazon.com
Hoskins, A. (2009). The mediatisation of memory. In *Save as... digital memories* (pp. 27–43). UK: Palgrave Macmillan.
Hoskins, A., & Reading, A. (2009). *Save as... digital memories*. Palgrave Macmillan. [Kindle DX version]. Retrieved from Amazon.com
Hwang, E. (2015). *100 million of the most interesting people we know*. Pinterest blog. Available at: https://blog.pinterest.com/en/100-million-most-interesting-people-we-know. Accessed 17 Jan 2017.
Internet Live Stats (2015). Available at: http://www.internetlivestats.com/ Accessed 17 Jan 2017.
Johnson, C. A. (2015). *The information diet: A case for conscious comsumption*. Beijing: O′Reilly Media, Inc..
Kampfner, J. (2014). *The rich: From slaves to super-yachts: A 2,000-year history*. UK: Hachette.
Krisel, J. (2011). Farm. Portlandia. IFC, January 21, Television.
Krotoski, A. (2012). *Untangling the web*. [Kindle DX version]. Retrieved from Amazon.com
Losse, K. (2012). *The boy kings: A journey into the heart of the social network*. [Kindle DX version]. Retrieved from Amazon.com
Lupton, D. (2014). *Digital sociology*. [Kindle DX version]. Retrieved from Amazon.com.
Maccarini, A. (2012). The emergent social qualities of a 'morphogenic' society: Cultures, structures, and forms of reflexivity. In *Late modernity* (pp. 49–76). Dordrecht: Springer International Publishing.
Maccarini, A., Morandi, E., & Prandini, R. (Eds.). (2011). *Sociological realism*. [Kindle DX version]. Retrieved from Amazon.com
Mayer-Schönberger, V. (2011). *Delete: The virtue of forgetting in the digital age*. [Kindle DX version]. Retrieved from Amazon.com
Nichols, S. (2015). *Coding academics are nonsense*. Tech Crunch. Available at http://techcrunch.com/2015/10/23/coding-academies-are-nonsense/. Last access 18 Dec 2015.
Noys, B. (2014). *Malign velocities: Accelerationism and capitalism*. [Kindle DX version]. Retrieved from Amazon.com
Pariser, E. (2011). *The filter bubble: What the internet is hiding from you*. UK: Penguin.
Pasquale, F. A. (2015). The algorithmic self. *Hedgehog Review, 17,* http://www.iascculture.org/THR/THR_article_2015_Spring_Pasquale.php
Porpora, D. V. (2003). *Landscapes of the soul: The loss of moral meaning in American life*. Oxford: Oxford University Press.
Porpora, D. V. (2013). Morphogenesis and social change. In *Social morphogenesis* (pp. 25–37). Dordrecht: Springer Netherlands.
Rainie, L., & Wellman, B. (2012). *Networked: The new social operating system*. Cambridge: MIT Press.
Rattansi, A. (2014). Zygmunt Bauman: An Adorno for 'liquid modern' times? *The Sociological Review, 62*(4), 908–917.
Reading, A. (2009). Memobilia: The mobile phone and the emergence of wearable memories. In *Save as... Digital memories* (pp. 81–95). Chicago: Palgrave Macmillan.
Rosa, H. (2013). *Social acceleration: A new theory of modernity*. New York: Columbia University Press.
Rosenberg, S. (2009). Say everything. How blogging began, what it's becoming, and why it matters, Crown, New York.
Sayer, A. (2011). *Why things matter to people: Social science, values and ethical life*. Cambridge: Cambridge University Press.
Seabrook, J. (2014). *Revenue streams: Is spotify the music industry's friend or its foe?*. The New York, November 24, 2014, issue http://www.newyorker.com/magazine/2014/11/24/revenue-streams

Shenk, D. (1997). *Data smog: Surviving the information glut.* HarperCollins.
Shirky, C. (2008). *Here comes everybody: The power of organizing without organizations.* Penguin.
Shirky, C. (2010). *Cognitive surplus: Creativity and generosity in a connected age.* UK: Penguin.
Smart, C. (2007). *Personal life.* Cambridge: Polity.
Stevenson, J., & Clegg, S. (2011). Possible selves: Students orientating themselves towards the future through extracurricular activity. *British Educational Research Journal, 37*(2), 231–246.
Stone, B. (2013). *The everything store: Jeff Bezos and the age of Amazon.* [Kindle DX version]. Retrieved from Amazon.com.
Sunstein, C. (2009). *Republic 2.0.* Princeton: Princeton University Press.
Thompson, J. B. (2013). *The media and modernity: A social theory of the media.* [Kindle DX version]. Retrieved from Amazon.com
Thomson, R., Bell, R., Holland, J., & Henderson, S. (2002). Critical moments: Choice, chance and opportunity in young people's narratives of transition. *Sociology, 36*(2), 335–354.
Vaidhyanathan, S. (2012). *The googlization of everything: (And why we should worry).* [Kindle DX version]. Retrieved from Amazon.com.
Van Dijck, J. (2007). *Mediated memories in the digital age.* [Kindle DX version]. Retrieved from Amazon.com
Van Dijck, J. (2013). *The culture of connectivity: A critical history of social media.* [Kindle DX version]. Retrieved from Amazon.com
Vance, A. (2015). *Elon Musk.* [Kindle DX version]. Retrieved from Amazon.com.
Walsh, P., Lehmann, D. (2015). *Problematic elements in the scholarship of Zygmunt Bauman.* Available at https://www.academia.edu/15031047/Problematic_Elements_in_the_ Scholarship_of_Zygmunt_Bauman
Wiley, N. (2006). Pragmatism and the dialogical self. *International Journal for Dialogical Science, 1*(1), 5–21.
Wilson, J. (2015). *Counting on Billionaires.* Jacobin. Available at: https://www.jacobinmag.com/2015/03/george soros philanthrocapitalism-millennium-villages/ Accessed 17 Jan 2017.
Young, J. (2007). *The vertigo of late modernity.* London: Sage.

Chapter 9
Corporations, Taxation and Responsibility: Practical and Onto-Analytical Issues for Morphogensis and Eudaimonia – *A posse ad esse*?

Jamie Morgan and William Sun

Taxation is not a glamorous subject. However, it is an important issue for human flourishing in a variety of ways. Tax is part of the cycle of spending flows into and out of the state. It has an important economic function, but its economic significance is broader than simply national accounting. Tax represents a commitment to a system. It gives one a stake in that system, and is a signal to others that one is returning a fair share as part of the maintenance of that system. What is paid and how it is paid is, therefore, indicative of the fairness of the system and, as a corollary, whether the system is broadly representative and operationally effective. These are all matters of human flourishing, since they are indicative of commitments to economic welfare, democratic practices, participation, and matters of justice. As such, they are indicative of a political economy, within which we live and through which we seek to flourish. Concomitantly, the capacity to influence how tax is paid and what tax is paid is a potentially significant issue for how human flourishing is developed. This extends to the particular issue of corporation tax.

Corporate tax avoidance is antithetical to human flourishing, broadly conceived. It is an *anti-social* signal that undermines the sense of fairness of the system, as well as the legitimacy of that system, in so far as corporations are able legally to avoid tax. That they are able to do so is a systematic issue. It speaks to the cumulative power of corporations and this can have many adverse consequences,

---

A posse ad esse: from possibility to actuality.

J. Morgan (✉) • W. Sun
Faculty of Business and Law, Leeds Beckett University, Room 520 Rose Bowl Building, Leeds, LS1 3HB, UK
e-mail: j.a.morgan@leedsbeckett.ac.uk

M.S. Archer (ed.), *Morphogenesis and Human Flourishing*, Social Morphogenesis,
DOI 10.1007/978-3-319-49469-2_9

intended and unintended. According to the OECD, globally between $100 billion and $240 billion in tax is avoided per annum. The range is because of the difficulty of tracking what is not paid. Moreover, this is likely an under-estimation. The European Commission estimates avoidance and evasion for just the European Union at more than € 1 trillion per annum. There are also the many adverse consequences of an international system that facilitates avoidance. Tax havens do not just store wealth to avoid tax. They provide a system to siphon wealth from vulnerable nations, and also to launder the proceeds of organized crime, including human trafficking. According to the United Nations Office on Drugs and Crime, between $800 billion and $2 trillion is laundered through tax havens every year. Corporate tax avoidance is, therefore, not just a problem for human flourishing, it is also part of a system of human harm.

Tax avoidance, however is just one issue consequent to the context and significance of corporations. The corporation raises a variety of onto-analytic issues for morphogenesis and the prospects for and meaning of a Morphogenic Society, first raised by Lawson in Volume 3 of this series. The corporation has emerged as a significant relational entity. As a relational entity it has shaped and been shaped by its environment. It has recognizably undergone changes and so has been in process within processes. More specifically, there has been an intensification of some aspects of corporate behaviour, which can be connected to Archer's work on relational contestation. The reproduction of the corporation and its legal person status has become something of a self-reinforcing tendency. The law accepts and works with the ambiguity and contradictions of a non-conscious immaterial entity that has legal person status. It does so in order to manage difference. There is, however, a difference between managing difference and preventing increasing disintegration of a system over time. The problem of disintegration creates issues regarding how one addresses specific problems of growing corporate power. Tax avoidance is one important area to address. Addressing tax avoidance is one way to consider how modern capitalism may be modified to become more 'pro-social' rather than anti-social.

Tax avoidance can be addressed in at least two ways. First, one can contest dominant ideas, which serve to reproduce the conditions for tax avoidance, providing an ideological resource for movements of opposition. Second, and relatedly, one can provide substantive alternative policy approaches, which deny the opportunity for some forms of out-of-control or irresponsible behaviour to corporations. However, though one might describe these activities as positive moves within 'situational logics of action', it may well be that the consequences are changes rather than transformations. One constrains and partially reshapes the corporation. It then becomes an open question whether the consequences are part of processes that lead to a Morphogenic Society, and the degree to which this contributes to transforming the conditions for human flourishing. We consider this in the conclusion.

The Social Positioning or Placement of the Corporation[1]

In his Volume 3 paper Lawson follows a long line of analyses and critiques of the modern corporation (e.g. Bakan 2005; Picciotto 2011; Veldman and Willmott 2013; the Corporate Reform Collective 2014). His focus, however, is ontology (the 'nature' of the corporation). Corporations are particular instances of a 'bizarre' social positioning or placement, one that has arisen based on historical contingency, subject initially to some degree of resistance and to offsetting control mechanisms (illustrated by their roots in British law). The corporation is the bearer of rights originally intended to apply only to human beings (natural persons). Those rights can be legal, and so a natural person also has legal status. This status was then extended to non-profit making forms of organization in the form of the legal person. These were so that they could own property and capital, and operate in perpetuity for some social purpose, which it was deemed would be enhanced by taking ownership out of the hands of the particular persons who occupied roles in the organization (churches, monasteries, schools etc). This legal person is artificial/fictitious or juridical. Such legal person status was carefully controlled for many years.

However, a key transition occurred when between 1600 and 1615 the East India Company successfully converted itself from a trade association to a joint stock company, and so became a legal person that was also a business entity. Despite some problems thereafter, as the industrial revolution developed, the perceived need for the organization of capital led to a series of acts in the nineteenth century that confirmed, constituted, and legitimated the legal person status of the commercially oriented corporation (whose characteristics have then been transmitted around the world). These included: a corporation could be created by a standardised process of registration rather than by special application for a charter, the owners of shares in such a joint stock company need not hold a significant position within the corporation, and the shares of the corporation could be freely traded. Perhaps most importantly, a corporation acquired limited liability. That is, the owners of shares, in addition to the value of the shares, were not liable for the debts of the corporation, nor were the corporations liable for the debts of the owners of the shares.[2]

The emergent result is Lawson's 'bizarre' social positioning or placement. In terms of social ontology, the corporation can be described as a form of organization (a kind of community) with an internal set of structures of relations, which express

[1]In the Volume 3 paper, 'The modern corporation: The site of a mechanism (of global social control) that is out-of-control' Lawson refers to positioning, but subsequently also uses the term placement. Note the term positioning may inadvertently be read as a passive term for what is a diachronically contested relational form. This passivity is not Lawson's intent, but neither are the dynamics involved explicated.

[2]One might also note the ability to demand the enforcement of contract law as a primary right acquired by the corporation as a legal person.

its form as an organization. Those relations involve the positioning or placement of persons in roles, which provide them with some of their scope for agency, and that involve sets of rights and obligations. These are also outward facing since the corporation is nested in broader frameworks (further communities, that create more sets of relations, which are significant for the corporation in a variety of ways). The corporation is emergent as an organization - a recognizable relational entity within and with reference to these broader frameworks. Legal person status is a key property of the corporation. But it is a curious one (see also Pagano 2010; Robe 2011). Strictly speaking no one 'owns' a corporation, one owns shares in it:

> Ownership, like friendship, has many characteristics and if a relationship has enough of them we can describe it as ownership. If I own an object I can use it, or not use it, sell it, rent it, give it to others, throw it away and appeal to the police if a thief misappropriates it. And I must accept responsibility for its misuse and admit the right of my creditors to take a lien on it. But shares give their holders no right of possession and no right of use. If shareholders go to the company premises, they will more likely than not be turned away. They have no more right than other customers to the services of the business they "own". The company's actions are not their responsibility, and corporate assets cannot be used to satisfy their debts. Shareholders do not have the right to manage the company in which they hold an interest, and even their right to appoint the people who do is largely theoretical. They are entitled only to such part of the income as the directors declare as dividends, and have no right to the proceeds of the sale of corporate assets — except in the event of the liquidation of the entire company, in which case they will get what is left; not much, as a rule. (Kay 2015)

At the same time, an unstable form of personhood is attributed to the corporation. As the Lord Chancellor of England, Baron Thurlow, put it at the turn of the nineteenth century, the corporation has neither sentience nor a material body (see Coffee 1981). It cannot have a conscience and relies on the natural persons in key roles within it to act on its behalf. Yet it can claim the right to fair trial, and can sue for defamation, both of which would seem to imply a sentient entity able to suffer. In a contradictory sense, the corporation is typically deemed not to be capable of, and hence 'guilty' of or culpable for, forms of activity that require intent. In this context it is held to lack sentience as an entity (as well as a material form that could be imprisoned).

Of course, the legal system is relatively comfortable with contradiction and ambiguity, despite the precision that is also built into the codification of statute and is applied to case law. The law accepts contradictions and ambiguity, it rules in accordance with them and so also develops them. It does so because the law is itself referenced to wider political, social and economic concerns within which these contradictions and ambiguities serve some identified purpose. Moreover, the law as an institutional form is often intended to serve a meta-role in terms of systemic integration, which is no more than to suggest that the law is one way in which society is bound together. At the same time, relations are always also power relations, and a highly generalised ideological claim regarding the meta-function of law does not imply that its practice and development is in any given case actually coherent or consistent as a means for such integration. In real historical time one often observes a process where few if any participants intend to reproduce institutional coherence or systemic integration by their activity in terms of the law (though the law is seemingly there to manage this integration). Participants can work with contradictions and ambiguities on the basis that these seem in some sense to *become* necessary, whilst they also serve to develop and foster different groups' concerns and interests, which may be purposive and yet ultimately, through cumulative effects, reduce integration.[3] This is one way to consider Lawson's bizarre social positioning or placement based on the legal person status of the corporation and its contradictions and ambiguities.

The Perpetuation of Tensions in Legal Person Status

Consider, it is the case that the corporation has been granted (has won) the right to sue. This requires that the concept of 'suffer' be metaphorically mapped onto a commercial framework, where sentience seems superfluous. Specifically, the entity suffers an actual or potential material commercial loss, which the law will seek to quantify, but only because 'suffer' has become a matter of quantities rather than state of mind. The presumption is that if this loss could not be in general deterred in the context of malicious or false accusations, then economic activity as governed within the territory of the state may be undermined - given the structures of economy that have developed (where corporations have a significant presence, and hence impact on the economy).

For similar systemic purposes the non-sentience of the corporation is emphasised in the context of behaviour (primarily in a criminal but also in some ways in a civil context). Natural persons occupying key roles within the corporation take decisions. If the corporation is held culpable for decisions made by key personnel, then the existence of the corporation is put at risk, again with economic consequences (given the structures that have developed). Here, a persistent struggle has arisen regarding the development of law to deter those natural persons from taking decisions that may be deemed criminal or reckless. The argument takes place at the level of the person within the corporation who is deemed to be the relevant representative actor on behalf of the corporation. Key recent areas of concern have been the validity of reported accounts (in the context of fraud), and also the specific problems created by finance organizations. For example, in the US the Sarbanes-Oxley Act of 2002 followed a number of widely reported accounting scandals (notably Enron and Worldcom). The Act stipulates that senior executives are held individually responsible for the accounts of the corporation.[4]

---

[3]'Seems necessary' is an operative term, since the role of ideas raises issues of false necessity, discussed for example by Heikki Patomäki in terms of corporate power and more generally by Roy Bhaskar in terms of TINA formations.

[4]Specifically, Section 906 states that the CEO and CFO are required to sign off quarterly financial reports, and in so doing they confirm that those accounts 'fairly represent' the material financial condition of the corporation. If they sign 'knowing' this is not the case they face fines of $1 m to

Since 2008, the global financial crisis has also produced legislative and regulatory responses intended to create deterrent effects. The 2010 US Dodd-Frank Wall Street Reform and Consumer Protection Act introduced new regulatory oversight for the finance industry, and imposed new obligations and potential sanctions on senior executives of financial corporations. In the UK, the Financial Services Act of 2012 created a new Prudential Regulation Authority (PRA) within the Bank of England, and part of its remit is to liaise with the Bank's Financial Stability Committee with a focus on deterring reckless or irresponsible behaviour within financial organizations.[5]

In all these cases it has been typical for lobbying by corporations to occur (see Drutman 2015).[6] This is both during the period in which the statute is developed and also after, in order to modify, repeal or limit the application of the law. The general context then becomes one in which the form and implementation of the law is

---

$5 m and imprisonment for up to 10 years or up to 20 years, depending on the specific nature of the offence (executives can also have pay clawed back in later years for related offences).

[5]In Dodd-Frank, three key issues were the elimination of moral hazard (perceived incentives to take reckless decisions because the gains can be immediate, and the possible detrimental effects are either long term, uncertain or will be likely suffered or covered by others), the strengthening of internal 'risk' management procedures, and limitations on certain kinds of activities (notably on direct ownership of hedge funds and private equity firms in what is termed the 'Volcker Rule', see Morgan and Sheehan 2015). In 2014/15 the PRA proposed a 'guilty until proved innocent' rule for senior bankers. If and when the organization for which they act manifests problems that may be indicative of some form of reckless behaviour or malfeasance then executives would be subject to a reverse burden of proof. That is, they would have to demonstrate they had sought to prevent the consequences - the assumption being this would foster a greater focus on creating and monitoring the formal systems within the organization, as well as its internal 'culture', since the latter may otherwise undermine the former.

[6]According to Drutman, corporations report spending approximately $2.6 billion per year on lobbying the US Congress and Senate, which is more than both houses actually cost to run; corporations spend around $34 on lobbying for every $1 spent by other forms of organization (unions, civil society groups etc) and 95 of the top 100 lobby groups are corporations or their industry representatives. Katz (2015) also makes the case that corporate lobbying has increasingly captured democratic spaces in the US to the detriment of other interest groups (notably labour). The EU has a transparency register for organizations seeking to influence EU bodies, but registration is not mandatory. As of December 2015 the register had 8981 registrant organizations. According to the campaign-working group, Corporate Europe Observatory, there are at least 30,000 lobbyists working in Brussels (compared to 31,000 EU staff), and there is a widespread problem of revolving door employment of MEPs, with large corporations, and many corporate interests, dominating consulting and advisory committees for EU policy. Patronage and influence also works on a personal level. For example, *The Sunday Times* published a supplement 'Power, Politics, Money and Influence: The Political Rich List,' April 19th 2015. It identified 197 people who had appeared on its general Times Rich List who were also significant political donors. These 197 contributed £82.4 m to the three main political parties (the majority to the Conservatives) between 2011 and 2015, and this constituted approximately half of the total donations of £174.7 m donated over that period. Seven of the top 10 donors were ennobled, knighted or received a CBE. Notable multi-million donors include Lord Farmer, founder of the RK Management hedge fund (made senior treasurer of the Conservatives); Sir Michael Hintze, founder of the hedge fund CQS, and Michael Spencer, CEO of ICAP.

diluted with regards to its original intent. Put another way the reality of law becomes an expression of the concerns of those it was intended to affect, and so is affected by them. There have been few actual prosecuted cases under the Sarbanes-Oxley Act.[7] Both Republicans and Democrats (including John Kerry) have consistently criticised the Act and have done so based on the centrality of corporate activity to the US economy, from a point of view that reinforces the interests and concerns of corporations.

Specifically, the core debate has concerned the rise in costs to corporations due to compliance (creating 'transaction costs'), and the claim that a counter-productive climate of fear is created among executives. Both have seemingly resulted in new corporations undertaking their initial public offering (IPOs) in the UK or Far East, where there is no Sarbanes-Oxley equivalent, and also some existing corporations deregistering in the US and reregistering elsewhere for the same reasons. For opponents, Sarbanes-Oxley is damaging the US economy and its capital markets. But for this to be a reason to repeal it one is effectively arguing that it is better to have low or no standards (in the absence of global standards) and so suffer the possibility of criminal behaviour with fewer possible (real) sanctions. One is taking the position of the corporation (and its senior executives) as dominant or natural. It becomes *the* primary economic imperative, rather than balancing this with the concerns of other groups within society (who may suffer from any actual fraud - though this also is an economic issue and a social issue). The argument is in any case a curious contradiction where the opposition see the Act as both too successful and also not effective enough - since it has been opposed, delayed and limited throughout its existence.

One might also note that new law is often only the beginning of a process - it empowers a body to make regulations and implement codes of conduct. So, Dodd-Frank empowered an initial five US government agencies. There is then great scope for further dilution of law as it is developed by each agency, not least because specifics are usually developed through consultation with those to whom they are applied, and who typically give an opinion regarding form and feasibility. For example, in the case of risk management and compliance, senior executives at large financial corporations succeeded in modifying their obligation under Dodd Frank to one in which they sign off that they *have* compliance procedures in place, rather than that they *are* in fact compliant, since this creates an entirely different sense for future liability.[8] Similarly, in the case of the UK PRA, lobbying on behalf of the City

[7]Section 906 of the Act is problematic, since 'knowingly' creates a standard of evidence that is difficult to establish. Only particularly egregious cases are prosecuted. Concomitantly, as of 2015 there have been fewer than 50 cases where the US Securities and Exchange Commission (SEC) has sought to claw back pay from executives, and the first case was only brought in 2007. Section 404 of the Act (which requires auditors to give an opinion on internal financial control mechanisms - something which may later create a source of evidence) has never been fully implemented (having been consistently delayed by the SEC).

[8]Much as Sarbanes-Oxley is affected by 'knowingly'.

and via the British Banking Association has succeeded in modifying and diluting the burden of proof mechanism for the current Finance Services Bill moving into 2016.[9]

The Out-of-Control Corporation

What does this all suggest? As noted, the focus in terms of potential criminality and the legal person of the corporation has often been at the level of the natural person who occupies a key role within that corporation. Here, the sentience or otherwise of the corporation has effectively been put to one side (or is addressed mainly indirectly). At the same time, the deterrent-focused struggle over the degree to which the individual is to be held responsible on behalf of the corporation for particular behaviours has typically taken the need to secure the concerns and interest of corporations (as a generic) as a major reference point. It has done so within a basic association between the economic concerns of the state and the reproduction of the corporation (a semi-fictitious alignment).[10] To be clear this has not required the two to coincide in all cases. For example, the universal banks in the UK have been subject to a long series of adverse rulings regarding the enforceability of historical practices and contracts (notably payment protection insurance, and also derivatives products sold to small and medium sized enterprises), which has cost them billions in fines in recent year (and both UK banks and US former investment banks, now incorporated in universal banks, have been forced to settle a series of claims - typically out of court and without admitting full liability, regarding conflicts of interest with clients in the lead up to the financial crisis - again concerning derivatives - as well as scandals such as LIBOR, see Colledge et al. 2014).

However, it has become 'common sense' for the state to be concerned with what concerns corporations because they have significant economic consequences. The fact that other recognizable groups (civil society organizations, organized labour etc) may have concerns and economic consequences is not ignored. Often it is recognized but held to be subordinate to the corporate point of view - reconciled to or expressed via it or with reference to it. This is clear if one considers the way social and political issues are engaged as problems of good corporate

[9]Rather than a 'presumption' (where one must establish one sought to prevent adverse consequences) there is now a general 'duty' of responsibility for the organization's conduct. In real terms this is little different from previously - since it is inherent in the role of senior executive that one is acting on behalf of the corporation. One might also note that the annual bank levy was reduced by then Chancellor George Osborne, and ring-fencing of investment bank components has been scaled back; and one might note that during the same period Stuart Gulliver CEO of HSBC has been engaged in a review regarding shifting its base of operations to Hong Kong (a two year review process creates some scepticism regarding the real purpose of this review - would it make sense to shift one's headquarters to a place where China would have significant influence? And what information could still be outstanding after 2 years?).

[10]Implying also that the state has been to some degree captured by the concerns of corporations and so the two become more aligned - a key claim made on behalf of neoliberalism and governance.

governance and corporate social responsibility (see below). As such, whatever may occur to the individual executive and in particular cases (some prosecutions, some fines) the reproduction of the corporation and its legal person status has become something of a self-reinforcing tendency (again, see Drutman 2015). It manifests itself synchronically as recognition of the significance of corporations, and diachronically as a growing power of corporations (including through the way corporations are able to resist or dilute attempts to constrain them or deter their activity).

So, the law accepts and works with the ambiguity and contradictions of a non-conscious immaterial entity that has legal person status.[11] It does so in order to manage difference. There is, however, a difference between managing difference and preventing increasing disintegration of a system over time. This is so if one fails effectively to address the cumulative consequences, as processes occur. As Lawson has argued in social ontology terms, and many others have argued in terms of the law or economy or some other disciplinary orientation (again see Bakan 2005; Picciotto 2011; Veldman and Willmott 2013; the Corporate Reform Collective 2014): the existence of a legal person that does not itself have materiality, awareness, conscience or a consequent sense of *personal* responsibility creates the potential for that entity to ‘act’ without conscience or responsibility. That is, others can act within it and on its behalf according to mechanisms that drive it and in the corporation’s case the core focus of its mechanisms is profit. A focus on profit in the context of cumulative power creates the possibility that a corporation becomes, at the extreme, one that seeks to augment its profitability in ways that are relatively indifferent to how profit is made, and where the corporation is captured by a minority of actors who concentrate those profits in as few hands as possible (see Morgan 2015). So, the corporation becomes an organization (as a community) that can be potentially harmful and indifferent to the harm it does, since it is not adequately shaped within or constrained from without in terms of how profit is made (and how this is situated in relation to how much is made via how it is made, and how it is then distributed).

To be clear this does not mean there is an absence of recognition, critique, discussion, or policies directed at these issues. It means they are not working effectively. The suggestion is that the corporation is not itself in general an effective source of restraint or right conduct in terms of its activities. It lacks the property of consciousness qua deliberation. A corporation can then become one that is

[11]This might also be considered in terms of versions of corporate manslaughter. Here the corporation can be convicted of the crime that its activity (or failures to act) leads to a person’s death. The criminal standard applied differs from civil litigation. A financial penalty is applied to the corporation, but the ultimate threat of imprisonment is directed at key executives; few countries have a version of this law. It does, however, exist in the UK as the Corporate Manslaughter and Corporate Homicide Act, 2007. The test applied in the UK is management failure (a breach in a management system akin to gross negligence). The concept of corporate manslaughter has been criticised as expensive (punishing innocent shareholders), unnecessary (given the existence of civil litigation) and senseless - given the corporation lacks sentience and will not be held accountable in any real sense beyond the pecuniary (For underlying issues see Coffee 1981; also, Wells 2001: Chps, 4 & 6; for more adversarial critique see Tombs and Whyte 2015).

'out-of-control'. Significantly, it is not the case that the natural persons who occupy key roles in a corporation deny that they have responsibilities. It is not the case that the corporation lacks obligations as well as acquires rights. It is rather a problem of how responsibility is situated. *Having* a recognized responsibility and *taking* responsibility are not the same things. Who one is responsible *to* is also significant in the sense that how one prioritises concerns and whether one integrates them is also important.[12]

In contemporary capitalism corporations articulate and notionally respond to a set of interlocking and yet poorly integrated frames of ideational reference. As noted, familiar points of reference include corporate social responsibility, as well as good corporate citizenship, the concept of the sustainable corporation, positive leadership and so forth. At the same time, corporations articulate and to some degree manipulate the concept of shareholder value. That is, the claim that maximising returns to shareholders is the primary and overriding concern of the corporation (a contemporary variant on theory of profit maximisation).[13]

There is, however, no necessary requirement that the corporation as a legal person maximises 'shareholder value', nor do they do so in reality. The legal person has a series of (apologies for using a term few like but everyone recognizes) 'stakeholders' to which it may owe or be ascribed duties (and what this means is a *shifting* point of reference as culture changes and as the law evolves by statute and case, see Tench et al. 2012; Bainbridge 2012). At the same time, what is often termed financialisation has created pressure for the corporation to articulate and reproduce shareholder value as a primary legitimating language (from which senior executives also benefit, since compensation is now tied to equity values, and executives are also often partly paid in freely given share options, see for example, Lazonick 2015; Williams 2000). The *primary* tendency is now focused on returns or profits and how these profits are channelled. When phrased this way, of course, it seems no more than some simple market 'logic', and a logic that is not new. But its *practices* and context are new. The existence of, and persistent calls for, corporations to be 'responsible' over the last two decades is widely recognized to have occurred *because* many corporations are 'irresponsible' in these terms. The scope for them to be so is expanding, and this has continued despite the proliferation of responsibility literature and concomitant

[12]For example: '"Saint" Antony Jenkins was brought in to clean up Barclays as chief executive after the Libor scandal, but profits suffered. He was cleared out and is being replaced with Jes Staley, an investment banker on a £10 million package. The lesson: ethics and profits don't mix.' (Aldrick 2015)

[13]Though phrased in terms of shareholder value the point is actually more general. The same pressures occur in terms of private equity finance, where the private equity firms create an investment fund run by a general partner (from the firm) on behalf of passive investors (termed limited partners), the fund is then used in conjunction with debt to buy companies (originally public or private, but turned into private companies for some duration - these are termed acquisitions). See Morgan 2009. Note also, one should not conflate the concept of the firm or recognizable entity with the corporation per se - since the corporation is a legal structure which may be constructed precisely to disaggregate the firm into many corporations.

policies, commitments, and agendas *driven by* corporations (see Tench et al. 2012; Haldane 2015; Ireland 1999: 32–33).[14]

To be clear, Lawson and many others are not arguing senior decision makers are necessarily amoral individuals or that they lack power as significant actors or that there are no attempts within law, society, academia and commerce to constrain or shape the corporation in potentially positive ways. The suggestion is that the weight of actual changes through time have enhanced the power and influence of corporations and reduced the actual constraints on them (Lawson 2015: p. 228).

Corporations and Onto-Analytical Issues

The social positioning or placement of the corporation raises a number of issues for the concept of a Morphogenic Society. As a first step in exploring these it makes sense to contextualise this social positioning in terms of the work developed in the first four texts in the *Social Morphogenesis* series. The corporation has emerged as a significant relational entity. As a relational entity it has shaped and been shaped by its environment. It has recognizably undergone changes and so has been in process within processes. More specifically, there has been an intensification of some aspects of its behaviour based on its positioning.

One might, for example, connect this to Archer's claim that corporations have become key components in the relational contests that have gradually undermined the initial unstable morphostasis that occurred in the developed democracies after World War II (Archer 2013, 2014, 2015). Corporate agency has been exercised to develop the productive-output aspects of corporations (long supply chains, outsourcing, offshoring, new network's of collaborations and connections) and this has occurred whilst also developing the scope and activity of financial corporations, which have then fed back into the ownership structures and capacity to act of all corporations. Both have reconfigured relations to states and to international and global organizations and regulatory bodies (the EU, WTO, IMF, World Bank etc), creating transnational effects and a potential transnational positioning for the corporation. This is despite the fact that the organization in its parts is also incorporated somewhere. Here, it is important to differentiate between the firm or recognizable larger entity and its parts. A corporation is a legal person and can own assets, and this includes legally separated entities - other corporations that form part of the recognizable larger entity. In one sense the corporation operates in specific geographic localities, each subject to regulation and law. However, it is the capacity to influence jurisdictions, whilst also being able to be in many places and

[14]For critique of the empty rhetoric of much of CSR see Porter and Kramer 2006, and 2011. For the growing extent of CSR projects, agendas and mission statements among corporations see the periodic KPMG survey. For example, 93 % of the world's 250 largest corporations reported on CSR in 2013, compared to 80 % in 2008 (KPMG 2013: p. 10).

in alternative places that imbues the firm, the primary unit of the corporation (via incorporation), and then its legally separated entities, with a form of disciplinary power within the systems it is otherwise a part of.

Law has helped to create this situation, as has technology. As Archer also argues corporations have benefitted from the technological transformations (hardware and software) of the last few decades. New corporations that have developed new technology focused around information use (and restructured business models) have come to constitute a recognizable economic sector at the same time as they have transformed the infrastructure and scope for activity of economies in general.[15] Yet corporations from Microsoft to Amazon to Facebook and the new wave of billion dollar start-ups have remained relatively conformist or traditional in so far as they are still tied to corporate models of ownership, income, and profits (and shareholders and dividends). They are, as Gorski reminds us, part of the longstanding mechanism of capital accumulation (Gorski 2015). As such they can be differentiated from other actors within the development of the same technologies; those who advance other agendas based on the potentials of the technologies - the creative commons and digital diffusionists more generally.

One might state, then, that the dominant tendencies within modernity locate the corporation as primarily within processes of morphogenesis. That is, elaboration of existing conditions within which they operate, both structural and cultural. However, the primary form of the elaborations seems to involve change in order to stay, in many respects, the same (consider again Sarbanes-Oxley and the initial examples provided). Particular tendencies are being reproduced. For the corporation, it is the reproduction of its capacity to act with minimal restraints and subject to augmentation of profit potential (and concentration). So, morphogenesis is also a type of morphostasis under a different description of the processes (that is, elaboration to resist transformation understood as resistance to shifts in power, even as relations develop). Within that reproduction there is also variation created, both in terms of the means by which interests are pursued, and in terms of the consequences for many other identifiable groups within societies. However, variation may also be described as a common set of responses. In a following section we are going to consider tax avoidance by multinational corporations. This creates and exploits variety but is also a common practice by contemporary corporations (multiple strategies to the same effect based on tax treaty disjunctions that offer opportunities).

[15]Noting also that technology is not fate - it is not deterministic but used and developed within social relations that give meaning and purpose to technology. Moreover, if one takes a Kondratieff wave approach to the diffusion of fundamental technologies, and the way societies reconstruct around them, and then consider past instances (the steam engine, electricity, chemicals, transistors, microchips etc.) this has taken decades to occur, so even if one accepts that the digital revolution is a fundamental change - it may well be too early to have a clear sense of what its fuller impacts will be (despite there already being clear consequences). One might also note that a focus on the digital may neglect the other major sources of technological change currently occurring (notably hydrogen batteries, new varieties of solar panels, nano-technology and synthetics - graphene etc.). See also Lawson 2014: 34–44, for link to systems and corporations.

Such commonality of variegation is also an intensification of underlying tendencies - the pursuit of capital accumulation by the corporation. As such, elaboration as a form of intensification can be recognizably disintegrative in its consequences.

Note, that a system can be disintegrated is no more than an observation - it carries no necessary implications for what follows, except in so far as it creates problems of organization for a system. Disintegration is not necessarily destruction, nor is it necessarily decay, nor an immediate trigger for profound change. It may be destabilising, it may lead to an overriding emphasis on one interest, concern, or tendential manifestation - its elaboration - creating a positive feedback loop that then becomes an identifiable crisis. Yet this can lead to fixes or responses of one kind or another that manage the problem in some way, to prevent both collapse and the translation of crisis into genuine forms of transformation that eliminate the original sources of the problem. Disintegration implies no more than that the coherence, compatibility and consistency of aspects of some object of concern is being undermined even as it is reproduced.

Here, it is important to bear in mind both a general ontological claim and a specific claim about the nature of contemporary societies explored in the Morphogenic Society project. Critical realism recognizes that societies are emergent. As such the processes within them have specific qualities. Humans are always and everywhere potentially reflexive, and societies are dependent upon human activity. Processes are not, therefore, simply matters of impersonal forces acting on and through automata. They are not simply analogous to physical processes. Nor are they analogous to biological mechanisms, including natural selection. They are more than this because humans cannot be reduced to any given role or socialised position. Humans are thinking entities with reasons for acting, even when they are reproducing the conditions in which they find themselves rather than transforming them. This does not mean power is irrelevant or that the scope for activity cannot be restricted, but it does mean that people remain sources of power and that there is almost always scope for activity in the sense that things can be otherwise. Societies are not simply places that include norms as some kind of way things proceed, which we simply describe, they involve the construction and contestation of norms as ways we should live. Moreover, the claim made within the Morphogenic Society project is that current processes are in some sense incomplete within a period expressing a social form. We are still within modernity.

Controlling the Corporation

Lawson makes the case that the corporation involves a bizarre social positioning or placement and that the current forms of legal person status contribute through process to the corporation as 'out-of-control'. The corporation is often irresponsible and typically lacks integrated ethical deliberation as part of its decision set (despite the existence of many discourses focused on corporate social responsibility etc). His main purpose is to provide a social ontology approach to a basic question that strangely is rarely asked (what is a corporation?), and to do so as a contribution to exploring issues of intensification and disintegration within modernity. In the conclusion he notes that the corporation is currently mainly affected by regulation as 'relational steering' (iterating interests rather than challenging adverse consequences), but that something more systematic might be done. He briefly considers what the way forward might be - noting that any attempt at constructive change is likely to be met by the full force of corporate lobbying power, but that it might begin from strengthening the 'powers of resistance of natural persons'. There is a great deal more one might say here, which then leads to matters of human flourishing or eudaimonia (which we will return to in the conclusion).

If there is a bizarre social positioning or placement of the corporation, then the reasonable point of departure is to seek to *reposition* the corporation. Since the attribution of being 'bizarre' flows from the tensions inherent in legal person status then one way forward is to address the tensions of that status. Clearly one cannot render the corporation sentient or provide it with a conscience. Nor is it likely that one can in a single transformative shift simply dispense with the corporation as an entity (legal personhood is the basis of ownership and the corporation is now powerfully embedded). One can, however, address the specific ways in which the tension is operative in order to reposition the options open to the corporation i.e. what legal person status allows. This is a matter of reshaping the environment in which the corporation 'acts'. This can be pursued in many ways. Note, 'specific' need not mean fragmented or without collective or broader intent or effects. One can have in mind strategic and potentially transformative changes. One can, following Archer's terminology, address the dynamics of 'situational logics of action' (see e.g. Archer 2012: p. 35).

A key issue for corporations is that the ethical-normative potential, which could be integrated into how those corporations 'act' is currently undermined by the dominant ideational positioning of the corporation. This is not just an issue of what the law allows but of how corporations approach the law (often as a set of explicit codes to be influenced by lobbying and also to be approached as opportunities for exploitation where possible). One can respond in two related ways here. First, one can restructure the ideological landscape within which the corporation approaches the law - seeking to encourage the corporation to be responsible (to take responsibility and to acquire and articulate genuine obligations). This can be more than a line of least resistance form of corporate social responsibility rhetoric (where 'encourage' is divorced from some degree of meso-institutional discipline or compulsion), because it can be situated within democratic and wider ideological processes as cultural positioning - which are beyond the capacity of the corporation alone to shape or determine (noting again that this has been a problem with the corporate social responsibility literature - since it has been driven mainly by corporations - creating group think and capture - rather than by social movements, critical discourses from activist experts, and from *the demos*). Second, one can, through policy, transform the structures within which corporations make decisions, and so prevent some kinds of adverse (out-of-control, irresponsible) behaviour. This may then promote a more constructive socialisation of the corporation. Both raise the possibility of the pro-social corporation. Though each also involves some degree of scepticism regarding the sufficiency of such changes within capitalism as is.

Democracy, Tax and Human Flourishing

Let us consider the contestability of the ideological landscape first and do so in terms of the problem of corporation tax, since this provides something specific to shape the argument around. Currently, multinational corporations have the option of structuring themselves as a series of legally separate entities, where some of those entities are located in particular places in order to create the potential to minimise corporation tax. The other separate entities involved in the organization are connected to these strategically located entities through particular forms of relation. Generically, the organization is able to apply transfer pricing. That is, it is able to ascribe values to transactions between its parts. This is intra-firm behaviour, but also involves inter-corporation activity (based on separate entity status) in a legal context. In a certain sense, since the activity is intra-firm, it is ordinary, but it is open to abuse in so far as the organization can maximise the value of transactions in locations of low or no taxation. One can shift where the majority of sales, income, revenue and profits are reported.

In terms of international tax law, rooted in the OECD model tax treaty (that forms the basis of most international tax agreements between particular states), an arm's length principle and test(s) is applied to such transactions. The arm's length approach seeks to identify what a market-based version of the particular variety of transaction would have been and compares this to the actual transaction. This has proved increasingly difficult for state tax authorities to apply. There are many millions of transactions, there is not always a clear reference group of similar transactions that are market based (and even if there are, it is unlikely they will be of a perfect competition variety, but rather will exist in real and hence uniquely - from this fictitious referent - 'distorted' markets), and a great deal of the modern economy involves issues of potentially unique valuations for intellectual property, branding and so forth in a digital economy. As such, tax authorities find it difficult to keep up with the sheer volume of possible contestable transactions, and similarly difficult actually to bring cases where they can effectively contest valuations. Corporations are thus in a position of great opportunity to engage in tax avoidance - that is, the *legal* minimisation of tax that could otherwise have been paid. This creates a divergence for any particular country between the actual percentage rates of corporation tax it sets and the real rate that corporations - based on their broader organization pay.

Moreover, many further strategies that develop on from transfer pricing are also open to the multinational corporation. By decomposing into many corporations in different tax jurisdictions the firm can shift reported income and profits to low tax localities. It can further expedite this through licensing its brands, patents, and various paraphernalia to its separated entities. The royalties or fee paid can pass the majority of revenue to an entity in a low or no tax jurisdiction; and this can be done in stages - passing first to a corporation within a co-operative state as the primary holder of licences within, say, a trade bloc, and then passing on further to an additional recognized tax haven - since one entity can be provided with loans from another entity in a tax haven, and interest paid can pass the revenue on (whilst also perhaps creating tax credits based on debt structures in various places along the way).[16] So, a reality of lucrative organizations generating multi-billion revenues can become a set of accounts that express minimal income or profits for tax purposes (see Sharman 2010). For this to occur requires some complicity from states (something Palan 2002, for example, describes as the commercialisation of sovereignty), as well as from the large accountancy and consultancy firms (see Sikka 2015); and the potentials have been exacerbated by technology and by financialisation - creating an instance of what Seabrooke and Wigan (2014) term global wealth chain effects.

Fundamental to the whole process of tax avoidance is the existence of separate entity status, the potentials inherent in an arm's length principle, and also the privileged status of debt for tax purposes (see Picciotto 2011). As previously noted, according to the OECD (which likely underestimates the effects), between \$100 and \$240 billion in tax is avoided per annum (up to 10 % of corporation tax globally).[17] Different states are being denied revenue that could contribute towards reducing deficits and/or improving investment and welfare.[18] One might respond that the problem is relatively minor since corporation tax typically constitutes only a small proportion of the total tax take in a modern state (for example, it was just 7.1 % of total taxation in the UK for the tax year 2013–2014). But this is to neglect the ideational aspect of processes and consequences. One reason why corporation tax is a small proportion of total taxation is that headline corporation tax rates have steadily declined across the advanced capitalist countries during the neoliberal

[16]Note the term tax haven should be used advisedly - any state can be a tax haven from the point of view of another; moreover, the generic use of the term tends to give the impression that only a particular and limited set of localities are problematic as havens (e.g. the Cayman Isles or some of the Swiss cantons). However, these are destinations, what matters are the processes, and there are many other expediting localities - not least the main financial centres, such as the City of London.

[17]The figures include all corporations and so also include those that are effectively domestic firms only (as organizations), which are unable to use the same strategies. Moreover, since many havens do not report (though this is changing) accounts and corporations are able to manipulate their accounts - it is difficult to provide a definitive assessment of what is avoided. This is one reason why country-by-country reporting will be a major (if limited in some ways) policy change; as is the growing pressure on havens (led notably by the US) to improve their transparency.

[18]However, the argument here is conditional on how one conceives the state and money creation.

period.[19] Corporations have successfully lobbied for lower rates, and states have also engaged in competitive reductions in tax rates. Tax is now positioned more as a tool of competition policy rather than primarily as a signal of commitment and contribution of the payee to the state in which it is paid. This is important because we have become used to thinking of tax as primarily a component in a type of economy (a technical issue of margins and incentives and revenues), rather than as something broader and more socio-political. This itself is political and positional. Corporations attract criticism precisely because what they do is legal - tax avoidance. The capacity provokes a profound sense of injustice. When called to account, however, corporations respond that what they do is legal - they comply with the law (they pay legally required taxes).

There is, here, a basic problem of corporate responsibility regarding how rights are pursued and obligations are recognized. Representatives of the corporation often use the discourse of shareholder value to imply that they are simply doing what is economically reasonable, in terms of general tax behaviour. In so doing they resist, in this case, and this is particularly manifest when called before parliamentary or congressional committees, placing their activity in ethical context. They do not emphasise the difference in what they pay from what they *could* (and so perhaps subject to deliberative determination *should*) pay; that is, at minimum, the difference between the real corporate tax rates they pay and the state's headline rate (what is avoided). And they respond in ways that are essentially forms of misdirection (creating a disjuncture between tax behaviour and the corporate social responsibility and related policies they may articulate in other contexts - raising a clear issue that they may recognize responsibility in some ways but do not accept or take it in

[19]For comparison note how corporation tax as a % of total tax receipts in the US has declined over the last century, whilst income tax has not:

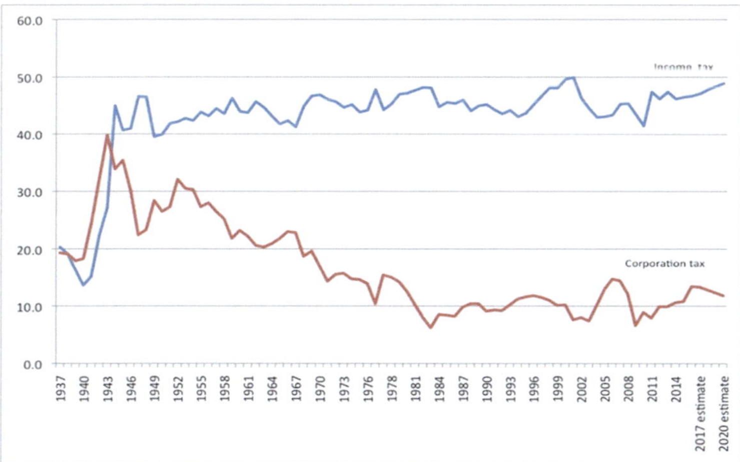

Source, Table 1: http://www.whitehouse.gov/omb/budget/Historicals/

others). Notably, there is a significant difference between the statements, 'we pay all legally required taxes' and 'we structure our activities to minimise the taxes we pay' (see Morgan 2016a).

Moreover, there is a further basic *legitimating* disjunction between how economic rationality is conceptualised (creating an unspoken supporting common sense notion of what is economic) and ethical as commercial behaviour. The economic theory of tax behaviour focuses mainly on evasion (where the law is broken rather than influenced, shaped and exploited), and is based on the seminal work of Allingham and Sandmo (1972). They adopt a form of rational calculation, based on a 'constrained expected utility optimisation' approach. Ethical considerations appear only as an ad hoc addition to the function based on the possibility of (unquantified) social pressure, rather than as an internal aspect of the deliberative socially relational human. So a form of tractable atomistic modelling is used to explore tax behaviour, one that marginalises concerns with ethics that might be explored in terms of institutions, justification, deliberation and genuine relationality. Most importantly this situates what it means to be economically rational. The basis of the model is an agent who calculates the probability of being caught evading tax in terms of the benefit of not paying the given sum. This may seem simply a neutral statement of what occurs, but it is actually an implicit set of assumptions regarding the behaviour of the *economically rational* agent. Specifically, it is permissible to break the law, and this is what one would do if not prevented (one is motivated to break the law). So, to be economically rational is to be criminal and subversive in terms of evasion. If translated into situations of avoidance, then the agent (the corporation) is manipulative and oppositional to the polity and society. Economic rationality becomes then tacitly anti-social.

In the context of observed multinational corporation behaviour, what one then has is an obfuscating context of economic theory. On the one hand, the point of theory is to identify and address adverse tax behaviour. On the other, the very terms of the behaviour occur in a context where there is a disjunction based on economic logic and theory: the corporation subject to pressures of shareholder value (sic) has an implicit duty to minimise tax, whilst the nature of economic rationality seems to position purely rational economic behaviour as extending this beyond paying the recognized rate of tax through the application of tax avoidance strategies. The problem, to be clear, is that economic theory fails to appropriately account for, describe and explain tax behaviour and then actually contest it in terms of 'being economic'. Argument is obfuscated based on the economics, and in order to address this one is required to move beyond the current economic approach - but this creates tensions and weaknesses - as though one were violating economic rationality by introducing ethical issues as part of the rationale. The point we want to emphasise here is that this is a problem all approaches to tax behaviour that draw on economics have confronted by since Allingham and Sandmo. Recent progress, for example, in the form of work on Tax Morale, is mainly rooted in behavioural approaches to economics and the law (Luttmer and Singhal 2014). These generally approach the problem by seeking to add 'non-pecuniary' components to the decision set of the agent. What they rarely do is contest the whole problem of ethical integration into economic issues based on the need for public deliberation and justification of actual practice (i.e. a frame of ideational-institutional reference in which the corporation is required to take responsibility). Economic theory has become part of the problem of context that affects the nature of the situational logic of action (and part of the problem is the ontology of economics followed by the developments and foci of the theory).

The broader problem or context here is the basic confusion over the nature of tax. This too is an ideational issue. As Richard Murphy, one of the founders of the Tax Justice Network, notes, a fundamental problem has developed in terms of how the concept of tax is positioned and perceived (2015). The standard way to think about tax is as a compulsory (compelled from the unwilling) contribution to the government, imposed on individuals and firms, where tax forms the basis of what the state can in the long term reasonably spend (as a trustee of what is essentially taxpayer's money). However, when one reflects on the nature of a modern democratic state, and also the reality of how money is created by the state (and in conjunction with the state through the banking system), all of this places taxation in a misleading context. Democratic government is not imposed on and resented by its citizenry, though there can be discontent, dissent and disillusion regarding the current particular state of democracy. Citizens recognize and value democracy and the protections, services and rights it provides. Taxation is recognized as an integral part of the existence of the state, and in general citizens pay tax willingly. The failure to pay is aberrational, encouraged by adverse socialisations, including via the concept of the self-interested economic agent. It is also rooted in the activity of think tanks, lobbyists, and professional specialists (within accountancy etc) whose agenda is to reduce the tax paid by interest groups (corporations and the wealthy). There is then a core problem that the failure of some to pay a fair share of tax corrodes the legitimacy of tax in general, and thus undermines the role of taxation within society, which in turn undermines the state and democracy, though curiously the argument is often made in the name of freedoms:

> When tax is defined as something we owe by compulsion to a government that is alien to us, out of property all of which is rightfully our own, then the claim can be made that tax avoidance and tax evasion are actions to prevent our own property being taken from us by duress. This affords cover to the tax abuser and those who assist them in their activities . . . [it] lets them claim they are doing a socially just act by preventing their property being taken from them - except for just one little problem, which is that such claims have very obviously been an affront to millions and millions of people in recent years . . . That is because most of us know that we are not alienated from government: the vast majority of us feel that to at least some degree our interests and its are closely aligned and that because of our power to participate in the democratic process, action to abuse the government is also action to abuse us. (Murphy 2015: pp. 43–44)[20]

[20]More specifically, Murphy argues that tax plays many key roles in a modern society, economy and polity. First and foremost, it gives citizens a sense they have a stake in society and the state (affecting legitimacy and consent, and affecting the degree of participation and sense of representation). Thereafter, it serves 5 other functions. Following modern monetary theory (and as the Bank of England now acknowledges), Murphy accepts that money creation is based on the

To be clear, Murphy's point is *not* that we fail to feel or express discontent with the actual state of government, but rather that the discontent derives from problems partly related to ideological misperceptions and practical consequences in terms of ongoing divisive policy and a consequent sense of antipathy. We are encouraged to be discouraged and to view the polity as an alien technosphere, which in turn creates greater scope for the structures of government to become technocratic and remote. This, however, runs counter to our underlying sentiment and to the interests of the majority. The real interest of the majority is to reclaim democratic spaces and to develop more effective participation and representation - to contest what is unjust rather than to conform to injustice by accepting a positioning of taxation that creates obfuscation. As such, revealing the problem is actually a resource that recontextualises our relation to the state and redirects our activity in regard of its failings. This is necessarily in opposition to those who would undermine the state's potentially productive role via greater participation and engagement, and this includes issues of tax avoidance and taxation.

So, there is then a whole range of resources available, which provide ways to contest the ideological framing of corporate tax behaviour. That contestation arises in ways that exceed the capacity of corporations to engage in capture or control (a recognized problem for much of the corporate social responsibility literature).[21] Moreover, these ideational resources are related to *existing* social movement activity and to activist-expert networks. Much of this is international in orientation, and focused on alliances and collaborations to construct benchmarks, or on persistent situated critique to reveal actual states of affairs, that otherwise may attract little attention (see Seabrooke and Wigan 2015, 2016). Over time this activity can be highly effective in creating spaces and potentials for alternatives. For example, the Tax Justice Network has done a great deal to maintain pressure on governments to address problems of tax havens and corporate activity. Richard Murphy has done a great deal to develop country-by-country reporting and this has now been adopted via the OECD by the G-20, to be implemented by 2017. Such reporting requires corporations to provide consistent full and detailed accounts for the territories in which they are incorporated. This will make it more difficult for corporations to engage in tax evasion and will create more information in order to address tax

---

state's capacity to spend in an economy, and the banking system further creates money through lending, which in turn creates matching savings (so it is wrong to assume that it is tax that creates the capacity to spend, and it is wrong to assume that it is deposits, which create the capacity to lend; institutional contexts rather limit the nature of spending and lending). So, tax serves the economic functions of: 1. Reclaiming money the state has spent in the economy (rather than creating the basis on which the state spends); 2. Legitimates the state denominated medium of exchange (the currency used), since it is the form used to pay taxes; 3. Provides a means by which the state intervenes in the economy to affect the levels of activity; 4 Provides a means for the government to engage in distribution and redistribution of income and wealth; 5. Allows the state to re-price goods and services for social purposes (encouraging some forms of socio-economic activity and discouraging others - taxes on petrol, smoking etc).

[21] Though this has not meant it has been conceived as necessarily anti-capitalist, anti the corporation etc.

avoidance. However, it does not directly address the context within which avoidance is made possible (separate entity status and reliance on an arm's length test). Here, members of the Network also advocate what is termed unitary taxation (see Picciotto in particular). This provides an example of policy that has the potential to transform the structures within which corporations make decisions, and so prevent some kinds of adverse (out-of-control, irresponsible) behaviour (the second issue we raised at the beginning of the section).

Basing taxation on separate entity status subject to an arm's length test encourages firms to decompose into a chain or circuit of corporations, some of which are strategically located to benefit from low or no taxation. Unitary taxation, directly addresses this problem (Morgan 2016a). Rather than simply taxing income, revenue and profit where it is reported, unitary taxation treats the entire multinational corporation as a single entity for tax purposes. The entity produces a single set of aggregated master accounts and these are reported to a designated tax authority. A proportion of the total income or profit is then allocated to the individual states, within which the entity is incorporated, based on some universally agreed formula. Crucially, the formula apportions on the basis of some measure of real economic activity or presence in the various states. Typically, the formula includes measures of sales, employment and non-financial assets. That is, the value of capital as a proxy for the scale of manufacturing or service delivery. The apportioned income or profit is then subject to tax in the given locality based on the rates the state applies. The primary advantage of unitary taxation is that it renders manipulative transfer pricing and also use of licensing (and potentially debt structures) redundant. Taxation is based on economic presence, rather than where income is shifted to for reporting purposes. This transcends the problems of applying an arm's length test and of contesting avoidance on a case-by-case approach, which simply encourages the mutation of strategies based on loopholes. One might note here that there are already several forms of unitary tax in existence within the US and Canada, and also advanced plans to implement a version of unitary tax within the EU.

Unitary taxation is an example of a policy that transforms the structures within which corporations make decisions. It prevents some kinds of adverse (out-of-control, irresponsible) behaviour. It thus creates a framework within which corporations may be encouraged to adopt more ethical approaches that are integrated into economic aspects of decision-making. However, it does not guarantee this, since there is a difference between denying an avenue for a given behaviour type and changing the perspective of the firm with regard to their behaviour. Unitary taxation cannot stand-alone.[22] For example, one must also address the degree of consent of corporations to the system within which they are active (a system in which one is compelled is operatively different from one to which one consents - as tax collection from the majority of ordinary citizenry indicates). However, one should not neglect that the implementation of unitary taxation potentially restores some degree of sovereignty to the state in respect of corporations, since it reduces the capacity of

[22]It functions best as an international (regional) or global system.

the corporation to trade off one state against another in order to capture reported revenues; though the problem may now recur in terms of lobbying for special treatment and exemptions within a unitary system. Whether it does so will depend to some degree on how democratic spaces are occupied by groups that oppose or resist this kind of activity (and this is something that is liable to have occurred to some degree based on the social movement momentum required to implement unitary taxation in the first place). Furthermore, it is worth remembering that neoliberalism began as a knowledge sharing and institutional project building-exercise. Any policy change that contests its current form must begin in the same way. This is precisely what it means to contribute to the construction and contestation of norms as ways we should live.

It may perhaps seem bizarre in quite a different way to refer to tax as an issue of human flourishing than it did to the social positioning or placement of the corporation. But this is to miss the point, it is the activity as a specific instance of a more generalised process that matters. Challenging corporate tax behaviour is an instance of constructive elaboration in response to the disintegrative tendency of current activity. It depends on reasoned intervention (activity), following forms of critique that recognize the significance of ethics (and are motivated by concerns with justice and fairness, pursued based on conviction qua virtues that are the emotive engine of those motives). *The very process thus embodies the kinds of activity recognized as human flourishing and is also directed at promoting human flourishing.* One may wince at the prospect of possible neologisms but this is more a matter of an unfounded philosophical superiority complex than it is a genuine substantive denial that there is a eudaimonic dimension to specific activity *of* human concern within the context of ultimate concerns.

Conclusion: The Morphogenic Society, *a posse ad esse*

As this and the previous volumes indicate, contributors to the 'From Modernity to Morphogenesis?' project explore and emphasise different aspects of possible issues for a Morphogenic Society. The main issue arising from this paper is whether capitalism is susceptible of modification such that it can be more 'pro-social'. Profit and the systemic dynamics of capital accumulation create at the very least a basic tension based on articulated interests. This has become a concomitant problem based on the social positioning or placement of the corporation. It invokes, for example, the kinds of issues Al-Amoudi and Latsis have previously addressed in terms of morphonecrosis (though perhaps with the possibility of Lazarus effects). One might ask, to what degree might one fundamentally change rather than simply seek to control the corporation? Clearly, there is no simple answer to this kind of question. It raises further issues regarding transitions that may be considered transformative in some ways but not others, and whether there are limits to reform. One might, for example, read any successful policies regarding corporations as forms of fixes that manage or temporarily reconcile disintegrations. There is, additionally, something of the problem of 'better-best' about the general issue of changing aspects of capitalism within and beyond modernity. Is the corporation improvable? Manifestly yes. Are there better ways to organize an economy and capital than the corporation, and capitalism as we know them? Many would argue yes.

It is worth noting here also that even if one takes a sceptical position, where the traditional corporation can only be controlled rather than transformed in some more basic sense, then there is still scope for considering the role of interventions as constructive in terms of the prospects for human flourishing. The corporation is a significant aspect within modern capitalism and modernity, and social reality remains one of process. As such, any shift in the character of the corporation that affects power affects also the relative situation of the corporation in relation to other and broader processes.

The end of a social form does not require any particular recognition of its end or coherent plan to bring about its demise. At the same time, particular purposive challenges to the current tendencies of parts of broader wholes may influence transformation, not least by reducing the capacity of significant parts, such as corporations, to effect changes around them to stay the same (the problem of elaboration to resist transformation, understood as resistance to shifts in power, even as relations develop). Furthermore, transformation and emergence are threshold phenomena, new forms *come into* being, but barriers to transformation can be in their own way as significant as the constituting components of what may come into being. Modernity has not simply dissolved or become 'liquid'. However, the most basic consequences of modernity and contemporary capitalism increasingly seem to demand fundamental transformations merely to ensure the reproduction of our species.

Modern capitalism is based on ecologically unsustainable practices. This is no longer in dispute, what is disputed is the timeline within which solutions can be implemented, what those solutions will be and who will take responsibility for implementation (Morgan 2016b). Modern capitalism also seems to be increasingly subject to a different kind of unsustainable tendency. Low or slow wage growth and increasing job insecurity have spread throughout economies. Moreover, an imminent technological transition based on robotics and 'learning algorithms' is widely recognized as likely to result in a new swathe of displacement of human labour. If this occurs within existing capitalism then there will be a further intensification of the problem of how a capitalist economy is reproduced, since the future economy may not require labour but it does require wage earners in order to consume what is produced. Growing inequality (within states) and the absence of employment (which may be different than mere unemployment) require solutions no less than do ecological problems. There are already arguments for de-growth and steady state economies, as well as technology induced forms of post-Capitalism (see Gillies 2015, on Mason).[23] It should also be noted that the problems arising are pervasive rather than particular. They do not stop at borders, but they are made more problematic by the existence of borders. More fundamentally, the need for solutions to problems, the addressing of which cannot simply be deferred indefinitely (because they are intrinsically problematic for the basic reproduction of societies) seem to require us to think and act differently *as a species*. Morphogenesis is in many ways a term for acting differently. One might then also argue that any response to the varieties of fundamental problems already embedded in our ways of living will need to be Morphogenic by form in order to be *both* pervasive and effective.[24] So a Morphogenic Society may well be increasingly likely, at least in so far as it is one defined by engrained elaborative responses to elaboration. Whether more and diverse morphogenesis is also a medium for human flourishing may be conditional in additional ways - not least how we deal with what seem to be imminent universal problems of technological transformation and environmental effects. Such problems speak directly to the need to respond to the world we have changed.

References

Aldrick, P. (2015). Business leaders must do their fair share to protect capitalism. *The Times* November 4th.

Allingham, M., & Sandmo, A. (1972). Income tax evasion: A theoretical analysis. *Journal of Public Economics, 1*(3–4), 323–338.

Archer, M. S. (2012). *The reflexive imperative in late modernity*. Cambridge: Cambridge University Press.

Archer, M. S. (2013). Social morphogenesis and the prospects of morphogenic society. In M. Archer (Ed.), *Social morphogenesis*. Dordrecht: Springer.

Archer, M. S. (2014). The generative mechanism re-configuring late modernity. In M. Archer (Ed.), *Late modernity*. Dordrecht: Springer.

Archer, M. S. (2015). How agency is transformed in the course of social transformation: Don't forget the double morphogenesis. In M. Archer (Ed.), *Social morphogenesis: Generative mechanisms transforming late modernity*. Dordrecht: Springer.

Bainbridge, S. (2012). *Corporate governance after the financial crisis*. Oxford: Oxford University Press.

Bakan, J. (2005). *The corporation* (new ed.). London: Constable and Robinson.

Buxton, N., & Hayes, B. (Eds.). (2016). *The secure and the dispossessed*. London: Pluto Press.

[23]Digital goods include all forms of product that are information basic - software and electronic games, research, novels, media, music, film, social media, etc. A digital economy is one where digital goods are distributed or transmitted, and includes platforms which serve as means for other forms of goods and services to be exchanged.

[24]However, there is no reason why this must be flourishing for all, it may simply be flourishing for the few. Some are already exploring the way current tendencies are encouraging various powerful actors to plan preservation solutions that are intrinsically militaristic, authoritarian, conflict-based and isolationist (Buxton and Hayes 2016).

Coffee Jr., J. (1981). "No soul to damn, no body to kick,": An unscandalized inquiry into the problem of corporate punishment. *Michigan Law Review, 79*(3), 386–459.
Colledge, B., Morgan, J., & Tench, R. (2014). The concept(s) of trust in late modernity, the relevance of realist social theory. *Journal for the Theory of Social Behaviour, 44*(4), 481–503.
Corporate Reform Collective. (2014). *Fighting corporate abuse: Beyond predatory capitalism*. London: Pluto.
Drutman, L. (2015). *The business of america is lobbying: How corporations became politicized and politics became more corporate*. Oxford: Oxford University Press.
Gillies, D. (2015). Paul mason's postcapitalism. *Real World Economics Review, 73*, 110–119.
Gorski, P. (2015). Causal mechanisms: lessons from the life sciences. In M. Archer (Ed.), *Social morphogenesis: Generative mechanisms transforming late modernity*. London: Springer.
Haldane, A. (2015). 'Who owns a company?' Speech, University of Edinburgh Corporate Finance Conference, May 22nd; Bank of England Publications
Ireland, P. (1999). Company law and the myth of shareholder ownership. *The Modern Law Review, 62*(1), 32–57.
Katz, A. (2015). *The influence machine: The US chamber of commerce and the corporate capture of american life*. New York: Random House.
Kay, J. (2015). 'Shareholders think they own a company – They are wrong,' *Financial Times* November 10th.
KPMG. (2013). *The KPMG Survey of Corporate Social Responsibility Reporting 2013* KPMG; accessed 7th Dec 2015; available at: https://www.kpmg.com/Global/en/IssuesAndInsights/ArticlesPublications/corporate-responsibility/Documents/corporate-responsibility-reporting-survey-2013-exec-summary.pdf
Lawson, T. (2014). 'A speeding up of the rate of social change? Power, technology, resistance, globalization and the good society' In M. Archer (Ed.), *Late modernity*. London: Springer.
Lawson, T. (2015). The modern corporation: The site of a mechanism (of global social control) that is out-of-control. In M. Archer (Ed.), *Social morphogenesis: generative mechanisms transforming late modernity* (pp. 206–230). London: Springer.
Lazonick, W. (2015). 'Stock buybacks: From retain-and-reinvest to downsize-and-distribute,' Center for Effective Public Management at Brookings, April; accessed 18th August, available at: http://www.brookings.edu/~/media/research/files/papers/2015/04/17-stock-buybacks-lazonick/lazonick.pdf
Luttmer, E., & Singhal, M. (2014). Tax morale. *Journal of Economic Perspectives, 28*(4), 149–168.
Morgan, J. (2009). *Private equity finance: Rise and repercussions*. Basingstoke: Palgrave Macmillan.
Morgan, J. (2015). Piketty's calibration economics: Inequality and the dissolution of solutions? *Globalizations, 12*(5), 803–823.
Morgan, J. (2016a). Corporation tax as a problem of MNC organizational circuits: The case for unitary taxation. *British Journal of Politics and International Relations, 18*(2), 463–481.
Morgan, J. (2016b). Paris COP21: Power that speaks the truth? *Globalizations, 13*(6), 943–951.
Morgan, J., & Sheehan, B. (2015). Has reform of global finance been misconceived? Policy documents and the Volcker Rule. *Globalizations, 12*(5), 695–709.
Murphy, R. (2015). *The Joy of tax: How a fair tax system can create a better society*. London: Bantam.
Pagano, U. (2010). Legal persons: The evolution of fictitious species. *Journal of Institutional Economics, 6*(1), 117–124.
Palan, R. (2002). Tax havens and the commercialization of state sovereignty. *International Organization, 56*(1), 151–176.
Picciotto, S. (2011). *Regulating global corporate capitalism*. Cambridge: Cambridge University Press.
Porter, M., & Kramer, M. (2006). Strategy and society: The link between competitive advantage and corporate social responsibility. *Harvard Business Review, 84*(12), 78–92.
Porter, M., & Kramer, M. (2011). Creating shared value: How to reinvent capitalism – And unleash a wave of innovation and growth. *Harvard Business Review, 89*(1/2), 62–77.

Robe, J. (2011). The legal structure of the firm. *Accounting, Economics and Law, 1*(1), 2–86.
Seabrooke, L., & Wigan, D. (2014). Global wealth chains in the international political economy. *Review of International Political Economy, 21*(1), 257–263.
Seabrooke, L., & Wigan, D. (2015). How activists use benchmarks: Reformist and revolutionary benchmarks for global economic justice. *Review of International Studies, 41*(5), 887–904.
Seabrooke, L. and Wigan, D. (2016) Powering ideas through expertise: Professionals in global tax battles *Journal of European Public Policy, 23*(3), 357–374.
Sharman, J. (2010). Offshore and the new international political economy. *Review of International Political Economy, 17*(1), 1–19.
Sikka, P. (2015). No accounting for tax avoidance. *Political Quarterly, 86*(3), 427–433.
Tench, R., Sun, W., & Jones, B. (Eds.). (2012). *Corporate social irresponsibility volume 4: A challenging concept*. Emerald: Bingley.
Tombs, S., & Whyte, D. (2015). *The corporate criminal: Why corporations must be abolished*. London: Routledge.
Veldman, J., & Willmott, H. (2013). What is the corporation and why does it matter? *Management, 16*(5), 605–620.
Wells, C. (2001). *Corporations and criminal responsibility*. Oxford: Oxford University Press, second edition.
Williams, K. (2000). From shareholder value to present-day capitalism. *Ecology and Society, 29*(1), 1–12.

Chapter 10
Networks and Commons: Bureaucracy, Collegiality and Organizational Morphogenesis in the Struggles to Shape Collective Responsibility in New Sharing Institutions

Emmanuel Lazega

Towards New Commons in a Bureaucratized Society

The current context for human flourishing is bleak: global warming and major extinctions caused by human action, triggering mass migrations, complex wars and the spread of global destructive capacity. Triumphant and ruthless capitalism armed with large bureaucracies (i.e. control, rationalization, technocracy and efficiency in mass and routine production), deregulated markets and a productivist growth mystique has led to predatory exploitation of the environment, to concentration of powers and to extreme levels of inequality in all domains. For example, the institutional framework of contemporary capitalist economies has been strongly influenced by liberalization policies initiated in the late 1970s: financialization of the economy, privatization of public services and withdrawal of the state, development of widespread, multilevel anormative regulation (Archer 2016). The prospect of being short of time for the transition to different kinds of societies, if not of big calamities and/or self-destruction by humanity going about its business as usual, is no longer fiction.

These contemporary challenges should lead to deep changes in civilizations. In other words they require institutional changes to begin with. Economists propose ever more markets to deal with the problem. There are not enough property rights on watersheds, biodiversity or traditional knowledge, for example, and therefore people do not care about them, overexploit them freely or let them disappear. Bring in more individual property rights. The market value for such goods will help individual or corporate owners price them properly and eventually protect them. Governments should make sure their dozy civil servants stay awake to regulate the quality and use

E. Lazega (✉)
Sciences Po, Centre de sociologie des organisations (CSO), CNRS. Sciences Po is a member of USPC, 19 rue Amélie, Paris 75007, France
e-mail: emmanuel.lazega@sciencespo.fr

M.S. Archer (ed.), *Morphogenesis and Human Flourishing*, Social Morphogenesis,
DOI 10.1007/978-3-319-49469-2_10

of these goods. Prices and inequalities will decrease, quality will increase, and of course this would not depend upon who governs. The purpose of this chapter is not to criticize this strange music that the world has listened to for too long. It is to ask whether sociologists can be more useful in thinking about institutional changes that are needed to manage local and global commons. For example, how such changes will be morphostatic or morphogenetic (Archer 2013), and why.

For current societies, a drastic decrease in the amounts of many kinds of resources for an increasing number of people, with growing inequalities in access and hoarding of opportunities, will make sharing increasingly difficult, even for non-rival goods. Bureaucratic mass markets having failed, who will survive which restrictions in energy, water, food and forests, as well as all the indirect costs that will come attached to such restrictions and/or the long list of horrendous events listed above? Many still believe in/hope for technological innovation as a possible solution for a smooth transition. But it is obvious that even with technological innovation, social innovation will be necessary. Social structures built for periods of growth and limitless resources will disappear. For the many the stakes are high. The proportion of losers in these upcoming changes is so high that the usual techniques for adaptation to incremental changes will probably not work. Deregulated markets may well be replaced by centrally -if not militarily- enforced quotas and parametrized commons. A great number and variety of new institutions, for example new forms of adaptable commons –including knowledge commons (Ostrom 1990; Hess and Ostrom 2007)– are needed, that can resist all sorts of enclosures and exclusivism and define their own form of collective responsibility.

The definition of commons used here refers to both shared resources in which members of a community have an equal interest, including the common pool resource institutions (Ostrom 1990) that are needed to manage these shared resources. Beyond Ostrom's formal approach, this institution includes the social rationality and the social capital on which this institution must count for its rules and conventions actually to work. Social rationality is encapsulated in shared kinds of appropriateness judgments (Lazega 1992) and the social capital of the community combines the social processes that help members manage the dilemmas of their collective actions (Lazega 2006): these social processes include bounded solidarity and exclusions, socialization and collective learning, social control and conflict resolution, and regulation and institutionalization (Lazega 2003). This social capital is shared by the members as a form of concrete social discipline that they recognize as legitimate. In this approach, common pool resource institutions can be local, or extend beyond the local, across boundaries, as in the case of the environmental commons or knowledge commons.

It may well be that militaristic responses of ruthless authoritarian regimes controlled by small coopted elites with their own private armies will help the few in managing freely their own commons and subject the many and their commons to destructive forms of collective responsibility. After all, the nation States have not been able to react to global financial crises in efficient and credible ways. They may not be able to manage worse crises, such as big environmental ones, more efficiently. This chapter looks at the possibility of a different solution, one that recognizes the many and their commons that are in danger of being left out of the system. It looks at how the rights of the many may be redefined – without idealizing future sharing institutions that may also be remote-controlled bureaucratically, and heavily taxed, by the predatory few.

The scenario is the following. Survival requires institutional changes. Among such changes, the bottom-up emergence of new cooperatives and commons became a legitimate goal at the level of the planet, and officially recognized by the United Nations at the turn of the twenty-first century. The number of organizations, public and/or private, set up for local collective management and collective responsibility in sharing scarce (re-)collectivised resources is increasing in most societies. Such commons operate based on what sociology calls collegiality, building on committee systems and consensus work among peers but also on diverse forms of social discipline that are considered legitimate by participants. These forms come attached to collective responsibility that is based on using personalized relationships to manage the dilemmas of collective action (Lazega 2001). Collegiality as an organizational form is based on self-governing by personalized relationships. The specific social discipline of collective responsibility that come attached to this organizational form have been described, for example, among professionals (lawyers, scientists, judges, priests, etc.). They have been studied in relation to collective action where tasks are non-routine (Waters 1989). In this form, which is not democratic,[1] coordination is carried out by 'peers' evaluating each other's legitimacy and governing themselves using networks and social capital defined as a set of social processes[2] (solidarity, control, socialization, regulation) facilitating collective action, all based on 'relational infrastructures'[3] (niches and status) (Lazega 2003, 2015a, b) and measured by social networks (Lazega 2001, 2012, 2016).

Indeed, as any form of commons is about collective self-management and sharing of collective resources, the outlook on such institutional changes is a neo-structural and organizational perspective on collective action (Lazega 1994). To measure and model the social capital of the collective, it is necessary to reason beyond 'embeddedness' studied in Granovetter's sense (1985). In organized settings, participation in non-routine collective action – for example, for team production, regulatory activity, or enforcement of previous agreements – requires personalized cooperation with others. This cooperation is expressed through personalized transfers/sharing or exchanges of various kinds of resources, as well as in commitments to exchange partners. These resources include, for example, information, coworkers' goodwill, advice, sometimes emotional support, and many other means that can serve individual and collective ends. From a neo-structural perspective, this means that

[1]"There is absolutely nothing 'democratic' about collegiality. When the privileged classes had to guard themselves against the threat of those who were negatively privileged, they were always obliged to avoid, in this way, allowing any monocratic, seigneurial power that might count on those strata to arise" (Weber 1978:362; see also Musselin 1990).

[2]For social capital as a set of relational processes and capacity for collective action, in particular for managing the conflicts and dilemmas of collective action, see Lazega (2001, 2006).

[3]For analytical definitions and methodological procedures to identify relational infrastructures in empirical work, see for example Lazega (2001, 2016).

specific local (uniplex or multiplex) sub-structures of social ties must be organized so that members can cooperate and exchange on an ongoing basis. Such cooperation is not based on purely moral virtue but on personalized interdependencies and the need to manage them strategically even in highly conflictual situations.

Creating a form of social discipline that is considered legitimate by actors relies on the stimulation of a social rationality[4] without which the fundamental social processes enabling collective action and the management of its conflicts and dilemma are meaningless for members involved. Social discipline characterizes both the individual and the collective level of agency. From the point of view of the individual, social discipline is the ability of actors to self-restrict themselves in the course of their negotiation with others, in the definition of their own individual interest and the scope of its claims, as well as in the exercise of their own individual power – notably their power to exploit. This self-restriction is an outcome of the politicization of exchanges in the relational infrastructures. Social niches and endogenous forms of status are structural forms that directly contribute to the management of interdependencies, to hoarding opportunities and to the durability of inequality. But they can also facilitate social mechanisms that help members manage the dilemmas of their collective actions in the organizational society. It is important to know that creation and maintenance of relational infrastructures (niches and status) trigger changes in social processes downstream, including regulation and institutionalization.

One of the ways in which the question of the nature of this social discipline can be addressed is by acknowledging that such changes take place in an organizational society that has been structured by two centuries of Weberian bureaucratization, i.e. governing by routinization of tasks (including by technology), hierarchy, valuation of impersonal work relationships, use of organizations as "tools with a life of their own" (Selznick 1949). This question can thus be translated into another: What kind of combination of this bureaucracy -the default organizational form- and forms of collegiality emerging with new commons can we expect? What is the nature of the interactions between bureaucracy and collegiality when solving particular problems of collective action and collective responsibility. How do these organizational forms mix and interact? Two kinds of combinations of these ideal-typical organizational forms have been examined empirically: Collegial boards of directors and executive teams at the top of (large) bureaucracies, and professional collegial pockets within large bureaucracies (Bosk 1979; Freidson 1986; Lazega and Wattebled 2011). Here I argue that bureaucracy and collegiality could drive each other's evolution in ways that may turn out to be morphegenetic in the sense defined by Archer (1995, 2013, 2015). In order to contribute to understanding these dynamics this chapter looks at an example of one articulation between bureaucracy and collegiality, leaving open the question of whether institutional changes ahead will indeed be morphogenetic.

---

[4]See Lazega (1992, 2014a) about the specificity of this social rationality, i.e. actors' reflexive and critical ability to contextualize their behaviour using appropriateness judgements that endogenize social structure and allow for building a real rapport with institutions, becoming institutional entrepreneurs experimenting with new solutions to the dilemmas of collective action.

Analyzing a potentially morphogenetic struggle between two organizational forms could help in trying to figure out what new sharing and taxing institutions may look like in the future. In particular, the collegiality of the commons of the many will have to interact with centralized bureaucracies dominated by the few and controlling the channelling of resources to local commons – if such a channelling takes place for co-optation purposes. Knowledge of these interactions may be useful when the many will try to protect themselves from the list of horrendous calamities detailed above by setting up new commons that may not be functional, viable and efficient if they do not interact in new ways with these centralized bureaucracies managed by the elites. The fact that common resources will be taxed by a centralized macro - level bureaucratic system raises the issue of effectiveness when the commons will in fact represent resistance of the many against the bureaucratic and military tools of the few.

Indeed the kind of collegial organization that many all too often idealize (in spite of the damages that hyper-personalized work relationships can create (Sainsaulieu 1977), including conflicts of interests, patronage and clientelism) and aspire to to some degree, is continually crowded out by markets and States (Lazega and Mounier 2002). One of the potentially tragic ironies here is that members often do not like the discipline of collegial organizations and are attracted to markets as a promise of escaping from this discipline. But they do so at the cost of exhausting the social capital and social trust that produce an alternative to the military path: from a sociological perspective, market emancipation and overkill can eventually lead to such a military path being taken. By the time we are facing this market plus/vs military question, might there be enough little seeds planted to help a cooperative third way, or balancing alternative, to emerge?

Answering this question requires, at the very least, a minimal grasp of what could be called organizational morphogenesis. It is interesting to use the model of collegiality to look at how the commons will be organized, and to try to reach that grasp, because collegiality is dual: it is both a specific organizational form and a tool for bureaucratic management. My purpose is to show that forms of collegial commons in an organizational society (that is already bureaucratized) help us think about morphogenesis. It is the endless struggle between collegiality and bureaucracy in framing social life that may be morphogenetic. An organizational approach to morphogenesis is proposed in which each model cannot exist without the other and in which the two models -that are actually two levels of collective agency (Lazega 2015b)- drive each other's evolution.

Collegiality: A Specific Form of Organization and a Tool for Bureaucratic Management

Organizations that coordinate the activities of peers, often experts and professionals, called upon to make decisions in situations of uncertainty and who spend much of their time accomplishing non-routine tasks, still represent a basic problem in mainstream sociology of organizations today. Max Weber's most systematic writings on the issue are centered on collegiality and are to be found, in the core of *Economy and Society*, at the end of the chapter on bureaucracy and in the section on division of powers in the chapter on types of legitimate domination. Those pages reflect his theory that rationalization and bureaucratization best characterize modernity and the specificity of the exercise of power and domination in modern societies. Weber presents collegiality as a managerial device, one tool among others, for bureaucratic rational-legal authority. The device consists in bringing experts together to work in committees, requiring from them that they build consensus and come to an agreement. The Prince or head of a bureaucratic organization applies that method to avoid depending on a single expert or on experts in general – whose authority they fear – and to test their loyalty and competence. At the same time, collegiality can also become a mitigating force in the face of a potentially arbitrary or autocratic, "monocratic" power.

Original neo-Weberian theses have recently listed an ensemble of formal characteristics that challenge this Weberian view of collegiality. They separate a collegial and "polycratic" form of organization from the bureaucratic and monocratic model and argue that collegiality is a fully fledged organizational form, not only a managerial device in the hands of the bureaucrat (Waters 1989). Such organizations use and implement theoretical knowledge. Their members are considered professionals and their careers divided into a minimum of two steps – apprenticeship and practice. Though performance-minded, these organizations encounter difficulties when obliged to evaluate and compare the quality of their specialists' performance, thus resolving to place them formally on an equal footing. The organizations exert formal self-control and are thus, to a large extent, self-regulating. They create at least one forum, the committee of the whole – that may rely on the input of a more or less complex and hierarchical system of committees and sub-committees – where decision-making is collective.

Waters' approach to the collegial form of organization remains a formal one. The neo-Weberian perspective also produced a theory of collective action among peers that accounts for the social discipline and collective responsibility observed in those entities (Lazega 2001). This social discipline helps rival but interdependent partners, who carry out non-routine tasks and manage the dilemmas of their collective action together. This cooperation among competitors is based on the uneasy management of personalized relationships and multiplex social exchanges among strategic individuals and sub-groups. Collegiality depends upon personalized relationships which, in the standard bureaucratic model, are considered "particularistic" obstacles to collective action (Perrow 1986). In an ideal-typical, collegial organization those personalized ties become, on the contrary, the source of a social discipline that helps close/distant members exchange, monitor, exert pressure, sanction each other, select leaders, or yet again negotiate precarious values for self-regulation.

The sociology of organizations has thus produced at least two approaches, one according to Weber's theory, whereby collegiality is defined as a means of bureaucratic management; the other according to neo-Weberian theory, where it is defined as an organizational form *per se*. Therefore, how the two approaches can coexist is a question that arises both in theory and in practice. The Weberian point of view is destined to evolve. In large bureaucracies, aside from the often collegial-like behavior of many top executives (Baylis 1989), the accent placed on cooperation between experts, the elimination of several hierarchical levels, or the generalization of project management have given rise to new work environments which promote what a bureaucrat might call "collegial pockets" characterized by the social mechanisms of survival and cooperation among peers.

The neo-Weberian point of view also evolves. It recognizes that the formal and social features of a collegial organization are precisely ideal-typical, like those of classical bureaucracies. Since routine and non-routine tasks are, in contemporary organizations and institutions, most often inextricably linked (Lazega 1993), bureaucracy and collegiality coexist in all modern structures of decision-making. In fact they do more than coexist. I argue that they challenge each other constantly, stimulating constant change in each other's implementation. The coexistence of both definitions of collegiality, one idealtypical, one empirical, indicates that collegiality and bureaucracy develop in a permanent if often unobtrusive, multilevel conflict, *i.e.* the result of a struggle between the top and bottom levels of an organization that brings together members who carry out non-routine tasks – whether in executive rooms where political negotiations are impossible to routinize or in collegial pockets of interdependent professionals and experts when they carry out work and cooperation that cannot be standardized.

As an example, this chapter looks at one possible combination of bureaucracy and collegiality in a Catholic diocese. This diocese is a bureaucracy in which the bishop is the absolute master of his organization. But the diocese cannot be seen exclusively as a bureaucracy. It is also a collegial setting because the priests consider each other as peers and are driven by different religious orientations and senses of professionalism. At the beginning of the twenty-first century, if a bishop does not try to understand how each of his priests is motivated by his *Beruf* or calling, the latter may simply leave.

Combining Bureaucracy and Collegiality in a Roman Catholic Diocese

Our setting is one of the largest Catholic dioceses in France. A diocese – which in France corresponds to a *département* – is a complex organization (Granfield 1988) with fuzzy borders due to the great number of associations, movements and groups that gravitate around it. It is composed of bureaucratically organized local communities complete with administrators, committees and a multitude of services all concentrated in one spot, the diocese. It is headed by a bishop nominated by the bishops of the given province and appointed by the Pope, Bishop of Rome. We think that it is possible to illustrate the conflict between bureaucracy and collegiality, i.e. managers and professionals, by the way the Roman Catholic Church, one of the most ancient and complex organizations in the Western world, functions; it should be added that the principle of collegiality among priests has no theological foundation.

It is no longer possible to describe a clerical organization of this type *before* it became a bureaucracy using Malcolm Waters' formal criteria. We will therefore examine how, in this diocese, collegiality as a form of organization was discernible in a collegial form of social discipline, both in the priests' various pastoral practices and in the organizational pressures of a bottom-up type that they create for collective action. This becomes possible if part of the priest's pastoral activity is understood as a form of expertise in specialized domains connected to various groups of believers (Gannon 1971). We will then proceed like archaeologists, looking for the markers of collegiality in an emerging structure (already partly redefined by the hierarchy) by analyzing their social networks. Analyzing the many areas of interdependencies and social exchange in a population of priests belonging to the same diocese reveals how part of the system of interrelations thus unveiled was organized according to a division of labor implying religious "orientations", among which it is difficult to establish any particular order and where the role of the Catholic chain of command is also somewhat wobbly. The social organization of the diocese, examined here exclusively from the priests' point of view, displays characteristics of a collegial organization, *i.e.* a specific organizational form. The fact that priests dedicated to different orientations interrelate makes it possible to build a consensus. All these elements substantiate that a bottom-up type of collegiality among priests exists.

But the Roman Catholic Church is also a bureaucracy in which the bishop, as an absolute master of his diocese, retains most of the power; his authority is monocratic in theory. Formally speaking, his power can be curbed from above, since the Bishop of Rome and the Roman Curia have the capacity to intervene should a disagreement arise (Gellard 1977; Schilling 2002; Vallier 1969); as well as – since Vatican II – from below through the councils, particularly with respect to finances (i.e. the existence of the Diocesan Council for economic affairs). It is the bishop's duty to appoint at least one Vicar General to assist him in directing the diocese. He is relatively free to organize the diocese as he sees fit, concerning, for instance, the meetings of the Episcopal Council, an equivalent to the "executive" power in the diocese. We shall be looking at the system of committees set up by the bishop in top-down fashion to cope with the pressures emanating from below that do not leave him much choice as to who should sit on those committees if he doesn't want his diocese to explode.

Let us start by describing priests' work, its routine and non-routine sides, the group of priests observed, and the variety of Catholic orientations they invent in order to adapt to their different clienteles – and the problems of identity and unity such diversity stirs up within the Church.[4] Seen through the eyes of the priests, collegiality represents a way to coordinate their activities, permitting the religious orientation they promised to create and represent to be built up, recognized and appreciated. We will next see how, since Vatican II, the bureaucratic organization of the Catholic Church has reintroduced elements of collegiality – such as the system of councils that frame the bishop's decision-making processes within the diocese or the creation of national Episcopal conferences. We shall describe how the Catholic hierarchy conceives of collegiality, institutionalizing and using it *à la* Weber, as a tool for management.

Bottom-Up Collegiality: Using Relations as Self-Management Tools

A neo-Weberian approach to collegiality begins with a description of actors' complex and uncertain work and the fact that they must collaborate in order to get a job done. A priest's activity occupies a double register, each of which creates specific conflicts and interdependencies: a relatively standardized, generalist register and a specialized register. The latter is the result both of the personal convictions at the root of a specific commitment and of the fact that a church is split into several religious orientations aimed at integrating different Catholic identities (Béraud 2006; Charles 1986; Gannon 1979a, b; Hervieu-Léger 2003; and Villemin and Caillot 2001). The specialized register opens up the possibility of bottom-up collegiality among priests. Individually, the diversity of persuasions and norms invested in their pastoral activity makes it difficult for them to accept a purely bureaucratic integration. Collectively, dividing pastoral activity into several different religious orientations makes it difficult for a monocratic authority to monopolize pastoral leadership. In this register, interdependencies between priests are more complex, more personal and collegial than in a generalist, impersonal and bureaucratic register. The various religious orientations that will be presented below – *activist*, *ritual* and *intellectual* for the main part – illustrate the variety of a priest's expertise and commitments and may explain the plurality of Catholic identities noted in and between parishes (Courcy 1999).

Priests' Pastoral Activity: The Collegial Construction of Religious Orientations

Generally speaking, the notion of "pastoral" work is vague and used for a multitude of activities which have no obvious relation to each other (Béraud 2006). Its collective and pragmatic side is in contrast to the "spiritual" and theological side. We defined it operationally as the activity that elaborates and implements all sorts of projects connected to a set of social and religious observances, aiming to religiously socialize and integrate all or part of a community – to uphold or reveal its religious specificity with respect to the behavior and significance of the non-religious environment. There is an intellectual dimension to that activity that turns it into what might be called "practical theology".

In our study, we considered that one of the main areas of uncertainty distinctive of a priest's work involves the relationship between the Catholic Church and its social environment: how to stop "exculturation" (Hervieu-Léger 2003) or, conversely, how to establish a possibly positive interaction with that society. In that respect, the most important resource in a diocese is the capacity to produce a "rational and systematic" discourse in which the diocese and French society intersect with a set of pastoral projects. Such discourse, rounded out by projects for secular as well as spiritual activities, aimed at believers as well as potential Catholics, is the raw material from which consensus is made. Discourses and projects rest on the identification of religious "needs", thought to be difficult to guess in advance and perhaps different according to the social group involved. Such discourse produces various religious orientations through which the diversity of Catholic identities noted among priests belonging to the same diocese is also expressed. Due to the complexity and variety of pastoral activities (Goudet 1997; Palard 1985), it is difficult for a monocratic authority and a hierarchy to control the many registers of an individual priest's activities, which also explains why it is impossible to prevent bottom-up collegiality from taking shape.

The notion of "religious orientation" refers to the principle of an internal division between competing approaches to pastoral activities. An orientation cannot be reduced to a segment of a 'catholic market' for parishioners. It is also the basis for these priests' commitment and expectations, for their conception of themselves and of their church. Between 1998 and 2001, we identified three different orientations – ritual, activist and intellectual – themselves stemming from two other orientations that had become nearly extinct: Catholic action directed at independent occupations and a specific orientation directed at the working class (*prêtres ouvriers*). Those orientations are part of distinct, historically ancient traditions updated at the local level and by the contemporary situation of each individual diocese. The plurality of religious orientations is not solely linked to religious logics. It also depends on the diversity of the groups of believers and their social evolution: for example the development of highly under-privileged urban areas (*banlieues*), and the disappearance of traditional working-class neighborhoods, the transformation of middle class attitudes to politics, or the quest for social distinction among the well-off bourgeoisie.

A *ritual orientation* typically reintroduces elements considered traditional into the religious activity of a parish (especially 'Adoration of the Blessed Sacrament'). This links up with young people's desire for religious leadership (*e.g.* the European scout movement), the demand for a Catholic identity in global society and implementing evangelical projects to recruit new worshippers. Among young priests, the three aspects are combined with emphasizing the emotional dimension clearly apparent in their affective involvement and resort to charismatic groups. The orientation conveys the vision of priest as holy leader looking to control and circumscribe discussion within a local community, particularly by making private confession a priority. The ritualists maintain ties to priests in charge of traditionalist associations.

An *intellectual orientation* is promoted by another group of priests who recruit, coach and collaborate more with lay persons than the priests representing the ritual orientation. Since World War II, it has been part of a permanent undertaking to discredit the pious form of Catholic identification and promote a thoughtful and liberal adhesion to Catholicism through theological learning. In the confrontation with contemporary thought, it suggests that Christian faith should be expressed in intellectually acceptable terms. Contrary to what prevails in the "*pastorale* of independent occupations" (from which it seems to have stemmed), the political dimension and sense of solidarity have evaporated to give way to the notion of believers finding fulfillment in their family and professional lives. The orientation is accompanied by a strong rationalization of pastoral activity (the project-based approach dissociating the organizational and the spiritual, a more sophisticated division of labour). Claiming a specific position for the priest, though still not fully guaranteed, is clearly pushed to the fore, at least his place as "intellectual leader and manager", and arbitrator in the definition of parish priorities.

The *militant* or *activist orientation* underscores the role of local communities in working-class contexts with high unemployment. This activist orientation is represented by priests who work in the *banlieues*. The oldest among them know the bishop directly. Their starting point is the observation that the pastoral and the social are united, which is prominent when giving priority to social intervention projects and inciting members of the congregation to participate in volunteer associations, religious or not. The idea is to claim Christian identity from that angle by being acknowledged as a social partner. It is also the starting point for a parallel activity aiming to enter into partnerships with local groups. A second perspective consists in provoking encounters with other religious groups, including communities of recent migrants, in particular Muslims, in order to clarify Christian identity. Putting the accent on lay responsibility, these priests constantly seek to downplay their own leadership and exploit the discrepancy between their own words and the traditional image of the priest. They stress their role as quasi social workers who work with many lay persons, almost *as* lay persons. Among them, the priests representing the catholic action in working class milieu (*prêtres ouvriers*) personify a shrinking orientation (in numbers), and they are slightly different in political discourse from the other militants, although the two are both activists and quite close. They stress catholic action oriented mainly towards very low revenue workers and the unemployed and their families.

Bottom-up collegiality among priests is based on the diversity of their commitments and on their need to jointly transform them into locally credible religious orientations and pastoral projects. The orientations reflect the fractioning of a diocesan clergy, thereby better able to respond to and socialize part of the several Catholic identities present. Bottom-up collegiality organizes cooperation between interdependent priests building up their religious orientations locally and wanting to remain in control of them. The top-down creation of the presbyteral council towards the end of the 1960s formally translated the hierarchy's reaction to that observable fact. At stake in this collegiality is the preservation of privileges, *i.e.*, in the present case, defending the specific authority of the priest with regard to lay people as much as with respect to the bishop.

Each of them represents a well known (to specialists in the sociology of religions) religious orientation, but also a social niche. These priests actually do not much like other priests defending a different kind of meaning and orientation. They criticize each other plentifully and many do not talk to each other. The question is therefore how does the bishop maintain some kind of social order in this institution which is so segmented and potentially so conflictual. The bishop's strategy is to identify in each of these groups/niches the most vocal persons, the priests who have some kind of status in their social niche, and invite these 'representatives' to become members of the episcopal committee. In exchange for participation in running the diocese from this committee they have to agree not to develop any form of oppositional solidarity or criticize each other in public. For example, the militant activists need to shut up about the traditionalists and the other way around. In exchange for this co-optation, the bishop does not want to hear any (collegially familiar) bickering that gets personal and destructive very quickly between opposed social niches – thus avoiding organizational drift. Observing exchanges between priests in their specific organizational context is a good way to grasp specific dimensions of bottom-up collegial organization, for it brings to light the relations existing in their specific social discipline and relational infrastructures, and thus in the joint production of their respective pastoral orientations.

The Relational Structure of the System of Social Exchange Among Priests

Our representation of the priests' exchange system illustrates the workings of bottom-up collegiality quite clearly. Before going into the details, it is necessary to present the general characteristics of the links we observed and the nature of the social resources exchanged.[5] The priests interviewed declared on the average 15.2 partners for collaboration, 5 partners for advice, between 6 and 7 for conviviality and 3 for personal support, with a considerable standard deviation (Wattebled 2004). Relations for possible teamwork involved, for example, collaborating within the same parish or deanery, or with the bishop's vicar to set up a parish team, or participating in a committee of the Presbyteral Council or yet again meeting with the person in charge of sacred art and liturgy to get a church altar ready. Counseling sometimes touched upon the same domains and involved sensitive issues (organizing the parish, celebrating the sacraments, resolving a conflict). In general, advice was sought out from members of the hierarchy or from members of a common social niche, or from other colleagues in the same deanery. Conviviality hardly ever respects the pecking order; rather it looks for groups where there is personal affinity, or a deanery, or yet again it entails outside relations. Personal support mainly combines hierarchical circles and personal affinity groups, as well as ties that extend beyond the established formal boundaries.

The system of social exchange between priests is sketched in Fig. 10.1. Within the context of a diocese and considering priests' relationships, a social niche can be defined as a space for dense exchanges that combines different sorts of resources: sharing advice, conviviality and personal support among priests with

[5]For a detailed presentation of the network study of this diocese and neo-structural analyses, see Wattebled (2004) and Lazega and Wattebled (2011).

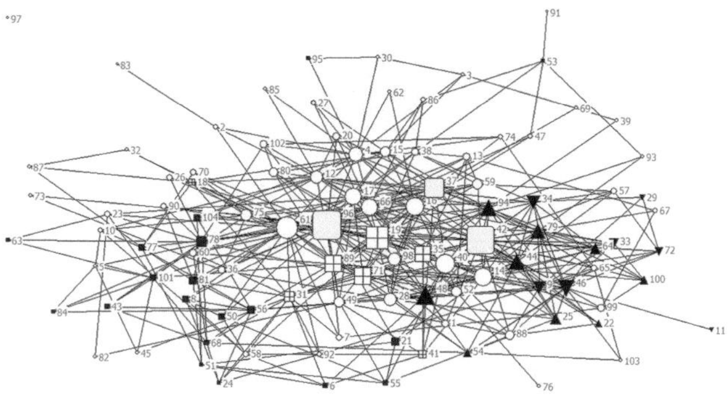

Fig. 10.1 Collegial pockets and linchpins in a bureaucratic structure: Religious orientations of the priests in a Diocese as mapped on their advice network

similar relational profiles and common attributes.[6] Local consensus develops among them and is maintained around a religious orientation. Activities are evaluated and members given credit for these activities by their peers. A social niche is thus also composed of teams of priests – whether informal or affiliated to a national or even international association (for a training period, collaborating in a journal, or even organizing a seminar). One nevertheless observes a trend among young priests at the time to constitute only informal, "unaffiliated" groups; in doing so, they are mainly espousing generational and pastoral affinities.

Legend: Representation of the advice network among the priests in the diocese. The size of the nodes represents the centrality of the priest in this network. Priests represented by white circles are uncommitted in terms of orientation. The three most central light grey rounded squares are the "linchpins", i.e. most central priests with an uncontroversial, declining 'Catholic orientation towards independent occupations', high popularity among the peripheral and uncommitted (in terms of orientation) priests, and high hierarchical positions close to the bishop. The white squares with a cross represent an intellectual orientation. The triangles represent activist priests, i.e. black upgoing triangles for priests sharing a militant orientation, and black downgoing triangles for priest sharing a working class orientation. The black squares represent the priests with the ritual orientation. For an interpretation of this structure, refer to the text.

Studying the bishop's formal system of integration does not mean that he cannot use less formal mechanisms, *e.g.* drawing on his own personal network. But since

[6]For the sake of clarity, Fig. 10.1 is built on the advice network among priests, but the other relationships measured in the diocese reflect the same underlying pattern, although in a more complexified way (Wattebled 2004; Lazega and Wattebled 2011). Centrality is measured as eigenvector centrality, a measurement that weighs the centrality of the person by the centrality of the contacts choosing that person. Highly central priests in this picture are priests who are sought out for advice by priests who are themselves sought out for advice. This measure represents with relatively good precision the pecking order between the priests as observed ethnographically.

the bishop did not wish to answer the network questionnaire, we are only able to examine the formal integration of the collegial pockets system. In the case in hand, the bishop did not originally come from the diocese; he had been installed recently and had little personal contact with the priests, which accounts for the important place occupied by the *Vicaire épiscopal*'s relations, himself being chosen for that position by the bishop because of his extensive familiarity with the priests.

The exchange system is organized in a series of social niches where each niche can be connected to a religious orientation. The system translates into an informal division of labour among priests. Three facets of the priests' activities explain these interconnections and the interdependencies between social niches in this system of niches. In the first place, redefining norms for religious activity and diocesan priorities requires building and maintaining consensus, even temporary. To do so, the social niches must not function separately and, as we mentioned above, priests must be able to extend their contacts beyond their own social niche in order to be able to operate as intermediaries or even spokesmen to the bishop. Secondly, the religious orientations described above prove complementary, addressing different populations of parishioners and in the end accounting for the diversity in the diocese. It is difficult for a bishop to choose among the different orientations and give precedence to one without running the risk of cutting himself off from a large part of the faithful, among whom the priests themselves. The fact that the priests fit into a system of social niches shows how complementary they are indeed and keeps the expression of radical beliefs and convictions in check. Lastly, young priests in particular share the desire to preserve the specific quality of their commitments which, as a collective concern, is likely to reinforce cohesion among priests beyond differences in pastoral and theological sensitivities. The bishop tries to deffuse the oppositions/conflicts between these constituencies by coopting members from all of them.

To understand the relational pattern in this system, it is also important to realize that it combines in quite a complex way a system of niches with a core-periphery structure. In this system the main social niches (each representing an orientation) represent the components of a semi-periphery in this core-periphery structure. In this core-periphery system, the core has representatives of several social niches, each representing an orientation/constituency (Wattebled 2004; Lazega and Wattebled 2011). In this pattern, we find the five main orientations present in the diocese, i.e. ritual, intellectual, militant, as well as the declining catholic action in independent milieux and catholic action in working class milieux. This informal division of pastoral work could only be identified by network analysis of the personal relationships of the priests among themselves. Priests developing the same orientation find themselves clustered in the same position because they share a common relational profile and have strong relationships with each other (which is the definition of a social niche).

However, as shown in Fig. 10.1, the most central members are priests who are administratively closest to the bishop and who often represent the declining orientation of the "catholic action in independent milieu". To understand this paradoxical situation it is important to add to the picture two additional characteristics of the diocese. Firstly, many priests are 'peripheral' in these networks: their relational capital is quite modest, they do not belong in any social niche and do not declare any specific orientation. These 'peripheral' priests tend to seek advice from the colleagues who represent older and declining –but uncontroversial– orientations. Three representatives of one of these declining orientations, precisely the catholic action in independent milieu, are the largest nodes in Fig. 10.1, who "benefit" from this situation. They are the *Vicaire general* and two *Vicaires épiscopaux* who owe their centrality to their administrative contribution and to the fact that they represent an unthreatening orientation; they are powerful individually but represent a spent force collectively. Secondly, it is important to know that the bishop himself had a militant and intellectual sensitivity. In order to pacify the milieu, he needed as deputies priests representing such an uncontroversial orientation. He found them, at the time and in this case, in these representatives of the catholic action in independent milieu. Structurally speaking these three persons became the linchpins or pivots of the structure. They were in a position to be trusted by the bishop and the many peripheral priests, as well as to remain on speaking terms with the traditionalists, intellectual and militants, i.e. the orientations that were the most creative in terms of adaptation to the environment, but also generating the tensions in the diocese. This linchpin position is thus complex; it is a mix of unthreatening popularity among the 'unaligned', brokerage between the 'aligned', and proximity to the bishop who backs them up while keeping them under close supervision.

The Endogenous Emergence of Heterogeneous Forms of Status Among the Priests

Developing cooperation among priests depends on a complex social discipline. But if each social niche becomes meaningful only within the broader system of niches, that is due to the fact that social discipline is not exclusively "local" and based on accomplishing presbyteral tasks: representatives of a pastoral orientation are in contact with colleagues who share the same commitments in other parishes and other dioceses. A reinforced allegiance to the bishop – a conception of the holy office shared by all the faithful and of the presbyteral office shared by all the priests – is also part of the social discipline typical of bottom-up collegiality among priests. Within the diocese, the priest is no longer looking to establish a local status (an attitude considered too "parochial") especially since, as of the 1970s, he has received his assignment for a limited period of time only. "Diocesan priests" theoretically occupy an intermediate position between the diocese represented by the bishop and the parishes mainly run by laymen and laywomen. That position incites them to try and create a diocesan status for themselves and aim for a formal title. Given the increasingly complex nature of pastoral activity and greater specialization of religious work, the large number of diocesan responsibilities – and small number of priests – this compels the latter to compete for those titles.

It is not easy to analyze status competition among priests: the subject does not explicitly appear in discourse (where it is censored by the values of fraternity and consensus), nor is it explicitly mentioned in the exchanges that they declared. As in the case of the three linchpins, we managed to analyze it by considering the priest in his position of middleman seeking to build a status for himself and having it acknowledged in the diocese and parishes. When analyzing priests' speech and exchanges, three levels appear to co-exist: the local level corresponds to the priest's traditional desire to make a place for himself at the heart of the parish community. Being appointed to a different parish threatens that place for he must rebuild it from scratch in a new community. The diocesan level includes that dimension: it supposes recognition of and commitment to diocesan preoccupations and consequently means lesser local commitment benefiting extra-parish exchanges with colleagues or lay people who have diocesan responsibilities in projects or councils. The extra-diocesan level concerns priests investing in activities or aiming for titles outside the diocese (the bishopry, a regional or national responsibility, academic notoriety). Each time, accessing a higher level in this multilevel structure demands a more selective reorganization of contacts at the lower level.

When considering the relational data collected – more exactly the centrality scores obtained by the priests in each exchange network – it is possible to calculate correlations, determine the degree to which the scores converge and identify forms of status (consistent or not). As suggested by the linchpins, rather than seeing a single chain of command emerging because of all the social resources being concentrated in the same hands, several profiles emerge when we combine our analysis of the exchange system and the priests' centrality scores. In the first place, members of the hierarchy, who all naturally have diocesan responsibilities, are very central in collaboration, advice and personal support. They declare few or no pastoral projects, having no parish appointment or if they do, doubtless no time to develop many. Secondly, about ten young priests are central in the different exchange systems, more especially for advice and particularly in their own social niche. Being identified with a religious orientation, they declare a large number of well-defined pastoral projects. They call themselves and are often called spokesmen ("loud-mouths") in the diocese. Though not always formally, they participate in at least one diocesan activity. Other priests, also approximately ten, young and less young, who also belong to a social niche, turn out to be relatively central most of all in matters of conviviality and personal support. Some of these priests are reputed to be "serious" or "wise", *i.e.* known to be good listeners and well-informed about the diocese. Most declare few projects and have no diocesan responsibility. Local stability and nearing retirement are two factors that allow us to detect priests whose status remains local. Parish priests in the large parishes present other characteristics: the large number of projects they declare (their parish being sufficiently well off for them to do so) does not encourage many interactions with their fellow-priests. They are busy either building a local status or one outside the diocese.

The relational structure and the interdependencies revealed in Fig. 10.1 shows why the diversity of religious orientations does not end in open conflict. It is the result of two relational strategies typical of collegial organizations: creating/looking for social niches, and peer competition for status. However, the more collegial the exchange system among priests, the more accessing a position such as, for instance, the bishop's vicar, demands being able to play the game of unity, and finding and coopting priests who want to accept positions of responsibility to promote their own beliefs. In turn, the bishop counts on status competition to identify the leaders he will co-opt and with whom he will negotiate an agreement on the most consensual positions and practices possible. Thanks to a few popular but weak linchpins, he manages to exercise control on the various coopted young spokesmen of controversial orientations. Thus the analysis of these interactions show which 'orientation' was embattled with another, but not that anyone clearly won. There was no clear winner out amongst these *tendances* at that time. A form of complex balance of Catholic orientations emerges that is able to present a collegial compromise based, firstly, on cooptation and neutralization of threatening centrifugal forces, and secondly on window-dressing an apparent consensus.

Top-Down Collegiality: The Complex Bureaucratic Management of the Diversity of Catholic Orientations

In short, this division of religious work in different orientations with an underlying complex relational infrastructure (social niches and forms of status) articulates the bishop and the exchange system in a way that creates a specific and local balance between bureaucracy and collegiality thanks to the distribution of diocesan mandates and co-optation in the episcopal committees. In the networks analysed in this diocese, the status and centrality of several priests from the unthreatening orientation, called 'catholic action in independent milieux', is mainly built on their popularity among the 'unaligned', their proximity to the bishop, their very general commitment to the construction of consensus and respect of collective responsibility in the '*sacerdoce presbytéral*'. In other words, they are the pivots/linchpins articulating the system of niches and the core-periphery structure. This system creates just enough cohesion between different orientations, between older and younger generations of priests, who accept the social discipline and compromise personified by the structural linchpins.

If bottom-up collegiality depends on a form of specialization in various domains – in conceiving of diverse and often opposed religious orientations for instance – which makes it easier to grasp the diversity of Catholic identities (Donégani 1993, 2000), then the risk that a church might explode is real (Willaime 1986, 1992). The story of the Catholic Church is punctuated by tensions with groups, movements or associations capable of provoking serious schisms. In order to manage diversity and preserve unity, the Church proceeded to establish an administrative and cultural bureaucracy by creating a chain of command that stands for unity even if it is only a front, and by standardizing symbols easy to communicate and identify. However, the contemporary context of the Catholic Church in France demands that priorities be redefined and new norms for religious activity negotiated. The bishop has the authority to make such decisions but there remains doubt as to their efficiency, both internally (their being obeyed) and with regard to the global society where democratic values prevail. In general, relations between the Church and French society seem uncertain and diminish the effectiveness of an organization and decision-making processes which are merely bureaucratic. Henceforth, the decision-making process is partly determined by the hierarchy's acceptance of relative autonomy for the rank and file and the search for consensus with the support of religious expertise. Organizing diocesan synods is the perfect example of the coexistence between the monocratic leader of a diocesan administration on one hand, and, on the other, the lower echelons coordinated in top down collegial fashion, whose largest possible participation in decision-making is only periodically sought.

Thus, the unity of the Catholic Church largely depends on the bishop's work and the complex balance of powers that he builds. The complexity of a pastoral activity divided into different religious orientations makes direct control by a monocratic authority difficult. The diocesan services contribute to elaborating the norms that govern pastoral activity and participate in the initial training and continuing education of religious actors. Their participation in defining the rules for religious activity can create conflict with the priests, who can criticize the bishop for treading on their toes – *e.g.* when it comes to catechism, deciding on the curriculum or the age for first communion. Relations between diocesan services and priests can be compared to the relationship between administration and professionals. The diversity and need for coordination translate into the fact that organizing diocesan responsibilities is primarily entrusted to priests. A bishop is supposed to represent the unity of the diocese even if his own convictions cause him to give one component of the diocese precedence over another. Nevertheless, it may be in his best interest to keep the show on the road and save his reputation intact by conferring diocesan responsibilities on the various representatives of religious orientations equitably. In so doing, he is promoting a hard-line, typically "Catholic" strategy that aims to integrate a maximum of diversity and obtaining in exchange, from the integrated elements, the toning down of the expression of their own convictions. On the other hand, a strategy of that sort – which we observed in this diocese – reinforces the interdependence between the bishop and the priests' exchange system, so that decision-making is necessarily collective, implying that the other religious actors – permanent deacons or lay people – also be included, in practice if not in theory.

In organizational terms, this is why it is crucial to identify the members who adopt one or several inconsistent forms of endogenous status, i.e. the linchpins. The bishop's co-optation of the most central colleagues in matters of collaboration, advice and personal support, puts the most visible representatives of the various religious orientations in a 'situation'. This means that collegiality is being transformed into a tool for management with help from structurally specific individuals who are able to manage the 'situation' created at the top, i.e. the structural linchpins. Formally, a bishop's action at the head of the diocese depends on his direct collaboration with three types of actors: the members of the Episcopal council – among whom figure the Grand Vicar and the district Episcopal vicars – the diocesan services and the diocesan councils. The latter are usually purely consultative, though voting procedures are applied *e.g.* during sessions of the Presbyteral council. They allow every type of actor – priests, deacons, monks and nuns, lay people – to participate to a greater or lesser extent in the bishop's decision-making.

The Episcopal council is where decisions are made and important diocesan orientations decided upon. The council includes Episcopal vicars who play an important role for they advise the bishop on parish appointments and the distribution of diocesan mandates. Theoretically, they oversee and evaluate priests' work. At the time of our research the diocese was composed of four pastoral zones whose borders had been traced in the 1970s. Each at that time was homogeneous from a social and professional point of view: one was traditionally bourgeois, one working-class, one a new town and one a rural area. Each pastoral zone was headed by an Episcopal vicar appointed by the bishop to organize the assignment of priests in the area and set up zone days during which most of the persons officially invested in pastoral activity met: priests, permanent deacons, lay members of the pastoral team or the chaplaincy. Those special days were built around themes such as the relationship to politics or to Judaism, or were opportunities for members of the pastoral team to exchange and compare their experiences. Each zone was composed of *doyennés* (deaneries, 16 in all), pastoral sections or groups of parishes. Every 3 years, each *doyenné* elected a dean from its ranks, theoretically to watch over his colleagues but in fact to be another relay for the bishop. This allowed the latter to summon the deans to yearly meetings. Pastoral sectors are what remains of the teamwork pastoral actors aimed to put into practice during the 1970s. Today they are the starting point for creating groups of parishes. At the time of our survey, the diocese was made up of 45 groups of parishes and 53 parishes.

A hierarchal system of committees – the Episcopal, presbyteral and pastoral diocesan councils in particular – is thus created top-down to allow the bishop to direct the diocese from above while translating into more general terms the priests' specialized, locally collegial approaches. The distribution of diocesan responsibilities is based partly on criteria connected to the priest's informal status: decision-making in the diocese and in the parishes is imbued with a modern rationalization that depends on profane competences and religious expertise (diplomas, experience). The creation and multiplication of diocesan services, supposed to be in the avant-garde of a religious domain composed of specialists (catechism, training, social work, etc.), is an example of how the demand for rationalization increases. Secondly, when one considers the way Episcopal zone vicars and deans are appointed, clearly the informal recognition of priests by their peers plays an important role, for the bishop nominates the dean or Episcopal vicar at the end of a consultative vote.

Top-down collegiality considered from that angle is precisely the way Max Weber defined it. It is adjustable and suits diocesan situations that involve bishop, linchpins, priests and lay people; for it does not mean that the hierarchy has eased its pressure on the lower ranks. For instance, at the time of our study, the hierarchy had installed a local "pastoral team", a collective managerial organ to replace the parish priest's individual leadership. It was comprised of the parish priest, often the vicars, and three to five lay members generally elected by the parish. The lay members are however designated by the bishop by way of an official letter of appointment and "installed" for a 3-year period by the zone's Episcopal vicar. That nomination procedure fuels the priests' fear that they will lose their traditional privileges and see a hierarchy parallel to theirs develop. Bottom-up collegiality among priests may then resemble a defense mechanism directed against top-down collegiality. They both play ball with the bishop (to publicize and share more widely their own private views about the nature of their religious and institutional commitments) and try to influence the decisions of the monocratic leader, thus bolstering their identity compared with lay people.

Micro-political, Morphogenetic Co-Constitution of Bottom-Up and Top-Down Collegiality

This case goes beyond just showing how the Catholic church's hierarchy finds a balance between its own goals and the goals pursued by priests working in local parishes, thereby revisiting the theory of institutionalization by co-optation. Making some headway on the problem of how two organizational forms – collegiality and bureaucracy – are interrelated, the duality of collegiality can be used to look at how the two definitons of collegiality are combined. Collegiality as a particular form of organization can be shown to be really a bottom-up type of collegiality, based on carrying out uncertain, non-routine tasks collectively among peers. In the case under study, it takes the form of conceiving and promoting religious orientations (conveying different conceptions of priestly professionalism), through an informal division of labour between orientations that are difficult to arrange in any hierarchical order among the organization's priorities. Such an informal division of labour creates interdependencies and depends on a specific social discipline that helps members keep up their active collaboration and commitment as well as certain forms of consensus. The priests' exchange system indicates and measures that social discipline and also reveals the fact that creating consensus is facilitated by forming a collegial oligarchy, in our case a limited number of priestly "spokesmen" for religious orientations and the linchpins who are also capable of playing the role of intermediaries with the master.

Our example of one articulation between bureaucracy and collegiality leaves open the question of whether institutional changes ahead will indeed be morphogenetic. Bottom-up collegiality is different from the one constructed by a hierarchy in an already bureaucratic context, *i.e.* collegiality as a tool for management, which we call top-down collegiality. In the best of cases, the latter identifies the social niches of bottom-up collegiality as "collegial pockets" that emerge in the organization. In top-down collegiality, the members of the committees assisting the official leader are chosen with an eye to gaining support for policies that can be decided autocratically as well as through collective deliberation. From the perspective of bureaucratic management, bottom-up collegiality is often an insignificant "micro-collegiality" responsible for problems of oppositional solidarity and integration that "macro-collegiality" can solve. In all more or less bureaucratic organizations calling upon expertise, *i.e.* in a large proportion of contemporary organizations, both forms of collegiality – bottom-up and top-down – coexist in that way.

But bureaucracy and collegiality do more than coexist in a context combining an endogenous system of niches and statuses on one side, and an absolute master, a hierarchical structure and a parallel administration on the other. They actually challenge each other in a potentially destructive way and can be said to drive each other's evolution in a potentially morphogenetic sense. If the structure of the network changes but the diocese survives, then the diocese as a system is morphogenetic. Each kind of collegiality thus represents a morphogenetic impulse pushing for change and creating variety on "the other side". The system can be morphogenetic because of the tensions between the groups and the fragile equilibrium that is unlikely to last without renegotiations. A bishop can try to ignore the problems of integration encountered in his diocese; the priests themselves may not feel obliged to welcome the different tendencies and conceptions of professionalism present; linchpins may not emerge. Everything depends on the social strength of the exchange system, perhaps on the priests' social origins (Bourdieu and Saint Martin de 1982), but also on the size, composition and structure of their network as a determinant of the social processes that together constitute their social discipline (Lazega 2012): a small number of isolated priests carry much less weight than a large number of priests united by their interdependencies and by certain forms of oppositional solidarity.

The portfolio of strategies available for coordinating bottom-up and top-down collegiality is fairly large. The first step is cooptation by choosing members of social niches to sit on executive councils. According to the level of rationalization implemented, the transformation of collegiality into a means of management may either constantly refine the relationship between the two types of collegiality, or forgo bottom-up collegiality, keeping only the rhetoric, thus paralyzing cooperation between experts/peers. The problem posed by the ubiquity of contemporary "bureau-collegiality" and related organizational morphogenesis concerns an increasing number of institutions: hospitals, universities, research institutes, political groups, etc. It is the renewed expression of an older and more profound question about the latitude and freedom of expertise and about professionals when they organize their work notwithstanding the many restrictions – economic or political – confronting them. But it is also a renewed expression of the issue of the relationship between the commons and the wider society. Indeed this example can be used as an introduction to the issue of the new commons as a potentially new and dual morphogenetic reality: that of the transformation of social discipline recognized as legitimate into violent and exogenous forms of collective responsibility.

Big Data and Digital Parametrization of Collective Responsibility in the New Commons

This case in point represents just one possible articulation between bureaucracy and collegiality, but there are many such combinations in a bureaucratized organizational society in which the commons emerge from attempts by the people to take control of the ways in which they want collectively to share common resources, locally and beyond. In many ways, the struggles between bureaucracy and collegiality that are described here are precisely the struggles to shape the institutionalization of the new commons. The organizational conditions under which the new commons can use social capital in collective responses to the bleak prospects of humanity and develop credible institutions that will resist the most destructive changes introduced by modernity, is a real political question. It is important to consider organized settings as sets of social mechanisms providing structural solutions to collective action problems. All the main social phenomena –such as solidarity and exclusions, social control and conflict resolution, learning and socialization, regulation and institutionalization – have a relational dimension and depend on relational infrastructures, established or emergent. Social capital is composed of social processes and relational infrastructure, and it is a form of social discipline that helps manage collective government of resources defined as commons.

A specialized, in this case ecclesiastic, institution cannot be a model for a democratic society (Where are, for example, women? Lay participants? Why should the meeting of bottom-up and top-down forces depend on the "generosity" of the absolute master willing to "share" some of his power? Etc.). In the context of the current transition, if democracy is itself threatened and paralyzed by its inability to deal with problems as horrendous as in the list at the start of this chapter, the morphogenetic dynamics illustrated by the case in point could be politically and morally much more inspiring than a morphostatic scenario in which society goes down a fascist path of collegiality among predatory elites abusing their powers without any checks and balances; sitting atop a police/military bureaucracy controlling civil society and uniform mass markets with quotas; and undermining any attempt to challenge their order by parametrizing the digital instruments on which local commons/communities count for self organization –thereby remote-controlling the many individually, by invading their privacy systematically; monitoring and using the risks associated with their health in order to threaten them; building relational infrastructures that promote stable forms of collective responsibility that neutralize institutional entrepreneurship or any changes sought out by potentially threatening bottom-up forces. Democracy must win, but there is also a lesson in an organizational morphogenesis forcing hierarchical, superimposed levels of oligarchs to accept changes coming from below.

The analysis of the two forms of collegiality provides leads for theorizing the social mechanisms that will institutionalize the commons, their collective intelligence and social innovation. Institutionalization of the commons cannot be construed as the top-down product of plouto-technocratic bureaucracies going down the military path. The latter are not able to create such new sharing institutions by *fiat*. It is reasonable to anticipate that they will try to coopt, control and "parametrize" them once they have emerged from much more bottom-up processes. In a ruthless capitalist society such a top-down parametrization will be for social control, imposition of vioent forms of collective responsibility, extraction of profits, and taxation. Given the current developments in technology, the process of top-down bureaucratization of the future new commons means their parametrization is likely to be their digitalization. Parametrization will be digital in the sense that it will rest on people's use of platforms, in particular network profiles and groups created on this platform and used by the people themselves to practice their daily social accounting of exchanges, management of meetings and coordination.

The bottom-up challenges to the legitimacy of top-down collective responsibility imposed by this bureaucratic parametrization to shape the institutionalization of the new commons will take the form of morphogenetic struggles to control this digitalization. Since there may not be any optimal stabilization of this struggle, society may also become a morphognenic system with an ongoing creation of new models. Digital parametrization of the new commons is part of contemporary morphogenetic institutional changes. This parametrization started long ago with widespread and gamified intrusiveness of platforms providing network profiles into individual privacy,[7] as well as the capacity offered to citizens to all become creators of online collectives. This digitalization may also undermine bottom-up institutional entrepreneurship. Indeed, in many online network services provided globally, individuals today can look at their list of contacts but not at the structure of their own network profile, even less at the profiles of their friends, and cannot reconstitute "communities" and organized social movements that are created by the hypergraph and concatenation of these profiles. They lack the capacity to zoom in and out of social networks that are, at any one point in time, the carriers of organized collegial action. Only ownership and control of the platform provide that capacity today, without any real checks on this new power.

Social digitalization as bureaucratic control of future new collegial commons is carried out as parametrization of the organization of collegial local communities and sharing networks. Such new commons may not be purely local but locality matters, even as geolocal grounding for these platforms. It makes it easier for ordinary citizens to resist when bureaucrats, party leaders, creditors, inspectors, etc. show up. The generic commons are for the neighbours' association, people sharing the same actual physical land resources. Locality creates a centre of gravity for them and for the sharing of resources or space that helps with their sustainability.[8] This social digitalization is based on monitoring, accounting for and making sense of exchanges, but also on shaping relational infrastructures (providing such actors with more centrality, such niches with more resources).

The morphogenetic process of institutionalization of new kinds of commons will use digital platforms and as such it may be a silent, invisible process of parametrization of these commons with bureaucratic algorithms as much as (if not much

[7]For an example of how bureaucratization of the future new commons could take place, recall 'social digitalization' as an indicator and substantive part of contemporary social morphogenesis, and see the use of devices such as body captors and network profiles and their influence on institution building (Lazega, Lazega 2015a, in Archer (ed.) *Generative Mechanisms Transforming the Social Order*).

[8]A purely online group is an effective way to organize for groups that are not limited / organized by a common locality, as when young innovators meet up to think up new codes in many areas (even in biology), work on projects together and start a business. These are not the same as commons with strong locality.

more than) an open political process of democratic (representative or participative) rulemaking. Social digitalization can be a new way of subjecting, homogenizing and taxing the diverse commons unobtrusively. As in the duality of collegiality, it may increase the rate of creation of new commons, but also end up subordinating them to bureaucratic control. The tools for creating the commons could also be the sources for their streamlining. Social digitalization will increase the rythm of creation of commons that existed before the emergence of these platforms. Research needs to flesh out the set of choices that these digital platforms make for citizens when they use them to build their new commons –i.e. choices that they are not aware of and that prestructure the unexpected ways in which these commons will be used to enforce collective responsibility.

If the meeting between bureaucracy and collegiality is now shaped by social digitalization bureaucratizing the commons in an organizational and morphogenetic process, platforms will organize civil society by parametrizing collective responsibility, within or without the framework of the/civil law. The social order that platforms thus develop will rest in part on online virtual social networks of interactions and organize the live offline relations that coordinate/emerge through these platforms. Since it creates the online context for live offline relations and exchanges, the multilevel architecture and the ownership and control of the platform itself deserve close sociological inquiry. This is even highly compatible with mass bureaucratized markets plus the military pathway to the bleak prospects outlined above. Such a digital structure can take over at the macro level and manage millions of collegial pockets that will try to protect themselves from both the environmental crunch and the violence of the military bureaucracy.

Creating institutions for the new local commons will be a dynamic multilevel process (Lazega 2013, 2014b) mobilizing networks, relational infrastructures, social processes and many other ingredients characterizing collegiality, including its vicious cycles (of patronage, clientelism and corruption). But the emergence of this institution will be parametrized by bureaucracy just as the bishop sets limits and conditions to his priests' participation and cooptation. It sheds light on the widening 'democratic deficit' that characterizes modern societies. This institutionalization raises the more general issue of the relationship between the democratic process and lobbying in pluto-technocratic bureaucracies. Tracing this regulatory process leads back to the determinants and proliferation of 'anormative regulation' (Archer 2016 volume; Al-Amoudi 2014; Al-Amoudi and Latsis 2014).

Behind any commons, there are communities mixing formal and informal rules, contractual and non market relationships (Coriat 2015) thanks to the relational dimension of social processes. In a world in which profit extraction and capital accumulation are violent, bureaucratization of the local commons can be seen as both a way to prevent local communities from closing off in oppositional solidarities, privatizing their resources in their collegial pockets; and a way to spread new digital and bureaucratic controls that will monitor, manage, tax and sanction, using collective responsibility, in potentially predatory ways these local communities. If elites with private armies prefer their current closure and the military pathway, then mechanisms must be put in place to challenge them and force them to equate survival and the interests of the many, not only the collegial and oligarchic few. Despots, even enlightened ones who are helped by big data platforms invading people's privacy, cannot achieve on their own the protection of a heritage that can be transmitted and without which the next generations will not have a decent life. Hopefully, democracy can be saved by new New Deals and new constitutions. It can be trumped by plutocracy and captured institutions. It can be destroyed by fascism; but it can be also weakened by parametrization of the new digitalized commons, i.e. transformed into an ersatz of democracy, using collegiality as a tool for management, just like the Catholic church, but with likely more brutal and forced forms of collective responsibility.

If morphogenetic processes only may be able to bring about the changes that are needed for collective survival, then mechanisms should be put in place that, based on better understanding of new forms of co-constitution of bureaucracy and collegiality, challenge closed elites and force them to equate survival and the interests of the many, not only the collegial and oligarchic few. By using for example dynamics of multilevel networks to identify forms of virtuous and vicious organizational morphogenesis, sociologists may increase their chances of making their discipline relevant again for institutional change and innovation. Indeed knowledge of organizational morphogenesis may help actors define the collegial social discipline that they find legitimate for their commons so as not to exhaust the social capital that produces an alternative to the bureaucratic and military path, and eventually understand how to create a protected heritage to transfer to future generations. A neostructural approach is a useful part of the intellectual adventure of contemporary social sciences if it helps identify in morphogenetic mechanisms what must change in the transition for the earth to be livable by future generations.

References

Al-Amoudi, I. (2014). Morphogenesis and normativity: Problems the former creates for the latter. In M. S. Archer (Ed.), *Late modernity: Trajectories towards morphogenic society* (pp. 193–220). London: Springer.

Al-Amoudi, I., & Latsis, J. (2014). The arbitrariness and normativity of social conventions. *British Journal of Sociology, 65*(2), 358–378.

Archer, M. S. (1995). *Realist social theory: The morphogenetic approach*. Cambridge, MA: Cambridge University Press.

Archer, M. S. (2013). Introduction. In *Social morphogenesis*. New York: Springer.

Archer, M. S. (2015). Introduction: Other conceptions of generative mechanisms and ours. In M. S. Archer (Ed.), *Generative mechanisms transforming social order*. Cham: Springer.

Archer, M. S. (2016). Anormative regulation in the morphogenic society. In M. S. Archer (Ed.), *Morphogenesis and the crisis of normativity*. Dordrecht: Springer.

Baylis, T. A. (1989). *Governing by committee: Collegial leadership in advanced societies*. Albany: SUNY Press.

Béraud, C. (2006). *Le Métier de prêtre. Approche sociologique*. Paris: Les Editions de l'Atelier.

Bosk, C. (1979). *Forgive and remember: Managing medical failure*. Chicago: University of Chicago Press.

Bourdieu, P., & Saint Martin de, M. (1982). La sainte famille. L'épiscopat français dans le champ du pouvoir. *Actes de la recherche en sciences sociales, 44*, 2–54.

Charles, F. (1986). *La génération défroquée*. Paris: Cerf.

Coriat, B. (Ed.). (2015). *Le retour des communs et la crise de l'idéologie propriétaire*. Paris: Les Liens qui libèrent.

Courcy, R. (1999). La paroisse et la modernité – lieu fondateur et arguments actualisés. *Archives de sciences sociales des religions, 107*, 21–39.

Donégani, J. M. (1993). *La liberté de choisir: pluralisme religieux et pluralisme politique dans le catholicisme français contemporain*. Paris: Presse de la fondation nationale des sciences politiques.

Donégani, J. M. (2000). Identités religieuses et pluralité des rapports au monde. In P. Bréchon, B. Duriez, & J. et Ion (Eds.), *Religion et action dans l'espace public* (pp. 211–224). Paris: L'Harmattan.

Freidson, E. (1986). *Professional powers*. Chicago: University of Chicago Press.

Gannon, T. M. (1971). Priest/minister: Profession or not profession? *Review of Religious Research, 12*(2), 66–79.

Gannon, T. M. (1979a). The impact of structural differences on the catholic clergy. *Journal for the Scientific Study of Religion, 18*(4), 350–362.

Gannon, T. M. (1979b). The effect of segmentation in the religious clergy. *Sociological Analysis, 40*(3), 183–196.

Gellard, J. (1977). Pouvoirs et stratégies dans l'administration d'un diocèse. *Recherches en sciences religieuses, 65*(4), 505–542.

Goudet, B. (1997). Qui parle ? Approche phénoménologique et analyse des formes et statuts de parole dans une assemblée synodale interdoyennés. In J. Palard (sous la dir.), *Le gouvernement de l'Église catholique – Synodes et exercice du pouvoir* (pp. 207–228). Paris: Cerf.

Granfield, P. (1988). Légitimation et bureaucratisation du pouvoir dans l'Église. *Concilium, 217*, 109–117.

Hess, C., & Ostrom, E. (Eds.). (2007). *Understanding knowledge as a commons: From theory to practice*. Cambridge, MA: The MIT Press.

Hervieu-Léger, D. (2003). *Catholicisme, la fin d'un monde*. Paris: Bayard.

Lazega, E. (1992). *Micropolitics of knowledge*. New York: Aldine-de Gruyter.

Lazega, E. (1993). Collégialité et bureaucratie dans les firmes américaines d'avocats d'affaires. *Droit et Société, 23*(24), 15–40.

Lazega, E. (1994). Analyse de réseaux et sociologie des organisations. *Revue Française de Sociologie, 35*, 293–320.

Lazega, E. (2001). *The Collegial phenomenon: The social mechanisms of cooperation among peers in a corporate law partnership*. New York: Oxford University Press.

Lazega, E. (2003). Rationalité, discipline sociale et structure. *Revue Française de Sociologie, 44*(44), 305–330.

Lazega, E. (2006). Capital social, processus sociaux et capacité d'action collective. In A. Bevort & M. Lallement (Eds.), *Capital social: Echanges, réciprocité, équité* (pp. 213–225). Paris: La Découverte.

Lazega, E. (2012). Sociologie néo-structurale. In R. Keucheyan & G. Bronner (Eds.), *Introduction à la théorie sociale contemporaine*. Paris: Presses Universitaires de France.

Lazega, E. (2013). Network analysis in the 'Morphogenetic Society' project: A neo-structural exploration and illustration. In M. S. Archer (Ed.), *Social morphogenesis* (pp. 167–186). Dordrecht: Springer.

Lazega, E. (2014a). Appropriateness and structure in organizations: Secondary socialization through dynamics of advice networks and weak culture. In D. J. Brass, G. (Joe) Labianca, A. Mehra, D. S. Halgin & S. P. Borgatti (Eds.), Volume on *Contemporary perspectives on organizational social networks* (Vol. 40, pp. 381–402), *Research in the sociology of organizations.* Bingley: Emerald.

Lazega, E. (2014b). 'Morphogenesis Unbound' from the dynamics of multilevel networks: A neo-structural perspective. In M. S. Archer (Ed.), *Late modernity: Trajectories towards morphogenic society* (pp. 173–191). Cham: Springer.
Lazega, E. (2015a). Body captors and network profiles: A neo-structural note on digitalized social control and morphogenesis. In M. S. Archer (Ed.), *Generative mechanisms transforming the social order* (pp. 113–133). Dordrecht: Springer.
Lazega, E. (2015b). Synchronization costs in the organizational society: Intermediary relational infrastructures in the dynamics of multilevel networks. In E. Lazega & T. Snijders (Eds.), *Multilevel network analysis for the social sciences*. Dordrecht: Springer.
Lazega, E. (2016). Joint 'anormative' regulation from status inconsistency: A multilevel spinning top model of specialized institutionalization. In M. S. Archer (Ed.), *Morphogenesis and the crisis if normativity*. Dordrecht: Springer.
Lazega, E., & Mounier, L. (2002). Interdependent entrepreneurs and the social discipline of their cooperation: The research program of structural economic sociology for a society of organizations. In O. Favereau & E. Lazega (Eds.), *Conventions and structures in economic organization: Markets, networks, and hierarchies* (pp. 147–199). Cheltenham: Edward Elgar Publishing.
Lazega, E. & Wattebled, O. (2011, November). Deux définitions de la collégialité et leur articulation: le cas d'un diocèse catholique. In *Sociologie du Travail*, 52/4: 480–502. English version: Two definitions of collegiality and their inter-relation: The case of a Roman Catholic diocese. *53* (Supplement 1), e57–e77
Musselin, C. (1990). Structures formelles et capacités d'intégration dans les universités françaises et allemandes. *Revue Française de Sociologie, 31*, 439–461.
Ostrom, E. (1990). *Governing the commons: The evolution of institutions for collective action*. Cambridge: Cambridge University Press.
Palard, J. (1985). *Pouvoir religieux et espace social. Le diocèse de Bordeaux comme organisation*. Paris: Cerf.
Perrow, C. (1986). *Complex organizations: A critical essay* (3rd ed.). London: McGraw-Hill.
Sainsaulieu, R. (1977). *L'Identité au travail*. Paris: Presses de Sciences Po.
Schilling, T. P. (2002). *Conflict in the catholic hierarchy: a study of coping strategies in the Hunthausen affair with preferential attention to discursive strategies*. Utrecht: Labor Grafimedia BV.
Selznick, Ph. (1949). *TVA and the grass roots: A study in the sociology of formal organization*. Berkeley: University of California Press.
Vallier, I. (1969). Comparative studies of roman Catholicism: Dioceses as strategic units. *Sociology Compass, 16*(2), 147–184.
Villemin, L et Caillot J. (2001). Mission de l'Église qui envoie. *Prêtres diocésains*, mars-avril, 1395, 161–189.
Waters, M. (1989). Collegiality, bureaucratisation and professionalization: A Weberian analysis. *American Journal of Sociology, 94*(5), 945–972.
Wattebled, O. (2004). *Discipline sociale entre prêtres: Bureaucratie et collégialité dans un diocèse français*. Doctoral thesis, Department of Sociology and Anthropology, University of Lille 1, France.
Weber, M., [1920] (1978) edition. In G. Roth & C. Wittich (Eds), *Economy and society*, Berkeley/Los Angeles: University of California Press.
Willaime, J. P. (1986). L'autorité religieuse et sa pratique dans la situation contemporaine. *Lumière et vie, 35*(180), 37–52.
Willaime, J. P. (1992). *La précarité protestante: Sociologie du protestantisme contemporain*. Genève: Labor et Fidès.

Chapter 11
Eudaimonic Bubbles, Social Change and the NHS

Tony Lawson

Eudaimonia or the 'good society' is a world or social system in which we all flourish in our differences. This is the conception I have defended elsewhere, both as a real possibility for humanity, and as the ethical goal of moral actions (see especially Lawson 2015, but also Lawson 2000, 2013). I have also suggested that whatever our differences, and of course each of us is unique in a multitude of ways, one factor common to us all is that our own flourishing requires that everyone else flourishes. It is impossible for any of us fully to flourish in a system that necessitates that others suffer.

I have also (and repeatedly) defended the idea that the path to eudaimonia is not about prediction, planning and control (see e.g. Lawson 1997). Rather it involves the imagining of forms of the good society (concrete utopias) identifying obstacles that lie in the path to reaching them, and seeking to remove such obstacles as are identified. Obvious examples of the later practice include identifying structures that allow/encourage the oppression of one group by another, say of those gendered one way by others gendered differently, or of immigrants by indigenous citizens, etc., and finding ways of transforming them.

It is important, though, that the manner in which we move towards the good society, in which we remove obstacles, is consistent with our vision of the good society. It is not an option to do harm to, or to disrespect, those who are ideologically blinkered or otherwise conditioned erroneously to resist emancipatory change, just because they are so blinkered.

I have also argued that there are tendencies to the good society everywhere in play that are rooted in the more fundamental features of human nature. These are ever present, and shine through repeatedly, not least in much spontaneous action, especially in the face of others observed to be in distress.

T. Lawson (✉)
Faculty of Economics, University of Cambridge, Cambridge, UK
e-mail: tony.lawson@econ.cam.ac.uk

M.S. Archer (ed.), *Morphogenesis and Human Flourishing*, Social Morphogenesis,
DOI 10.1007/978-3-319-49469-2_11

These are, though, frequently offset by countervailing tendencies, the latter being usually grounded in ignorance/lack of criticality and fear. Whether the good society is ever reached is of course an open question; we are quite capable of destroying life on the planet, ourselves included.

But tendencies to the good society, even when efficacious, are just that: tendencies. They take time. As it seems very likely that capitalism is itself a major obstacle to generalised human flourishing, and there are few signs of it being supplanted in the near future, the question obviously (and repeatedly) arises as to whether it is possible for any of us in the meantime to flourish, if not fully then at least along one or more axes of our concerns.

By this I mean can we provide (sub) communities in which certain sets of needs at least are adequately met, and met in ways that are not harmful to others. An organising principle that, where applied, appears to be an at least necessary condition of it is the following: that the allocation of society's resources and possibilities be made on the basis of the maxim 'from each according to her or his abilities to each according to her or his needs, in the pursuit of generalised flourishing in our differences'.

Can we achieve conditions *within* capitalism that allow this? Assuming we only live once, and that most of us are not likely to outlive the system, this is a question of significant continuing interest and bearing.

Because I am considering these matters as a participant in a project that is studying processes of social change, and where a specific focus is social morphogenesis, it is also of interest here to question whether morphogenetic processes have a bearing on reinforcing/inhibiting not only tendencies to full, or fuller, flourishing in the longer run (an issue I partially addressed in Lawson 2014) but also, and in particular, in establishing/inhibiting situations both of increased or partial flourishing in the short run, and even the here and now.

Defining Some Terms

The first matter I want to stress is that most of the central terms I am using do not, and could not sensibly, have fixed or absolutist meanings. There is much relativity involved including context and technological possibilities. I take it that everything social and much that is human is evolving and that the future of more or less everything social or human is open. This includes many aspects at least of human nature, technology, assessments of the meaning of, as well as the possibilities for, human flourishing and so on.

In taking this stance I clearly presuppose there is such a thing as human nature even if it is always in process, just as I presuppose that notions of greater and/or less flourishing of human beings are meaningful and relevant. Let me elaborate.

Though a rock may (pace Spinoza) be unaffected by its placement in one context rather than any other in which it endures, I doubt this is true of human beings. For humans, survival or endurance is not enough. As is very likely the case with all sentient beings, there are conditions that must be in place for us to realise ourselves as the sort of beings we are. There are conditions of human well-being or flourishing. We all do clearly have needs. Some are common to all of us, such as that of realising our capacities to enter competently into both social and non-social being, to acquire language and so forth. Others will be specific to us as members of particular communities - for example the need at a certain stage in life to speak a given set of acquired languages. Others will be unique.

A reason for optimism that, despite the differences in human needs, a form of society is possible in which all, or the more fundamental, needs can be compatibly met, is the recognition that any given need can be met in a multitude of ways. For any need can give rise to an array of wants, with each want in turn being potentially being met from any of a multitude of satisfiers. It is thus in principle easy to realign wants and (so) satisfiers, to achieve generalised compatibility of activities, and yet meet the different underlying needs.

If, for example, a (in this case likely shared) need is for respect, only under certain systems will this be manifest as desires/wants for status possessions, and only under even more specific conditions still, will the latter be satisfied by flashy cars and yachts and so forth achieved at the expense of the majority having relatively little. The latter are simply unnecessary for the meeting of real needs. There are, of course, communities and scenarios, both actual and imaginable, where respect is achieved simply by wanting to, and finding specific ways to, care for others.

In any case few things are fixed. Certainly fixity is not a trait of most aspects of human nature, in particular those that have been contextually conditioned (like a need to communicate with others in a specific language), but even less is it a feature of technology, and possibilities of restructuring societies and creating conditions of flourishing. As I say, more or less everything social and much that is human is open to future development. The good society is nothing if not a social totality in process.

The position I am sketching I have elsewhere defended under the heading of *critical ethical naturalism*, an orientation presupposing or incorporating a *moral realism* (see Lawson 2015, also 2000, 2003, 2013). This position is a *naturalism* in that it is quite consistent with the best findings of the non-social sciences and of naturalistic social theory; it is a form of (moral) *realism* in that the issue of whether or not our actions lead us towards the good society rest *not* on our (always fallible) *assessments* but on the truth of the matter; it is *critical* in that it goes beyond most other ethical naturalisms, the majority of which fail to recognise that the generalised flourishing of all (as opposed to some bare consideration of others) is a condition for any significant flourishing of each.

Unfortunately, I cannot defend these positions here without the paper becoming inordinately long. So I take the positions elsewhere defended (in particular see Lawson 2000, 2013, 2015) as given, and question the possibilities for achieving a degree or form of flourishing, at least along one axis, or a set of axes, in the here and now. For those who reject my premises, this topic may still be of interest, even if the question posed does not seem as pressing as I myself believe it to be (and the current way of organising society not as de-humanising as I interpret it to be).

So if the demise of capitalism is not around the corner, what can we do meanwhile? This is a question that is regularly posited. What, if anything, can we do of value in conditions that militate against generalised flourishing? If the organising structure of the wider community in which we live is of a nature that participants are constrained to act in ways that in part at least are harmful (whether to themselves or others), and if that structure is beyond being easily dismantled by individual participants or restricted sub-communities, at least for the time being, what, if any, are the available options for a practice that is effective and morally defensible?

Eudaimonic Bubbles

The sort of answer I here want to explore I have, over the years, often discussed in Cambridge meetings, like those of the *Cambridge Social Ontology Group* (see Pratten [ed.] 2015).[1] But I have not previously developed some of these ideas on paper. That answer I defend or explore involves the creation of wider-community-specific flourishing-facilitating contingently protected sub-communities that I refer to as *eudaimonic bubbles.*

As the metaphor suggests I mean relatively advantageous, if often precarious, conditions in which sub-communities can insulate themselves, relatively speaking, from specific sets of dehumanising or oppressive features characteristic of the wider community within which they are located.

Clearly all sub-communities share much of the social structure of wider embedding communities. But in some cases a sub-community or bubble may emerge that is successfully oriented to achieving a specific set of goals that are perceived as essential to, or highly consistent with, human flourishing, that are difficult and usually impossible to achieve consistently in the wider community. If they emerge at all they will frequently do so, I suspect, precisely in conditions where the concerns or needs in question are particular ill-served and individuals are suffering much harm. But there is no reason that this has to be the case, especially if the goal of generalised flourishing is a motivating feature of all of us.

Obvious examples are close friendships, partnerships, many families, refuges, perhaps certain monastic communities, possibly some retreats, and even various study groups. In these situations, interactions are or can be based in the main not on competition, oppression, unnecessary hierarchical power, and such like but on cooperation, love and care. If there is an organising principle for all such bubbles, a eudaimonic principle even, then ideally it is indeed that allocation of resources and opportunities accord to the maxim ‘from each according to her or his abilities to each according to her or his needs, in the pursuit of generalised flourishing in our differences’.

[1] Also see http://www.csog.econ.cam.ac.uk/

Are these scenarios exceptional? I believe they are more common than appreciated, and continually emerging and re-emerging, just because they are more authentic in the sense of being more in tune with our humanity, than alternatives. But maintaining them is difficult, just because (by definition) they emerge within and into communities organised by structures and (their) mechanisms that are essentially oppressive and militate against bubbles of any significant persistence or scope. I am thinking here of structures like capitalism, patriarchy, some forms of institutionalised religion, racism, nationalism, intellectual dogmatism, and so on.

If despite everything eudaimonic bubbles of relatively localised, if usually precarious and often temporary, flourishing keep appearing, my question is what governs their emergence and relative survival. Are there conditions common to successful cases? And given the wider project to which I am contributing, how, if at all, do processes of morphogenesis contribute? My suspicion is that there is no systematic answer, and that much depends on context.

Previously I have identified various factors that underpin or reinforce eudaimonic tendencies. I indicate the nature of these in the following section. I shall argue that the same factors are necessary and supportive of (though we shall see are insufficient for) eudaimonic bubbles. In order to convey the sorts of factors I have in mind I do though need first to elaborate a bit more of the critical ethical naturalist position I defend.

Critical Ethical Naturalism as a General Presupposition

Elsewhere (in particular see Lawson 2015) I argue that the ethical naturalist including moral realist positions I have briefly sketched above (or positions very similar to them) are not only coherent but also actually presupposed by the doings of us all. I thus believe that the conception sustained is as much descriptive as prescriptive in character; that it expresses in effect not merely a need but also a tendency for us all to be authentic, i.e., to become as coherent as possible with who we already really are.

As an illustrative indicator I might note that many cultures and religions have their own version of the parable of the Good Samaritan (Luke 10:25–37). The relevant matter here, of course, is not that the parable and others like it relate a true account (whether or not it is true is not the issue), but that we all appear to recognise the moral worth of the Samaritan's actions, or more generally of the moral goodness of helping other beings in need, in particular human beings. In other words, we often, and spontaneously, go to the help of others because we recognise, and act upon, what is good for them; we recognise or perceive their value or worth existing independently of us (or at least independently of our own willing) and we can and do act on it. And if we are ourselves somehow in fear of helping the other-in-need, and often become self-critical in the process, we usually judge as morally good the actions of those others who do so go to help.

And we can revise our assessments, recognising they are fallible. It is noticeable, in this regard, that a significant number of those people who in 2003 supported the invasion of Iraq now view it as having been morally wrong.[2] Clearly, if such criticism can coherently be made of an action, there must be a position from (or standard by) which it is done. In the case of the Iraq War those involved presumably revised their whole understanding of the actions taken in terms of the actual, and threats to, the wellbeing of the very many people involved and especially those who have suffered directly or indirectly as a result of the invasion. It is the survival and flourishing of some relevant party that allows us to determine whether (or which) actions in a given context qualify as morally good. The moral worth of an action is derivative of the good or flourishing of some being(s).

I am suggesting, then, that the widespread experience of certain (other-helping) actions which many individuals in appropriate contexts undertake, presuppose (as a condition of their intelligibility) a generalised regarding of others as worthy, of value, involving a willing of their generalised flourishing, and that such actions are assessed to be morally good just because of this. In other words, the moral worth of actions is derivative of how these actions relate to the survival and flourishing of forms of, but typically of human, being. It is being as being that is of (or is invested with) intrinsic worth, and the sought-after flourishing of which grounds our (always fallible) moral deliberations (for a lengthy discussion see Lawson 2015; also see Collier 1999).

A Tendency to the Good Society

Why did I earlier suggest that there are tendencies towards the good society at play, that there are mechanisms of sorts at work in the social world tending to bring us closer to it? Seemingly, without some such ethical mechanisms to give us a perpetual prodding towards the good society, moral deliberations may yet be largely pointless, if meaningful. But where are they? In what do they consist?

An account of such mechanisms and tendencies is implicit in the outline already elaborated, in the thesis that we are all in effect critical ethical naturalists, including moral realists. In other words, the mechanisms lie in the drive basic to all of us to work, ceteris paribus, to remove obstacles to the flourishing of all others, as well as ourselves.

This is a feature of our basic human nature and being, even if our specific positioning in society leads us to be frequently mistaken and/or weak and so also to act in ways that are inconsistent with ourselves.

This is a thesis I have defended at length elsewhere (see especially Lawson 2015). Here I want to suggest that the tendencies in question, and the factors reinforcing and inhibiting them will likely to be in play in producing, maintaining and resisting eudaimonic bubbles too.

[2]When I last googled the passage "the Iraq war, I was wrong" in June 2013 I found 141 million entries.

But more I think is required for the emergence of concrete eudaimonic bubbles in the here and now. In particular the following two additional conditions seem essential: 1) that a significant level of generalised awareness or clarity prevails on the part of participants allowing authenticity to rise above blinkering forces of background ideology; and 2) that protective (possibly highly contingent and fortuitous) material support is available of a degree that allows projects based on authenticity and caring to be relatively insulated against wider-societal mainstream counterforces (seeking to undermine and impose conformity with prevailing ideology).

I want to illustrate the importance of these two seemingly necessary conditions for eudaimonic bubbles by considering factors that have been in play in grounding the phenomenon that in the UK has perhaps been the most significant eudaimonic bubble of the last century. I refer to the *National Health Service*. Many regard the National Health Service as an established, virtually unassailable, almost nation-defining, institution. In 1992 Tory Chancellor Nigel Lawson, in his book ***The View from No. 11***, observes (critically) that "The National Health Service is the closest thing the English have to a religion"[3] (Lawson, N.). A decade later in Michael Moore's 2007 film ***Sicko*** (highlighting the dire state of US health provision compared to others, and especially to the NHS) Tony Benn speculates that attempts to abolish the NHS would trigger a revolution (in the sense of a popular uprising).

And yet, as I write, the NHS may well be, if not on the way out as a eudaimonic bubble, then under serious attack from forces that want it to burst. Why do I suggest this? And if I am correct, how could such a scenario have come about? In particular, is it due to the forces that are sometimes characterised as morphogenetic and is the implication that eudaimonic bubbles, at least of a significant sort, are untenable in a morphogenic world? These are the questions I now pursue.

The National Health Service

The National Health Service is formally the healthcare system of England.[1] From the outset it has been publically funded, primarily through taxation, and it constitutes the largest single-payer healthcare system in the world. It is also the oldest, having

[3]Adding somewhat sarcastically: "with those who practice in it regarding themselves as a priesthood. This made it quite extraordinarily difficult to reform".

[4]The four countries of the United Kingdom each has a publicly funded health care system referred to as the National Health Service (NHS). The terms National Health Service or NHS are also used to refer to the four systems collectively. However, only the NHS in England uses this name officially. The four separate services were founded in 1948, based on legislation of 1946 for NHS England and of 1947 for NHS Scotland. NHS Wales was part of the same structure as England until powers over it were transferred to the Secretary of State for Wales in 1969. Responsibility for NHS Wales were passed to the Welsh Assembly (later the Welsh Government) under devolution in 1999. Each system operates independently and it accountable to its own political authority, though there is inter-service cooperation, especially where one service lacks a particular facility.

been proposed in the 1946 National Health Service Act, and brought into effect on July 5 1948. It constitutes a system of health care treatment available all members of the community, one that has been in place now for more than 65 years.

The principles upon which it was established are:

- That it meet the needs of everyone
- That it be free at the point of delivery
- That the provision of its services be based on clinical need, not ability to pay
- That it be financed through taxation

The system is available to every legal resident in the United Kingdom, with many services (for example treatment of emergencies or infectious diseases) free to all, including visitors to the UK.

Clearly, this system was basically established in accordance with the organisational criterion I am calling the eudaimonic principle, namely: 'from each according to her or his abilities to each according to her or his needs, in the pursuit of generalised flourishing in our differences', at least where the prevailing taxation system is progressive.

As such the NHS does not fit comfortably with the basic workings of the capitalist system in which it emerged. This is regularly observed by critics. In fact, it is a commonplace amongst supporters of the market system, especially (though not only[5]) in the US, to dismiss the NHS as communist, with the latter considered to be a pejorative term. How then did the NHS emerge, and how has it been maintained so far?

The Second World War was pivotal. Healthcare prior to the war had comprised an unsatisfactory mix of private, municipal and charity schemes; and there was a widely recognised need for a decent healthcare system to be created well before the actual establishment of the NHS[6].

It is unsurprising, then, given the contingencies of war, that right at its outset in 1939, an Emergency Hospital Service was introduced, providing free treatment to casualties and war evacuees. This centralised state-administered service employed doctors and nurses to care for those injured by enemy action and arrange for their treatment in whichever hospital was available (see Addison 1975). From the start

[5]It is even a view expressed by Anthony Browne, the health editor of the supposedly left-leaning UK Observer published online in the *Guardian* on Sunday 7 October 2001, and downloaded on 21/10/2015 from: http://www.theguardian.com/politics/2001/oct/07/comment.comment

[6]The view that access to health care was part of the structure of a civilized society was voiced back in the 19th century of course. Various municipalities, such as the London County Council, had the goal of running hospitals as well as utilities. Hospital charities had been supported by the benevolent while left leaning intellectuals like the Webbs argued for a state system or the insurance principle of paying in advance when well to provide any care needed when sick. During the the First World War army medical services had demonstrated the benefits of organisation and transport, with the result that, after the war, numerous reports were produced on how a health service might be organised, and caring activities be pursued by local authorities (with the result under the Local Government Act, 1929, local authorities took over poor law hospitals that now became municipal hospitals serving ratepayers, not paupers).

2378 hospitals were allocated to the scheme, and 35,000 beds were requisitioned from mental health and mental deficiency hospitals. Some were allocated forms of X-ray apparatuses, laboratories and operating theatres. Hutted hospitals were built providing thousands of beds (see Webster 1988, p. 328). Numerous hospitals were removed from cities into the country, with the scheme including provision of an ambulance service for moving patients from one place to another.

So a working centralised model based on need was in play from the start of the war, and was found to be both effective and popular. Against this background, (and encouraged by heavy canvassing by Arthur Greenwood, the UK Labour Party's deputy leader and wartime Cabinet Minister with responsibility for post-war reconstruction), a report on Social Insurance and Allied Services was commissioned in 1942. The committee that produced the report, chaired by economist and social reformer William Beveridge (the report is commonly known as the Beveridge Report), introduced the idea of a National Health Service.

Beveridge identified five 'giant evils' in society: squalor, ignorance, want, idleness, and disease, and proposed wide ranging reform to the system of social welfare to address these. It also promised recompense for the sacrifices undertaken by everyone during the war.

The war time coalition government accepted the idea of a National Health Service in February 1943. A White Paper followed in 1944. And in July 1945 Clement Attlee's Labour government found itself in a position actually to create the NHS as part of the "cradle to grave" welfare-state reforms following in the aftermath of the Second World War. It was Aneurin Bevan, newly appointed to the recently upgraded post of Minister of Health, who took the lead in the task of building the National Health Service.

Needless to say, the NHS proved hugely popular with the majority of community members throughout the UK, and set out the basis for the post-war reforms known as the Welfare State.

This is not to say that in the war and early post-war period there was no resistance along the way, including prior to the NHS being inaugurated. Opposition was voiced both by consultants and doctors (fearful of a decline in their employment conditions) and of course by the Conservative party (who have never come to terms with the NHS) and others enamoured by conceptions of the market system and 'private enterprise'. The Labour Cabinet too was divided on various issues, with Herbert Morrison arguing that local councils rather than government were better equipped to run health care.

But ultimately Bevan managed to get his way by dividing and cajoling the opposition; and on 5th July 1948, at the Park Hospital (now known as Trafford General Hospital) in Manchester, Bevan inaugurated the National Health Service proclaiming that it provided for the country "the moral leadership of the world".

There afterwards the National Health Service, free at the point contact, based on needs and financed via taxation, a veritable eudaimonic bubble in terms of care provision, became perhaps unsurprisingly the country's most popular institution. Even the Tory government of 1951 reluctantly accepted that the principle of a free health service for all, paid for out of general taxation, had been, for the time being at least, securely established if not universally embraced. As already noted many observers even came to compare it with a religion, and most still view it in this light and so as seemingly indestructible. And yet there is reason to suspect that it may soon be undermined and conceivably even replaced by something like a US style national insurance scheme. Why do I suggest this?

The Demise of the NHS?

Until 1990 the NHS was a unified organisation, albeit one that had become rather complexly structured. NHS facilities were centrally planned and funded, and delivery services were organised through a system of regional and district branches of the central NHS management. As already noted, its performance throughout was widely positively assessed, with its success deriving from the principles of providing for the needs or wellbeing of all in a manner based on an ethics of caring and trust rather than profit seeking.[7]

In 1990, however, all that was about to change. In 1989, following a review of the NHS commissioned by Margaret Thatcher a year earlier, two white papers *Working for Patients* and *Caring for People* had emerged. These outlined the introduction of an organising structure that was termed the 'internal market'. This was to shape delivery of health services for the near future. Despite widespread opposition, not least from the *British Medical Association*, though not really noticed or appreciated by most of the general public, the internal market was introduced.

The 1990 National Health Service and Community Care Act (in England) formulated a notion of the 'internal market' as a system in which Health Authorities ceased to run hospitals. Instead, the latter authorities were required to purchase care from their own or other authorities' hospitals.

For this, most NHS bodies were formed into trusts. Some, the NHS hospital trusts, provided services; others, the primary care trusts, purchased them. The former were run by boards of governors and chief executives; the latter purchasers included many GPs who were made "fund holders" and were able to pay for care for their patients.

These changes, of course, encouraged competition, as hospitals were forced to vie with each other for business; they also inevitably increased local differences. They were 'justified' as an attempt to reduce red tape and costs; instead, the changes replaced a culture of cooperation with one of opposition and antagonism, and actually markedly raised costs, not least with the large increase in administrators and managerial staff that inevitably followed (see Bloor et al. 2005, Paton 2015).

[7]As the Centre for Health and the Public Interest (CHPI) put it in a recent report "Good performance was achieved through line management but relied implicitly on trust, which in turn rested on a service ethos grounded in a shared commitment to prioritising the wellbeing of patients" (Stoll and Butta, 2015, p. 8).

Private firms were not yet involved. But a structure was now in place that facilitated their easy introduction. Although Labour came to power in 1997 with the Blair government promising to remove the internal market, abolish fundholding, and inaugurate instead a system of 'integrated care' based on fairness and partnership, it did just the opposite; it actually extended and reinforced the internal market. In this it encouraged outsourcing of medical services and support to the private sector. Thus 'New Labour's' NHS Plan (2000) and NHS Improvement Plan (2004) allowed the internal market to expand into an extensive market.

The primary goals were to create openings for private companies to provide health care for NHS patients on a regular basis; to reorganise NHS trusts and other entities into competitive businesses; and to prepare the NHS workforce for being transferred into private sector employment (involving new lucrative contracts involving 'merit awards' for consultants and GPs, but with no protection for others who were transferred to worsened conditions compulsorily).

With the fortress breached, market competition, oppositional interests, payment by results systems and related structures quickly took the place of cooperation and trust.

The Blair government revealed no signs of sharing the vision or concerns of its early post war predecessor, as expressed by Aneurin Bevan:

> Danger of abuse in the Health Service is always at the point where private commercialism impinges on the Service; where, for example, the optician is paid for the spectacles he himself prescribes, or the dentist gives an unnecessary filling for which he is paid. Abuse occurs where an attempt is made to marry the incompatible principles of private acquisitiveness with a public service. [. . .]The solution is to decrease the dependence on private enterprise (1952)

Rather the Blair government encouraged such dependence, and so abuse. By 2009 almost 150 private hospitals, 'treatment centres' and clinics were treating patients 'on the NHS' and using the NHS logo (Leys and Player 2011). And with the doors to private enterprise now wide open, by the time the Conservative-led Coalition Government's 2012 Health and Social Care Act came into effect, private providers were competing to provide NHS clinical services, using legally enforceable contracts.

With the latter 2012 Act, Clinical Commissioning Groups (CCGs), took over the Primary Care Trusts' purchasing role, and were obliged to put contracts out for competitive tender to the private sector. As I write many tens of thousands of contracts likely hold between NHS England and the private sector (see Stoll and Bhutta 2015).

Mostly these developments have increased costs for the NHS, whilst only a fraction (so far an average of 85%) of contracted services are actually delivered (see El-Gingihy 2015, p. 8); but more importantly the eudaimonic culture has been severely undermined.

The recent history, put briefly, is one of corporations muscling in and profiting hugely from tax-payers money that should have funded nothing but health care for those in need. It is a period that has witnessed ever spiralling costs and worsened outcomes for patients and hospitals.

The 2012 Act is somewhat obscurely formulated, and I certainly cannot address all its details here (for these see El-Gingihy 2015, and the contributions in Davis and Tallis [eds.] 2013). But amongst other things, the 2012 Bill in fact devolves the obligation of a National Health Service from the Health Secretary to the newly created CCGs. This in itself is significant. But at the same time the obligation itself is much reduced. In fact, it appears that the CCGs are not actually required to provide health services for all, even in a given area, but only for those on GP patient lists. So the principle of care for all is broken. CCGs can also decide which services are free at the point of delivery. So the principle of each according to their needs, and without paying, was abandoned (see Pollock et al. 2012). In fact, the only legal requirement placed on the CCGs is to provide emergency care and ambulance services.

Overall the vision is one of health care rationing, and insurance enclaves that can exclude the poorest and sickest. The outcome is uncertain. But the NHS is already a market-based system in most of its doings.

Currently, a trade agreement, *The Transatlantic Trade and Investment Partnership*, (TTIP), is being negotiated between the EU and the US that could not only accelerate these trends but ensure they are irreversible. The agreement under the mantra of "removing barriers to market access" is designed to eradicate all protective regulation that international traders regard as unhelpful to pursuing greater profits and control.

A particular proposal is for the creation of a new supra national court known as the Investor State Dispute Settlement (ISDS). This would be used by overseas companies and speculators to sue governments and even the EU over any action or legislation that they deem harmful to their money making activities. In particular, and this is a prominent focus of many concerned about the agreement, were any US private healthcare firm prevented in any way from buying up part of the NHS it would be able to go to the ISDS and, at the very least, claim millions of pounds in compensation from the UK government.

In short, the TTIP (the details of which are being negotiated in secret behind closed doors), representing the biggest bilateral trade deal ever negotiated, is potentially set to make the sell-off of the NHS irreversible by giving profit seeking activities of corporations precedence over national concerns and even lawmakers.

Currently there are various close observers who believe that all this is foregrounding a complete demise of the NHS and its replacement by something like a US style insurance system favouring the rich, is likely and not far away (see especially Youssef El-Gingihy 2015, or Colin Leys and Stewart Player, 2011).

Whether or not the worst fears of these close observers are realised, it is clear that, at the very least, if the NHS is still something of a eudaimonic bubble, it is an extremely precarious one, and that the confidence that many have in its indestructability is misplaced. As many NHS campaign groups recognise, the situation is such that if the NHS is to be preserved as something worth having, this requires significant positive collective political activity.

My question is how did we get into this situation and are forces that might be termed morphogenetic a feature of the explanation? What does explain the NHS's precarious current state, and seemingly likely impending demise?

Explaining the Current Precariousness of the NHS

Let me first note some possible explanatory hypotheses that do not withstand critical scrutiny.

Most fundamentally, perhaps, the tendencies noted in no way reflect any obvious decline in popular enthusiasm for a National Health Service. As always I am cautious about relying on survey data. But surveys regularly carried out do seem consistently to point in one direction. By all accounts, and despite a continuous campaign by the Murdoch press and others to render the NHS unpopular, survey results unswervingly suggest that the service remains as positively valued as ever by its users.

As an example, I note that a British Social Attitudes Survey published in 2013[8], reported that 65% of those asked said they were satisfied with the NHS. Commenting on this survey in that same year – for the US based Business Insider[9] (in an article headed "The British Are Surprisingly Satisfied With Their Controversial Socialized Health Care System") - Adam Taylor compares its findings with those of a comparative study published in the 2013 Health Affairs Journal[10]. The latter study "found that just 28.9% of U.S. citizens felt that their health care system "'works pretty well, and only minor changes are necessary to make it work better'". Taylor notes that in this same study the "figure for the United Kingdom was 61.3% — almost exactly the BSA result."

As I say, these survey findings and others (including those mentioned below) must, like all empirical claims, be interpreted cautiously. But there is certainly little apparent evidence of any kind that the British public want the NHS to be replaced.

Moreover the popularity of the NHS is seemingly not unconnected to support for its founding principles. In 2013 in an article entitled "The NHS: even more cherished than the monarchy and the army", Sunder Katwala reports that "New polling [. . .] shows that while attitudes to the NHS have fluctuated, commitment to its founding principles has remained remarkably consistent". Though speculating that support for the NHS may go "beyond the politics of healthcare" the author infers from the findings that "the NHS represents a now deeply entrenched fairness ideal - that healthcare should not depend on the ability to pay".

Nor is the NHS especially costly to the public, at least when compared with heath schemes elsewhere. Indeed, the NHS remains relatively inexpensive, despite corporate profit-taking increasingly sucking out resources[11].

---

[8]On 25/10/2015 this report can be downloaded from: http://www.bsa.natcen.ac.uk/media/38925/bsa32_health.pdf

[9]On 25/10/2015 downloadable from http://www.businessinsider.com/british-satisfied-with-nhs-2013-9?IR=T

[10]On 25/10/2015 the relevant report in Health Affairs Journal can be downloaded here: http://content.healthaffairs.org/content/32/4/734.full

[11]Thus according to the *OECD Health Statistics 2014 - Frequently Requested Data* the UK spending on healthcare in 2012 was 9.3% of GDP. This compares with EU-15 average of 9.9%,

So do morphogenetic factors form the basis of the explanation? The answer I believe is that they do not *if* we consider these factors somewhat abstractly and divorced from context. That is, I think the demise of the NHS, if that is what it is, has little to do with the pace of social change considered as an abstract phenomenon, whether in terms of change "speeding up" or "accelerating",[12] or of intensifying morphogenesis, or of morphogenetic processes coming to dominate morphostatic ones (if they are).

Rather, if the pace of generalised social change is relevant at all, it is the manner in which, or the background against which, these changes are occurring that is significant, or so it seems to me.

I say this, not least because, at the relevant level of abstraction, the sorts of features just noted are not so different from those in play during the period when the NHS was actually established. The early post Second World War period was also chacterised by significant social transformation, or morphogenesis, also taking the form of widespread austerity, substantial technical change, significant international migration, housing shortages, increasing demands on healthcare services, large national indebtedness, and so on; just the sorts of conditions that in the UK currently prevail.

However, the manner and context of the developments have been very different in the two periods. The single most important factor marking a difference between current developments and those in which the NHS was established, I believe, though one with numerous causal conditions, is the (lack of) political awareness of the contemporary community that is the UK. Following years of ideological conditioning by the right-wing media, contemporary UK society is highly atomised, fragmented and depoliticised. Participants are encouraged to think primarily in terms of material benefits, and then mainly for themselves and their immediate contacts; authenticity is swamped not merely by worries about increasingly uncertain material conditions but also by the continuous stream of alienating market-oriented dogma.

In contrast, in the mid-1940s, following a period of sustained wartime cooperation, the UK constituted a community for itself, as well as in itself. Its participants were far more aware of the generalised needs of all members of the community, and of the principle that all needs deserve to be met, not just those of the powerful few, and a recognition that if united in seeking such outcomes they can be achieved.

The Second World War was of course a time of declared national unity, where people of different classes and genders were not only not dissuaded but required to join together and cooperate as a united community in resisting the incursions of

---

and, according to the World Bank data, a US figure of 17%. Only 5 EU-15 countries allocated a lower share of their GDP to health expenditure (Greece, Italy, Finland, Ireland and Luxembourg). However, as marketization has increased throughout the current century this figure marks a relative movement in the rankings (in 2000, for example, only Ireland of the EU-15 had spent a smaller portion of GDP on health care than the UK).

[12]See e.g., Rosa, Hartmut, 2003; Rosa, Hartmut and William E. Scheuerman (eds.), 2009, and for a critique see Lawson 2014.

a declared common enemy. Under such conditions, the usual forces that work to redistribute from poor to rich were not only put in relative abeyance, but efforts were made to meet the expressed needs of the poor and so keep everyone on board. The emphasis was on inclusiveness, so that the needs of all were acknowledged and regularly met.[13]

Such conditions, as with any of generalised participation oriented to the common good of a community, facilitated rising political awareness, the prioritisation of authentic human qualities, and the pursuit of ways of meeting needs over competition, individual power and profit seeking.

Against this background proposals for a National Health Service always had a chance of being accepted. In fact, these same conditions, including mass participation and so rising political awareness not surprisingly saw a massive swing, in the 1945 elections, to a Labour Party that had canvassed on a manifesto promising a revolution in Health Care.

Fundamental in all this was the sharing of suffering and sacrifice. This inevitably allows participants to recognise that the needs of each of us is bound up with those of others, and that those with the power to do so have an obligation to provide basic health care, more equal rights, and conditions that better facilitate wellbeing more generally. All members of the community can better flourish if each knows that all have access to these conditions, especially to good medical treatment when in need.

[13]Unsurprisingly, then, the war years saw great improvements in working conditions and welfare provision for all, improvements which paved the way for the post-war welfare state.

There was, for example, an expansion in infant child, and maternity services. In June 1940 grants of fuel and of subsidised milk to mothers and to children under the age of five were made by the Official Food Policy Committee (chaired by the deputy PM and Labour Leader Clement Attlee), leading during the following 5 years to a 50% increase in the proportion receiving milk (rising to 73% in 1945). Also the 1940 Board of Education made free school meals more widely available. Free vaccination against diphtheria was provided for children at school.

Supplementary pensions for the elderly were introduced in 1940, with further improvements in rates and conditions for those in receipt of supplementary pensions and unemployment assistance in 1943.

Food prices had been stabilised in December 1939, initially as temporary measure, but rendered permanent in August 1940, while both milk and meals were provided at subsidised prices, or free in those cases of real need.

In July 1940, increased Treasury grants led to an increase in the supply of milk and meals in schools, with the number of meals taken doubling within a year and increased school milk increasing by 50%.

The proportion of children eating at school rose from a mere 3.3% in 1940 to about 33% in 1945. Those taking milk increased from about 50% to roughly 75%.

Wartime rationing actually led to significant improvements in the diets of poor families. The poorest third of the population of Britain who, in 1938, were chronically undernourished, had their first adequate diet in 1940 and 1941 (a development that led to the incidence of deficiency diseases and infant mortality falling markedly; see Timmins 2001).

Moreover, the fact of large numbers of civilian casualties from bombing raids necessitated that free health care treatment be provided. This meant that large numbers gained access to a health care of a form they had never previously experienced. Once experienced, of course this was not a facility that many wanted later to lose.

Aneurin Bevan, who took the lead in establishing the NHS had recognised this all along, observing in his 1952 book *In Place of Fear*, how:

> Society becomes more wholesome, more serene, and spiritually healthier, if it knows that its citizens have at the back of their consciousness the knowledge that not only themselves, but all their fellows, have access, when ill, to the best that medical skill can provide (Bevan 1952, p. 79)

If the reason that the NHS emerged when it did clearly owed much to the prevailing conditions and raised political and moral awareness of all members of the community, this rising state of political and moral awareness was hardly restricted to the UK of course. And nor of course was the focus merely on healthcare services. The rights of women in particular took a huge step forward as the contribution of women to the war effort, and their share in the suffering, were recognised (in France and Italy, for example women got the vote). But the benefits were widespread.

Thus, in January 1941 US President Roosevelt made a 'Four Freedoms' speech recognising a generalised demand for a new and more just world, with freedom of speech and expression and of religion, and freedom from want and fear. Of course this never worked out over the long term, despite some positive developments.[14] But it all reflected the climate of cooperation that prevailed.

In contrast, the modern world, certainly the contemporary UK, has largely lost the knowledge and confidence that comes with prolonged cooperative and unselfish collective practice. More so than ever before, perhaps, with the exception of pockets of critical participation and resistance here and there, the typical individual is today blinkered by, largely because relentlessly subjected to, an ideology or narrow self-interest and individualism.

All contemporary societies that fondly refer to themselves as democratic, have ruling elites whose power rests not only on the legalised use of force and aggression, but also on mechanisms for dumbing down the population. In the UK, at least for the last few centuries, the latter mechanisms have been the more powerful or anyway active; over the last 50 years or so they have been dominant indeed.

That said, a population can yet become politically aware and dynamic reasonably quickly where conditions arise that are unsettling and promote insecurity, or even where active participation is encouraged by those with the power to do so. In recent years we need only to look at events during and especially in the aftermath of the 2014 'Scottish referendum' (on the question of independence from the rest of the current UK), or recent developments in Greece as a result of the country's debt crisis (and the election of the left wing Syriza Party), or the national and international shows of solidarity and concern for others in the wake of bombings and other atrocities in major cities during the present century.

I am suggesting, then, that the level of generalised awareness relating to politics, real societal possibilities, our humanity and our connectedness, was different in the

[14] Such as widespread acceptance of the notion of a common humanity possessing the same universal rights, an idea later reinforced by the establishment of the United Nations in 1945, the International Court of Justice in 1946 and Universal Declaration of Human Rights of 1948.

two periods here being compared, and that a raised awareness of all these issues (currently lacking) is fundamental to the establishment and sustaining of eudaimonic bubbles.

But, vitally, the material conditions that have prevailed in the two periods are also very different in the promise they hold. I have already noted that both are/were periods of austerity, very significant technological change, housing shortages, high rates of immigration, and so on. There though the comparisons end. Following the war there were high expectations of improvement via post war reconstruction. In the current period few see any prospect of such demand led programmes of regeneration either being introduced, or working if they were.

A significant feature in all of this is the nature of technological change. In the early post war period technological developments were mostly designed for the direct benefit of consumers. Under the stimulus of war, governments had poured resources into developing new medicines like penicillin and consumer technologies like microwaves and computers.

In comparison, recent developments in technology, as I have elsewhere argued at length (see Lawson 2014), are significant in their capacity to render capital more mobile. Of course, new developments in production technology are always adopted with the intention of rendering the skills of workers redundant with the aim either of replacing workers or reducing their bargaining ability. With capital increasingly mobile, any resistance to the worsening of conditions of the UK workforce can be, and is increasingly, met by capital threatening to locate elsewhere, not least (currently) in countries like China, Brazil and India, and increasingly countries of Africa, with little history of worker resistance. Against these background conditions, the UK manufacturing sector continues to shrink, and measured productivity growth stays relatively low, as productivity inducing investments are located elsewhere.

Set against these two sets of background conditions (level of general awareness and specific technological/material developments), it is not so surprising, perhaps, that the eudaimonistic bubble that is the NHS has become highly precarious. It is understandable that a fragmented, atomised workforce, who receive healthcare that is still (largely) free at the point of delivery and is focussed on fears concerning job losses, reductions in skill statuses, and rising insecurity, etc., will have missed the significance of the complicated, piecemeal and sequential developments in the NHS that have been going on in the main out of view. It is also understandable that the few that are critically aware and informed feel helpless in the face of such developments.

The situation is only made even worse by those most responsible continuously and cynically reproducing an empty rhetoric of the NHS being safe in their hands.[15] Indeed, so cynical is much of this rhetoric that many close observers are moved to interpret developments, and in particular the manner in which the NHS is being dismantled as if by stealth, as reflecting something of a conspiracy (see e.g. Colin Leys and Stewart Player 2011; Lucy Reynolds and Martin McKee 2012;

[15]Indeed, the latter activity by relevant Tories, not least Prime Minister Cameron and Health Secretary Hunt, is truly remarkable.

the numerous contributors in Jacky Davis and Raymond Tallis (eds.) 2013; or El-Gingihy 2015).[16] Of course there is little doubt that most Tories and the interests they support have been concerned to dismantle the NHS from the beginning[17] and replace it by a market based system advantaging the well-off; critical self-awareness (or who we all really are) and/or trust in humanity have never been features of supporters of market competition. But only relatively recently have moves to undermine the NHS been pursued behind a rhetoric that departs so radically from the reality; wherein changes from a system based on need is replaced by one based instead on profit and greed are presented as mainly administrative and coherent with the values of the NHS shared by all.

This has all been aided by the fact that, with the exception of the creation of foundation trusts, legislation has not been required to effect any of the moves that have transformed the NHS into a healthcare market, providing entry points for privatisation. Rather the various transformations effected were simply presented as administrative adjustments; and were largely hidden in documents with homely titles (see Leys and Player 2011[18]).

---

[16] Although I myself am not a conspiracy theorist by nature (not least because the world is open and bringing plans to fruition, whether conforming or opposed to human authenticity, is difficult enough at the best of times), there are, as I say, numerous close observers of recent developments that do see a conspiracy, and they do make a plausible case

They point to instances like the following. Back in the 1980s, before the changes to the NHS really kicked in, the pro-market *Centre for Policy Studies*, published a series of studies exploring how the NHS might be quietly dismantled. In one of them, John Redwood, who had just become a Conservative MP, and Oliver Letwin, then merely an activist but later the Tory Minister of State at the Cabinet Office, put forward the following suggestion for transforming the NHS:

> But need there be just one leap? Might it not, rather, be possible to work slowly from the present system towards a national insurance scheme? One could begin for example, with the establishment of the NHS as an independent trust, with increased joint ventures between the NHS and the private sector; move on next to the use of 'credits' to meet standard charges set by central NHS funding administration for independently managed hospitals or districts; and only at the last stage create a national health scheme separate from the tax system.

For a fuller discussion see e.g., Leys and Player, 2011, El-Gingihy (2015), or Reynolds and McKee (2012).

[17] Why? Mostly due to the uncritical acceptance of a naïve belief in the idea that it is good for some (themselves and their friends) to gain power and wealth at the expense of others. It is ultimately based on failure to recognise their own humanity, or to lose sight of the latter under the sway of the prevailing ideology in support of the validity of profits and greed. Some, like Hayek, do genuinely seem to suppose that a market-based system is the best framework for achieving wider 'freedom'. Hayek of course believed that state planning reflecting the preferences of some (possibly benevolent) dictator was the only alternative to the market, and never developed an understanding of human needs. Rather he thought that preferences were somehow all that mattered, and that each individual knows best what they are (ignoring the fact that most producers commit the highest proportion of their outlays to advertising and marketing, attempting to convince people to take their products and brands, whether they need them or not, and no matter how harmful they might truly be).

[18] According to Leys and Player (2011) in fact "Misrepresentation, obfuscation and deception have been involved at every stage" (Leys and Player, 2011, p. 2).

Whether or not the case of those who see conspiracy is plausible, the NHS as a eudaimonic bubble is, if to repeat, in a highly precarious state. The reason for it is simply that it is being steadily attacked and abused in a situation where the conditions essential for its assured survival are largely absent. These, to recall, are 1) that a significant level of generalised awareness or clarity on part of participants allowing authenticity to rise above blinkering forces of prevailing ideology, and 2) protective (possibly highly contingent and fortuitous)) material support is available of a degree that allow projects based on caring and being true to ourselves to prevail (or be insulated against) mainstream counterforces (seeking to undermine and impose conformity with prevailing ideology).

So my answer to the question of whether morphogenetic forces or any other forms of social change are consistent with eudaimonic bubbles, is that it depends on their nature and content. Social change is an ever-present feature of all social being. Those forces for change that operated during and after the Second World War period are qualitatively different to those currently in operation, and so supported different outcomes. For those of us living in the West, the forces currently in play seem likely only to further undermine conditions consistent with humanity or authenticity. Not only do such conditions augur badly for the NHS but are likely to facilitate any of a number of misguided somewhat foolish responses, whether taking the form of racism, abandoning commitments to human rights legislation, giving up on responsibilities to support welfare provision in general and so on.

At the heart of these developments, are forces increasing the marketization, or better commodification, of everything, harnessing ongoing developments in technology to render capital ever more mobile and effective in plundering the resources of the planet. With capital increasing mobile, workers' resistance along with other forces more consistent with human development are continually weakened.

On a more positive note, and again as I have argued elsewhere (Lawson 2014), these developments, if currently mostly destructive, do presumably hasten the day when the globe is fully industrialised and capital no longer has any new location to which it can run; the conditions are being laid whereby more progressive forces everywhere can effectively unite in enlightened resistance, and collectively remove these obstacles to eudaimonia.

Meanwhile how about the NHS as we have come to know it? Can it be saved in the meantime?

Possibly. But the parties concerned to maintain it need to push in one and the same direction, and they need additional support. Somehow various obstacles that lie in the path of rescuing it need removal. These include those factors that are frustrating our natural/human sensitivity to the shared conditions of our flourishing, as well as those impeding recognition of forces seeking relentlessly to undermine the NHS. At the same time, the NHS requires funding. The UK is still a relatively wealthy country and currently the share of resources devoted to the healthcare is relatively low. That share could be significantly increased. But such a redistribution requires once more a rise in community-wide political awareness, the removal of our atomistic blinkers, in order that priorities are rendered more coherent with our needs as human beings. Such a prospect does seem less than likely in the current political environment, especially with media outlets perpetually working to reinforce the blinkers (for an analysis see Oliver Huitson 2013). But that said, the eudaimonistic tendency is always operative at some level; and the world and our future are forever open.[19] If despite everything we are able to act together, if a form of conscious resistance comes to be sparked, and there clearly are critically aware, active groups of this sort scattered throughout the country,[20] the future of the NHS remains in our collective hands and action. As Aneurin Bevan observed over 60 years.

> A free Health Service is a triumphant example of the superiority of collective action and public initiative applied to a segment of society where commercial principles are seen at their worst (Bevan 1952, chapter 5)

The challenge is to find ways to reclaim those early conditions.

---

[19]As I write (October 2015) Jeremy Corbyn, a Labour MP whose stance reveals more critical awareness than is usual of Labour MPs of recent years, has been elected Party leader. And Caroline Lucas, a Green Party MP, has a Bill (National Health Service Bill 2015–16), also supported by a cross party group of MPS, going through Parliament and due for a second reading in March 2016, that is trying to restore some of the benefits to the NHS system. Amongst other things, it seeks to re-establish the Secretary of State's legal duty concerning the National Health Service in England and to make provision about the related duties of the Secretary of State in that regard. In summary, the Bill aims to restore the NHS as an accountable public service by reversing 25 years of marketisation in the NHS, abolishing the purchaser-provider split, ending contracting and re-establishing public bodies and public services accountable to local communities. The Bill certainly looks in the right direction; it remains to be seen if it is a direction in which Corbyn's parliamentary colleagues allow him and the Party as a whole also effectively to push.

Addendum to the foregoing footnote added March 18, 2016. The latter Bill was due to be debated in Parliament on March 11 2016. However, a group of Tory MPs filibustered, meaning that they purposely talked so long on the Bill that was tabled just before the NHS Bill that they succeeded in reducing the time left to debate the NHS Bill to 17 min, ensuring that it was shelved without a vote. Of course, this fits with the view of those that see a conspiracy at every turn. Certainly, it reveals a Tory party full of people with little critical awareness, fearful of informed debate and discussion, being naively more concerned with profits and greed than their own and everyone else's flourishing. The Labour Party though did not publicly back the bill, even though its individual members claimed to. In fact, I write a day following a budget in which the Tory Chancellor Osborne made £650 million of so far unnoticed or 'secret' cuts to the NHS. See http://www.independent.co.uk/news/uk/politics/nhs-cuts-budget-george-osborne-secret-stealth-privatisation-a6938441.html

[20]As an illustration, one highly active group or set of groups is located in Bristol. See e.g., (all downloaded on March 18 2016): https://protectournhs.wordpress.com/tag/bristol/

https://www.facebook.com/groups/277576572316379/?fref=ts

http://www.bristolpost.co.uk/pictures/Hundreds-Bristol-city-centre-protest-changes-NHS/pictures-28869984-detail/pictures.html#mMYTCOIh68vQP2J9.01

https://www.opendemocracy.net/ournhs/caroline-lucas/tories-stole-nhs-bill-debate-from-public-but-bill-to-save-our-nhs-is-not-going

Final Comments

I have focussed, via the notion of eudaimonic bubbles, on the possibility of achieving a degree of flourishing, along one set of axes at least, in the here and now, something that is sufficiently eudaimonic as to be worth having.

I have noted that if processes characterised as austerity and fast technical change and so forth can support factors that undermine eudaimonic bubbles, they can also support, and have supported, factors that lead to their emergence. The context, content and quality of change is fundamental in effecting any outcome. I assume this observation applies whether or not morphogenetic process are intensifying.

That said, a specific tendency that is ever present, I believe, because reflecting the sorts of beings we really are, is the continuous push towards a society, a set of communities, in which we all flourish in our differences. The moral objective in the face of such a tendency, if such it is, and given who we really are, is to identify obstacles that lie in the path to the good society and seek to transform or remove them.

This usually requires a level of human criticality and joint participation. Whether intensifying morphogenetic forces, or their dominance, are more of a help or a hindrance is something about which I feel unable to generalise. But even if, as I suspect, very much does depend on context, this conclusion is not without implication for action, and nor is it lacking in grounds for optimism. For it reflects the fact that the future is truly open and is always something for us to make. The conclusion requires too that, as best we can, we stay ever alive to opportunities that may be thrown up for achieving progress, and that in pushing towards the good society we are never doomed to inevitable short or long term failure, especially if we act collectively.

References

Addison, P. (1975). *The road to 1945: british politics and the second world war* (pp. 178–181). London: Jonathan Cape.

Bevan, A. (1952). *In place of fear*. New York: Simon and Schuster.

Bloor, K., Harvey, E., & Maynard, A. (2005). *NHS Management and Administration Staffing and Expenditure in a National and International Context*, York University: unpublished paper (embargoed by the Department of Health).

Browne, A. (2001). "Why the NHS is bad for us", the Guardian, published online (and observed on 08/10/2015) at: http://www.theguardian.com/politics/2001/oct/07/comment.comment

Collier, A. (1999). *Being and worth*. London: Routledge.

Davis, J., & Tallis, R. (Eds.). (2013). *How the NHS was betrayed – And how we can save it*. London: Oneworld Publications.

El-Gingihy, Y. (2015). *How to dismantle the NHS in 10 easy steps*. Alresford: Zero Books.

Huitson, O. (2013). 'Hidden in Plain Sight' in Jacky Davis and Raymond Tallis (eds.) 2013, chapter 5.

Katwala, S. (2013). "The NHS: even more cherished than the monarchy and the army", *New Statesman*, Jan 14. The report by Katwala can (25/10/2015) be downloaded here: http://www.newstatesman.com/politics/2013/01/nhs-even-more-cherished-monarchy-and-army

Lawson, N. (1992). *The view from No 11: Memoirs of a tory radical*. London: Bantam Press.
Lawson, T. (1997). *Economics and reality*. London/New York: Routledge.
Lawson, T. (2000). Evaluating trust, competition and co-operation. In Y. Shionoya & K. Yagi (Eds.), *Competition, trust and co-operation – A comparative study*. New York/Berlin/Tokyo: Springer.
Lawson, T. (2003). *Reorienting economics*. London/New York: Routledge.
Lawson, T. (2013). Ethical naturalism and forms of relativism. *Society, 50*, 570–575.
Lawson, T. (2014). A speeding up of the rate of social change? power, technology, resistance, globalisation and the good society. In M. S. Archer (Ed.), *Late modernity: Trajectories towards morph genic society*. Dordrecht: Springer.
Lawson, T. (2015). Critical ethical naturalism: An orientation to ethics. In S. Pratten (Ed.) (2015) pp. 359–387.
Leys, C., & Player, S. (2011). *The plot against the NHS*. Pontypool: Merlyn Press.
Paton, C. (2015). *At what cost? Paying the price for the market in the English NHS*, Published by the *Centre for Health and Public Interest*.
Pollock, A. M., Price, D., & Roderick, P. (2012). Health and social care bill 2011: A legal basis for charging and providing fewer health services to people in England. *British Medical Journal, 344*, e1729. Published 08 March 2012. Downloaded from http://dx.doi.org/10.1136/bmj.e1729, Oct 2015.
Pratten, S. (Ed.). (2015). *Social ontology and modern economics*. London/New York: Routledge.
Reynolds, L., & McKee, M. (2012). Opening the Oyster: the 2010-11 NHS Reforms in England. *Clinical Medicine, 12*(2), 128–132.
Rosa, H. (2003). Social acceleration: Ethical and political consequences of a desynchronised high-speed society. *Constellations, 10*(1), 43.
Rosa, H., & Scheuerman, W. E. (Eds.). (2009). *High speed society: Social acceleration power and modernity*. University Park: Pennsylvania State University Press.
Stoll, L., & Bhutta, M. (2015). *The contracting NHS: Can the NHS handle the outsourcing of clinical services? Published by the Centre for Health and the Public Interest*, March.
Timmins, N. (2001). *The five giants: A biography of the welfare state, (revised edition)*. London: Harper Collins.
Webster, C. (1988). *The health services since the war*. London: HMSO.

Chapter 12
The Will to Be: Human Flourishing and the Good International Society

Colin Wight

Introduction

Terminology matters, and there are good reasons why terms such as the 'good society', and human flourishing do not figure prominently in the discipline of International Relations. Despite much evidence to support the thesis that violence in the contemporary world is on the wane (Goldstein 2011; Krause 2009; Pinker 2011), at the international level, human suffering and not human flourishing is still perceived to be the most pressing problem. In December 2015, there were four ongoing conflicts that meet the definition of major wars (those involving more than 10,000 deaths a year); Afghanistan, Iraq, Syria, and Nigeria. In Afghanistan, estimates suggest that there had been more than 2,000,000 casualties since the outbreak of major conflict in 1978 when the Soviets first invaded. Since then, despite brief periods of peace, any attempt to apply the concept of human flourishing to the Afghan people, and or Afghan society more generally would seem not only to be misplaced but to be a perverse misuse of the term. Unless the great powers can reach some accommodation, the conflict in Syria could soon overtake Afghanistan at the top of the death-by- war league. As of December 2015, annual deaths in Syria have been approximately 75,000 a year. In total, there have been over 250,000 casualties in the Syrian conflict, with more than 12 million people displaced. In addition, to these major wars, there are also currently fourteen ongoing conflicts that kill between 1000 and 10,000 people a year, and a further 22 ongoing conflicts that produce casualty figures of 100–1000 (Security 2016).

C. Wight (✉)
Department of Government and International Relations, University of Sydney, Sydney, NSW, Australia
e-mail: colin.wight@sydney.edu.au

M.S. Archer (ed.), *Morphogenesis and Human Flourishing*, Social Morphogenesis,
DOI 10.1007/978-3-319-49469-2_12

Of course, when compared to the carnage of World War I and World War II arguments about the decline in casualties from war clearly have some salience. Salience, however, is not evidence of a causal law and certainly not enough to legitimise talk of the 'good international society' at this point in time. Moreover, the resurgence of Russian assertiveness, and the rise of China suggest that great power politics may yet reemerge as a major factor in global politics, and when placed within the context of the inequities of global capitalism, the migration crisis, international terrorism, human trafficking, torture, global infant mortality figures, domestic violence, and the threat of global environmental catastrophe, then talk of the 'good international society' at the global level seems misplaced. There may be pockets of the 'good society' across the international system, but it is not yet a notion that can be globalised. Moreover, what pockets of the good society that there are tend to be concentrated in the affluent parts of the Western world. Under global capitalism, the good society is defined in terms of dollars. At the international level, the 'good society' is expensive, life, it seems, is cheap!

That said, I think there is much that could be said about the *possibility* of the 'good international society'. What would such a society look like? What are the conditions of possibility for such a society? How might the international system be reformed in ways that enable human flourishing rather than human suffering? How exactly would the 'good international society' be structured? Answers to these questions inevitably take us into the realm of speculative utopian theorising. But engaging in this form of theorising in the discipline of international relations has more often than not brought about the premature end of one's career. Utopian theorising is derided in the discipline as idealism: an idealism that confronts a harsh Hobbesian world at every turn. Set against this idealism are various forms of realism. What separates such realisms from idealism is that they all resolutely refuse to engage in utopian theorising.

Indeed, Hans Morgenthau argues that values have no place in either the practice or theory, of international politics (Morgenthau 1978). According to Morgenthau, values and idealism should be kept out of international politics for four main reasons. First, the concept of the good is not universal. What is good in one part of the international system may not be good in another part. Second, since there are no universal moral 'goods', the attempt to impose 'our good' onto the 'other' cannot in itself be good. Third, those who propose universal values at the level of the international system will inevitably meet with resistance. Hence however well-intentioned the idealists may be, they produce more conflict not less. A recent example here might be the invasion of Iraq in 2003. Setting aside for the time being all counter arguments, one of the main reasons often cited by both George W. Bush, and Tony Blair for the invasion was that the removal of the vicious dictator Saddam Hussein was a good outcome for the Iraqi people, and that the bringing of democracy to the region would also be a positive development both for the people in that region but also for international society itself. Bush has even been credited for the so-called Arab Spring (Rosen 2011).

Yet, as many have pointed out, even if the reasons for the invasion were well-intentioned, the outcomes have been anything but good (Ricks 2006). And this brings us to Morgenthau's fourth reason for why values should be kept out of international politics. According to Morgenthau what motivates states at the international level is always the acquisition of power relative to other states within the system. Hence, even when state leaders claim to be acting in pursuit of the good, Morgenthau maintains that what they are actually seeking is power. This kind of reasoning, of course, underpins many of those critics of American foreign policy, such as Noam Chomsky, for example (Milne 2009).

Hence, the concept of the 'good international society' is not only contested within the discipline, but the possibility of such a thing is not even acknowledged. Perhaps the main reason for this is that international relations as an academic subject is actually about the study of how we deal with difference (Rosenberg 2015). Differences that is, which often ultimately settle on competing notions of the good. And in the absence of a universal standard of the good that applies to all places in all times then there would seem to be little prospect of anything approaching the 'good international society' at this point in time. In the absence of a notion of the 'universal good', it appears that we cannot even imagine what the good international society might be.

What this means in practice is that in order to imagine the possibility of the good international society we have to theorise the possibility of the universal good and this takes us into the difficult philosophical terrain of the universal versus the particular. Philosophers have long struggled with this issue, but I suggest that its resolution is dependent upon three things. First, is moral realism, for without it conceptions of the good are always going to be embedded within particular social and cultural contexts (Shafer-Landau 2003). And at the international level, this leads to a debilitating moral relativism. For in the absence of such realism, what is good and right is deemed to be culturally determined. Second, is that when considering human societies this moral realism has to be cashed out in terms of the notion of what it means to be human (Pinker 2002). In this respect, there has to be something about the human that is of value irrespective of social and cultural contexts. And as Phil Gorski demonstrates in this volume, attempts to push beyond the human go too far if the very nature of the human is left behind (Gorski 2016). Third, and as a resolution to the complex issue of the universal versus the particular, I suggest that what is universal about the human is its particularity (its individuality). What makes us human is our unique sense of self; a self that it not the other. This is something that all humans feel and it is an important part of what it means to be human, hence this particular characteristic is a universal characteristic of all humans. No human is reducible to another human or to the collectives in which they reside.

This chapter will proceed to unpack these issues and engage in some explicit utopian theorising about what the good international society might be. Admittedly, at this point in time, it will be only a figment of our imaginations. But given the way societies are socially constructed we cannot construct what we cannot imagine.

The Morphogenic Society

In many respects, this chapter can be considered as a set of concluding reflections on the four previous chapters I have written in this series. As such, this is an opportune moment to reflect on my position regarding the morphogenic society. How should we use that term and how does it relate to any attempt to imagine the 'good society'? Change is not just an aspect of social life, it is constitutive of it. But then again, so is continuity (Wight 2001, 2013). As such, all societies are structured by both mechanisms of morphogenesis and morphostasis (Wight 2004, 2015). The contrast between morphogenesis and morphostasis is clear. According to Archer, morphogenesis refers to 'those processes which tend to elaborate or change a system's given form, structure or state', and morphostasis as 'those processes which tend to stabilize and recreate a system's given form, structure or state' (Archer 2015: 1). Hence, morphogenesis and morphostasis are reasonably clear when considered as analytical concepts, and potentially, at least, understandable in an ontological sense as actually existing mechanisms that produce change or continuity. But what then, is a morphogenic society?

The term, of course, stands in a relationship to others, such as the Risk Society, Late Modernity, the Postmodern Society, or perhaps the catchall leitmotif of the day, globalization (Bauman 2000; Beck 1992; Young 2007). However, what is it about the morphogenic society that provides us with both an improved theoretical vocabulary and set of concepts that enhance, or improve on, these alternatives? My understanding is that a morphogenic society is one in which the change-driving (morphogenetic) mechanisms of society prevail and overcome the stability-enhancing (morphostatic) mechanisms, such that rapid and turbulent change not only appears to be everywhere but is everywhere. Thus, a morphogenic society displays substantial structural change rather than continuity or equilibrium. This is an ontological statement, not just an analytical one. It is an ontological claim about the world today. The problem, as I outlined in my chapter in volume One of this series, is that we lack a coherent theoretical framework within which to discuss change (Wight 2013). Moreover, while the perception of change may be prevalent, without a clear way to operationalise the concept it may just be a perception rather than a reality. In this sense, I will admit that I am sitting somewhat on the fence. I consider the concept of the morphogenic society to be useful in terms of providing a set of analytical tools with which to theorise change, yet I remain agnostic as to whether ontologically speaking the world today can be considered to be morphogenic.

Indeed, I would think it is possible to construct a philosophical argument that humans are predisposed to experience change rather than continuity. Hence, the appearance of change might be simply that, an appearance and not a deep underlying reality. The belief that we are witnessing a period of fundamental and substantial change may be illusory. And indeed, just as one can point to indicators of change, one can also point to significant areas of continuity. So for example, war can be said to be changing, but the fact of armed conflict among social groups continues.

The nation state is said to be changing but it still remains the most powerful actor at the international level. Patterns of inequality might be changing, and not in the direction we might wish, but inequality itself continues. Globalization is often said to be changing everything, but nationalism, sexism, and racism continue.

Moral Realism and the Human

By moral realism I mean to suggest that entities in the world can have value independent of that given to them by individuals or human communities. How can this be? Is not the concept of value in itself a human construct? The basis of the moral realist argument is that the meaningfulness of moral language presupposes the objective existence of moral properties. Moral claims are statements that can either true or false. If, on the other hand, value is simply a human imposition on the world then when we make a claim, such as, 'killing people is wrong', what we are really saying is that I, or this community, 'believe killing people is wrong'. What we are categorically not saying is that killing people is objectively wrong. Likewise, if there is a planet somewhere in the universe that also sustains life, the moral sceptic cannot ascribe any value to that life, or indeed that planet, independently of the value that they, or the community, ascribe to it.

Moral realism also implies a form of universalism. If it is wrong to destroy our planet for reasons that go beyond its instrumental value to us, then it is wrong to destroy any planet. But this should not be understood in terms of the Kantian categorical imperative. Ethical knowledge is practical in nature, its object being to guide an individual's, or a community's conduct in *particular* circumstances. Circumstances vary and individuals are unique. Hence, principles within the realm of practical ethics are always contingent and context dependent. There can be no such thing as an abstract understanding of the human good unless we first understand the many concrete forms of it, and any understanding of this concrete form must begin from a consideration of the human being itself. In this way we have to begin with the concrete then move to the abstract, only to return once again to the concrete in a never ending dialectical spiral of ethical consideration.

The Human

All social theories have embedded within them some notion of the human. Insofar as theories or theorists make judgments about what is good for people, they will already tacitly, or explicitly, presuppose a certain view of what it means to be human. There is no escaping this, and even those theories that reject the concept of the human will implicitly invoke it as soon as they enter the terrain of moral critique. Without a concept of the human, moral discussion in the human sciences and society at large would be redundant. Yet, the concept of the human is rightly treated with deep suspicion in the social sciences. Ideas of the human meld with those of nature and seem to suggest that there are right and wrong ways of being human. Yet, despite the well-meaning and often theoretically well-grounded arguments against human nature there are problems with its rejection. We are both biological beings and socio-cultural artefacts. These two aspects of our 'being' cannot be separated. Every human being is born into a socio-culture that plays a crucial role in forming how that human develops, but the notion of being physically born requires a biological substrate that can then be subject to the effects of culture (Brown 1991).

From the material problems of how to get from X to Y to the very basic requirements of food and shelter and other human needs, navigating the material world is an aspect of everyday life. Yet the post-positivist turn in international relations theory, and social theory more generally, has tended to lead to a position that suggests that nature, or materiality, does not matter, and along with it the concept of human nature (Pinker 2002). Yet, the denial of human embodiment in material structures is empirically unsustainable. We need social ontologies that can show how material and ideational factors may interact, without necessarily knowing in advance how they do so. The separation of the material conditions of possibility for social life from its ideational manifestation is a serious error.

Morphogenesis and critical realism advocate a non-reductionist relational social ontology that can demonstrate how reductionism in either downwards or upwards forms is an error (Archer 1995). Approaches that see either biology or materiality as being the sole determinants of social outcomes are to be rejected. In this respect, an important concept is that of emergence. Through emergence, we can articulate a notion of what it means to be human without embedding our explanations exclusively in terms of 'human nature.' What it means to be 'human' is, in part, to be social; and the social is that realm that emerges when humans interact. Moreover, as an emergent reality, the social has its own properties that causally affect what humans can do (and will do) and which cannot be explained in a reductive manner. As members of the human species, we share some common basic needs, desires and wants. But these are the seeds of what we are, not what we do. Hence, questions of the human can remain at the level of what we are (ontology) without straying into matters of how we value what we do (axiology). Any conflict between the universal and the particular is resolved in the concreteness of the human, which is both a particular socially constructed individual who is at the same time part of the universal that is the human species.

The myriad ways in which humans satisfy their basic needs and desires negates any attempt to specify a normative program for humanity based on biology, or the material facts of our interactions with nature. Nonetheless, the mere existence of this shared 'species being' allows us to situate a critique of those practices that block, bar, and impede the fulfillment of human flourishing in all its forms. At a very basic level, the physical and biological limitations of the human require us to be concerned with meeting our basic needs: food, shelter, psychological and social well-being, etc. The requirement to meet these needs has shaped our interactions with one another, but equally, the social and cultural context in which these needs are met also plays a crucial role in how we pursue them. Thus, for example, antediluvian societies tended to have a direct experience of food production and acquisition, whereas in highly developed and industrialized societies food production and acquisition is mediated through a complex supply chain. In both types of societies the basic need to 'eat' remains constant, yet the means of meeting that need differs. Indeed, the meeting of basic human needs and the differing ways in societies did so, forms the basis for historical materialism (Anderson 1983; Marx et al. 1972).

What of those other human characteristics that are often thought to be at the heart of international relations: self-interest and/or altruism? What seems obvious is that humans can be both at the same time. Indeed, the determination of any judgment as to whether any particular act derives from self-interest or altruism depends on social context; the act in itself has no meaning outside of that context. All that we have are forms of human behavior, and setting aside the intentions behind that behavior, how it is understood depends upon the socio-cultural context in which it takes place. What does this all mean for concept of the 'good international society'?

First, my position rejects the complete decentering of the human (Žižek 1999). Second, in rejecting a decentering of the human, I also reject the understanding of agency that is embedded in the new materialism, such that talk of the 'post-human' becomes permissible (Bennett 2010; Coole and Frost 2010). The new materialists decenter the human by attributing agency to natural objects; hence, the distinction between humans and nature is elided. Yet, in doing so, they confuse agency with power. Agency is a very distinctive characteristic of social life that necessarily involves specific assumptions about the human individual in order to be instantiated. What distinguishes agency from power is the reflexive (intentional) moment involved in any social act such that we are able to distinguish it as an 'act' rather than a mere behavior (Archer 2000, 2003, 2007). Raising one's hand would be behavior if doing so was simply the desire to stretch. It would be an 'act,' and instance of agency, if the intention was to signal. As such, the vast majority of meaningful social life happens only insofar as it is mediated through human agency; hence the indispensability of the human. In addition, of course, the radical decentering of the human and the move towards the transhuman that one finds in the new materialism may not always lead to the positive outcomes suggested by the new materialists (Gorski 2016 in this volume). Third, and despite this insistence on the specifics of human agency, intentionality does not provide an exhaustive account of social action. Here it is important to see that although humans form intentions, their ability (power) to act in social settings is not reducible to their intentions, but is derived from their placement in the social field. As such, the human being is also a social being; human nature is social all the way down. This claim should not be misunderstood, and its opposite is equally true, the human is also a biological being; human nature is also biological all the way down. In this sense human being is both biological and social all the way down.

We can consider two broad and conflicting views about the concept of nature, and hence, by extension, the human; these are the philosophical realists, on the one hand,

and the constructivists, on the other (Soper 2001).[1] Although oversimplifying in the extreme, the distinction between these two positions should be clear; and although there are variations and differences among each of them, the two approaches are representative of the extremes of the debate. Realists insist on the independent reality of a natural domain or mode of being; constructivists, on the other hand, suggest that there is no ‘nature’ in this sense and that everything we refer to as natural is, in one way or another, a construct of culture. Realists about nature are keen to reject the idea that ‘it is language that has a hole in its ozone layer’ (Soper 2001, p. 55) or in an IR context, that ‘language possesses nuclear power.’ An important distinction in terms of these extremes is that between ‘deep’ and ‘surface’ forms of realism (Soper 2001, p.56). This distinction is necessary since it allows us to see how nature – as that we experience and interact with (nature-surface) – has indeed been shaped by human practices, whereas those practices do not alter or change the laws of nature (nature-deep), or (typically) produce that which is shaped. Certainly humans produce nature of a kind, but even the concept of ‘production’ relies on materials that limit how that human product (nature-surface) can be produced.

Of course, environments can be destroyed, grown, shaped, and distorted by human practices, yet trees, for example, pre-existed humans, and humans can only produce trees if certain material conditions can be met (soil, seeds, water, etc.). Hence, the realist insists on the fact that whatever the human concept of nature is, it includes within it some things that existed before the emergence of humans on the planet and will endure after we have brought about our own destruction. As such, although nature can only be an object of discourse in and through language and other conceptual tools, the discourse of nature can, and often does, refer to entities or processes existing independently of their representation, and in some cases also unaffected by that representation. Constructivism comes in many, often conflicting, forms. Some forms of constructivism simply focus their attention on social construction of knowledge, which is an acceptable position since all knowledge is indeed socially constructed.

Others forms of constructivism, however, extend this to argue for the social construction of reality itself. ‘Reality,’ however, is a very slippery term in this context, and it is again important to differentiate between ‘experienced reality,’ which is socially constructed, and ‘deep reality,’ which is not. Constructivists, however, seem too ready to deny or disregard this deeper realist account of nature, as a realm of materiality that sets the conditions of possibility for the social. Underpinning most forms of constructivism is an admirable normative commitment that aims to expose everything considered to be ‘natural’ actually to be ‘constructed,’ hence, potentially at least, subject to change. Commendable as this position is, and while accepting the ethico-political necessity of challenging all ‘naturalist’ claims, as a species we have had far more success in dealing with the problems nature throws at us than we have had in dealing with the ones society

[1] The discussion in the following section is strongly shaped by Soper’s excellent analysis.

gives us. Hence, there is no reason to think that 'nature' implies fate/determinism and 'construction' freedom/change. Indeed, the idea that simply because something has been socially constructed it can be changed may be misguided.

Hence, while everything we directly experience is given meaning through processes of 'cultural construction' we can still preserve the idea of nature in the realist sense of causal powers and processes, enabling and limiting the socio-cultural work. Thus, violence, inequality, torture, death, disease, etc., and any attempt to deal with them, only make sense in the context of some material facts about the entity suffering from these practices/phenomena. Indeed, any attempt to place emphasis on the variable and culturally relative quality of human malleability requires recognition of the more constant and universal features of our embodied existence if it is to be meaningful. The concept of 'human differences,' then, requires some notion of the continuity of the human for differences to be meaningful. Without it, we could not recognize difference, only otherness.

However, although we operate within a relational ontology (Donati and Archer 2015) we also accept the view that an entity is never fully defined by its relations; it is frequently possible to detach an entity from one particular set of relations and insert it into a different set of relations, with different entities. For every entity has certain 'properties' that are not defined by the set of relations it finds itself in at a given moment; rather than being merely an empty signifier, the entity can take these properties with it when it moves from one context (or one set of relations) to another. At the same time, an entity is never devoid of some relations. So in terms of social agency, we have the biological entity (the human) embedded within sets of social relations that define it as a social actor of a particular kind. But this human agent can, at various moments in time, move from one set of social relations to another, while still remaining essentially the same human individual even as its place in the social field has changed.

Put differently, no entity can be absolutely isolated because it is always involved in multiple relations of one sort or another, and these relations affect the entity and, potentially at least, cause it to change. But this is not to say that the entity is entirely determined, or constituted, by these relations. On the one hand, the entity has an existence apart from these particular relations, and apart from the other entities with which it is in relation. On the other hand, what the entity is, is not just a function of its present relations, but of a whole history of relations that have affected it over time. Hence, we need to distinguish between the properties an entity possesses (which are what it takes with it to another context - the human) and the capacities of that same entity (its potential to affect, and to be affected by, other entities - the socio-cultural human) that it acquires as a result of the relations in which it finds itself embedded or embeds itself.

Accepting the limitations placed on us by our 'species being' does not entail that we are determined by it. But equally, when placed in the context of the account of agency developed here, we have no need to reject the idea that our 'species being' plays some role. Because of our 'species being,' we need to fulfill basic needs. This means that human interactions with nature have been shaped by our 'species being' and vice versa, by what we can and cannot do. Our interactions with nature would be very different if we had the ability to move from place to place instantaneously, or if we did not require the consumption of resources in order to sustain ourselves. Equally, because we are limited (but not determined) by our species being, and the material conditions we are embedded within, both will play a role in how societies are constituted.

However, they will not determine the social order, if only because material conditions will differ across time and space, and one of the properties of our 'species being' is an almost infinite potential for creativity. This means that there are innumerable ways of dealing with both our 'species being' and the material conditions we inhabit. But equally, understood this way, our 'species being' provides a necessary ethical standpoint from which to judge social practices: How far do existing social practices and conditions enhance, preserve or promote our species being? It is only if we have an understanding of what we are as a species – what we are capable of and what our limitations are – that we are able to say any practice is wrong. And this is a necessary starting point for any discussion of the 'good international society.'

Human Flourishing

Accepting then, that the concept of the human, or species being is an essential aspect of every theory, whether explicitly admitted or not, and that such a starting point is a necessary aspect of any attempt to specify the good, then how do we reconcile this concept with the socio-cultural world which is also a necessary aspect of the human? We begin by recognizing that the concept of the human is prior to that of human rights and that the concept of human rights is itself prior to any notion of human flourishing. Moreover, the move from one to the other is dependent on the prior condition first being met. Thus human needs are prior to human rights, and human rights are prior to human flourishing. This firmly places my position within a more socialist orientated political theory. The concept of human flourishing can only be realised when basic human needs are met.

In addition, we need to differentiate clearly the concept of human flourishing from emancipation. Hence, for example, when Bhaskar discusses absence as the general category that frames his discussion of emancipation, it is emancipation not flourishing that is the central category.

> Insofar as an ill is unwanted, unneeded and remediable, the spatio- temporal-causal-absenting or real transformative negation of the ill presupposes universalizability to absenting agency in all dialectically similar circumstances. This presupposes in turn the absenting of all similar constraints (Bhaskar 1993, p. 663).

Thus, it is clearly within the concept of emancipation that Bhaskar defines the transition from unwanted, unnecessary and oppressive determinations, to wanted and/or needed and empowering sources of determination. Emancipation is essentially the freeing of oneself, or by someone, from unwanted constraints and structures (Bhaskar 1986, p. 171). But human flourishing represents more than this, and only once one is emancipated can one flourish. In effect, to flourish represents the 'will to be'; emancipation represents the process of freedom. But simply to be free is not the same as flourishing. Hence, although related the two concepts are quite distinct.

An understanding of the good society then, requires first and foremost knowledge of what kind of living thing a human being is and knowledge of how human beings achieve their goods; knowledge of how what I have called generic goods and virtues are expressed in the normative paradigms and illustrative narratives of one's society and culture; knowledge of who one is; and knowledge of the concrete situation in which one's conduct takes place. Knowledge of these factors is also a process and not something static. One is learning all the while; so, it may be more accurate to say that in these matters we work along a continuum. We often start with established opinions and slowly see these opinions become knowledge after successfully meeting challenges from contrary accounts and beliefs. Ethical truths emerge out of our practical engagement in the world. What is most important to notice here is that the kind of knowledge that matters most is not the theoretical or universal, but the practical. Trying to put all of the forgoing considerations together into a coherent whole in order to determine the appropriate course of action for a person in a concrete situation is crucial, and this helps explain why practical wisdom of what is possible is itself an ethical good. Hence, for example, knowing that it is practically not possible for Western governments to intervene to stop internal conflicts across the globe is itself an ethical good.

Simply put, we need to be able to differentiate between knowing what is true and good, and when it is possible to achieve what is good. If the world is populated with different types and kinds of realities, one of the gravest intellectual errors, indeed ethical errors, would be to confuse abstraction with reality. This is because abstractions are tools for grasping reality, as well as a process for rendering modes of thought intelligible to others' modes of thought, but our theoretical abstractions are not what are real, although of course, they are a reality in and of themselves. Whatever may be true, be it in physics or in the human ontological landscape (both psychologically and socially), the truth is always more complex than our abstract models can capture. Circumspection about the formulation of propositions in strict universalistic terms is, then, the only sensible posture for the realist theorist to take, but nonetheless a minimal universalism is already embedded within this approach through the concept of the human.

Recognizing the moderate realist view of abstraction and realist ontology liberates us from the prescriptive model of ethics so prevalent in much modern ethical and political theory. Instead of seeking to organize and force people to conform to ethical norms prescribing common patterns of behavior, we would think instead of principled inducements to flourishing based on our minimal concept of the human. This approach, because of its inherent openness to diversity and the critical need for practical wisdom on the part of the agent, makes respect for others a consequence of the approach, and is, I suggest, the only possible ethical way forward in the realm of international politics. For, given that this realm is defined in terms of differences we have to find a way forward that recognises those differences but equally places the value of those differences firmly in terms of how they provide for basic human needs, themselves understood in terms of what it means to be human. A widely shared conception of the human provides a better support for the idea of human flourishing and the kind of political community in which we want to live.

Thinking about the Possibility of Human Flourishing in International Relations

But how does this principle then translate to the realm of international politics? In this section, I intend to engage in some speculative utopian theorising that suggests ways in which the international political system might be restructured, at least to open up the possibility of a commitment to human flourishing and the coming of a yet to be 'good international society'. Admittedly, perhaps even the conditions of possibility for such a society are not yet in place, hence, what I present here should in no way be understood as a programme to institute change. The commitment to practical wisdom in concrete circumstances entails that I accept the fact that any attempt to construct a moral framework with the intent of implementing such changes is a chimera. The conditions of possibility for the good international society are not yet in place. But if they were, what would the good international society look like?

First, given that the meeting of human needs is a necessary condition for human rights, and that human rights are a necessary condition for human flourishing, then it stands to reason that the good international society would not be capitalist in orientation. We know this from two facts. First, capitalism as a mode of economic organisation is centuries old (Appleby 2010; Morton 2005; Neal and Williamson 2014). Second, during the whole of capitalism's existence it has been unable, and perhaps even been a barrier to, the provision of basic needs for all humans. Since capitalism has patently failed to provide the basic requisites for human needs, then the conditions of possibility for human rights and human flourishing cannot be met under capitalism. Of course, alternatives to capitalism have been tried, although it is doubtful in a highly interconnected economic system whether those alternatives ever genuinely had a chance to succeed. Nonetheless, what the recent crises in capitalism demonstrate is that it may be a system in terminal decline (Kaufman 2013; Žižek 2012). Moreover, as realists, we can ascribe some tendencies to capitalism as a particular social-economic form and say with a fair degree of certainty that capitalism produces inequality and a competitive environment that structurally tends to set human communities against other human communities.

Third, is the problem of which form political organisation should take? At the heart of this issue, of course, is the problem of the state. A typical answer to this problem is to suggest the possibility of a world state or world government. Brilliantly articulated of course, by Aldous Huxley in his novel *Brave New World*

(Huxley 1932), the idea of a world state has been seriously discussed in international relations. Towards the end of *Politics Among Nations* (1978), Morgenthau considered the possibility and came to the conclusion that there can be no permanent peace without a world state. But, he suggests, ‘there can be no world government until there is world community, and a sense of world community cannot form unless national decision-makers resolve or ameliorate world tensions through a return to a wise diplomacy’ (Speer 1968: 1). More recently, Alexander Wendt has suggested that a world state is inevitable (Wendt 2003).

Wendt’s argument rests on a particular understanding of the human desire for recognition. According to Wendt, ‘a global monopoly on the legitimate use of organized violence — a world state — is inevitable. At the micro-level world state formation is driven by the struggle of individuals and groups for recognition of their subjectivity. At the macro-level this struggle is channeled toward a world state by the logic of anarchy, which generates a tendency for military technology and war to become increasingly destructive’ (Wendt 2003: 491). Thus, for Wendt, states will come to recognise that in a world where wholesale destruction of all is a technological possibility, that a world government is the only thing that could prevent global wholesale destruction. In this sense, even state survival itself rests on the possibility of a world government. Attractive as the concept of a world government is to many, would it necessarily contribute to human flourishing and the good international society? I will admit to being a sceptic on this issue.

The history of states does not supply a great deal of confidence in this notion of a world state. In fact, while theoretically states are meant to protect their citizens, in practical terms the reverse has often been the case. Moreover, would a world state lead to less conflict, the eradication of injustice and inequality, and a system that would meet basic human needs, which are a precondition for human flourishing? Moreover, would a world state lead to a borderless world, or just a world where borders are administered from one source rather than many? How would democracy function in such a political configuration? In fact, the more one thinks about it, the more problems one can see in the concept of a world state. For the time being at least, and despite claims to the contrary, the state is not withering away (Spruyt 2002) and will probably be with us for some time, and may be the optimal form of political organization to enhance the prospects of a human flourishing.

Indeed, states, for all of the problems we encounter with them, have in many senses the potential to provide those resources, structures and protections necessary for basic human needs to be met. From a causal powers point of view (Cartwright 2007) states are perhaps the only entities in the international system with the power to provide for basic human needs. Thus human flourishing may depend on the existence of the state. That empirically many states have been a threat to their own citizens, and continue to be so does not mean that the state must take that form. Hence, what the good international society would need is a collective means of controlling only the excesses of state power, not a pattern of interference into all the affairs of state. We already have such a body and what we need to do is to empower it so that it can react in ways that force errant states to change their behaviour.

Skepticism towards the UN, of course, is rife. But when viewed historically it is a relatively young organization and one that has had a number of remarkable successes. The UN is not perfect, its structure, and, in particular, the place of the Security Council in that structure is a major barrier to it fulfilling its remit. However what the UN needs is reform, not replacement. And if the UN is both preferable to a world government and necessary for the promotion of human needs then given it is a collection of states then states are also necessary. For there can be no UN without states.

A mediating mechanism between states and the UN, however, might be more powerful regional organisations such as the EU. Again, the EU is far from being a perfect organization, suffering mainly from a lack of democratic mechanisms to link it to the populations of states. But whatever its problems the EU has the virtue of providing an alternative identity for all the citizens of Europe as well as a constitutional framework that enables it to represent those peoples at the international level. In this sense, regional organisations such as the EU can incorporate difference into their policies and provide mechanisms at the international level for those different views to be articulated. Thus, in fact, rather than being a threat to the sovereignty of individual states it is better to think of the EU as providing an additional framework through which difference can be articulated. Hence, if the problems of the democratic deficit could be dealt with, the citizens of each European state would have two political bodies through which to articulate their claims.

In addition, there is no doubt that cooperation among states is on the increase as the nature and scale of some of the global problems they face require coordinated action among them. In addition, a range of non-state actors is now pushing agendas in these areas. From the role played by *Médecins sans Frontières* in providing medical care to the needy, to the activist networks built by Greenpeace, and the humanitarian efforts of the Red Cross and the Red Crescent, we can see new actors playing a major role in shaping the global politics. Indeed, despite the fact that international politics could be said to be the paradigmatic example of the Nietzscheian 'eternal return', there are signs of moral progress in the international system. Nothing can guarantee that this progress will continue, but if it does it will depend on the continued efforts of non-state actors to keep the immense power of the modern state in check and to remind it that its primary function is to provide for the security and well-being of its citizens. If the state cannot fulfill this function then we may well question if it remains fit for purpose in the morphogenic age.

Conclusion

There is no doubt that the concept of human flourishing is a deeply problematic notion in the field of international relations. Indeed, some consider it to be a problematic issue in any domain (Porpora 2016). Because this field of enquiry by definition deals with the problematic issue of difference, our ethical sensibilities are always primarily tuned to allow for difference in all its forms. This, in part, explains why realists and postmodern IR theorists have settled into a curious peace and take up a common cause of criticising liberal humanitarian interventionism. For Realists, difference needs to be protected because it is only by prioritizing difference that we can protect our own difference. It is a form of ethical apartheid. For postmoderns, the valorization of difference is the ethical good in itself.

But both positions are unable to speak to situations where there are extreme human rights abuses. Both adopt of a form of moral relativism that can provide no grounds for any action orientated towards the dealing with a difference we find ethically questionable; fascism for example. The morphogenetic and philosophically realist position I have outlined above doubtless also has its problems, but it has the virtue of giving us at least one universal standpoint on which to base moral critique: namely, Moral realism allied to a commitment to the human. Certain forms of social practice are just wrong, and not merely because we believe them to be wrong. What a thing is, is essential to its flourishing, and the 'will to be' is what makes a thing what it is. Social practices that fail to supply, or impede, the basic needs of our species being are barriers to human flourishing. This might be a small step, and there is a long road yet to travel, but unless we start the journey it cannot end.

References

Anderson, P. (1983). *In the tracks of historical materialism*. London: Verso Editions.

Appleby, J. O. (2010). *The relentless revolution: A history of capitalism* (1st ed.). New York/London: Aufl/W. W. Norton.

Archer, M. S. (1995). *Realist social theory: The morphogenetic approach*. Cambridge: Cambridge University Press.

Archer, M. S. (2000). *Being human: The problem of agency*. Cambridge: Cambridge University Press.

Archer, M. S. (2003). *Structure, agency, and the internal conversation*. Cambridge: Cambridge University Press.

Archer, M. S. (2007). *Making our way through the world: Human reflexivity and social mobility*. Cambridge: Cambridge University Press.

Archer, M. S. (2015). Generative mechanisms transforming the social order. In M. S. Archer (Ed.), *Social morphogenesis*. Springer: Dordrecht.

Bauman, Z. (2000). *Liquid modernity*. Cambridge: Polity Press.

Beck, U. (1992). *Risk society: Towards a new modernity*. London: Sage.

Bennett, J. (2010). *Vibrant matter: A political ecology of things*. Durham: Duke University Press.

Bhaskar, R. (1986). *Scientific realism and human emancipation* . London.Verso

Bhaskar, R. (1993). *Dialectic: The pulse of freedom*. London: Verso.

Brown, D. E. (1991). *Human universals*. London: McGraw-Hill.

Cartwright, N. (2007). *Causal powers : What are they?: Why do we need them?: What can and cannot be done with them?* London: Contingency and Dissent in Science Project.

Coole, D. H., & Frost, S. (2010). *New materialisms: Ontology, agency, and politics*. Durham: Duke University Press.

Donati, P., & Archer, M. S. (2015). *The relational subject*. Cambridge: Cambridge University Press.

Goldstein, J. S. (2011). *Winning the war on war: The decline of armed conflict worldwide*. New York: Dutton.
Gorski, P. (2016). Human flourishing and human morphogenesis: A critical realist interpretation and Critique. In M. S. Archer (Ed.), *Morphogenesis and the good life*. Springer: Dordrecht.
Huxley, A. (1932). *Brave new world*. London: Voyager Classics, 2001.
Kaufman, C. C. (2013). *Getting past capitalism: History, vision, hope*. Lanham: Lexington Books.
Krause, K. (2009). War, violence and the state. In M. Brzoska & A. Krohn (Eds.), *Securing peace in a globalized world* (pp. 183–202). London: Palgrave Macmillan.
Marx, K., Engels, F., Lenin, V. I.′i., & Borodulina, T. (1972). *On historical materialism: A collection*. Moscow: Progress Publishers.
Milne, Seumas. 2009. US foreign policy is straight out of the mafia. The Guardian. http://www.theguardian.com/world/2009/nov/07/noam-chomsky-us-foreign-policy. Accessed 19 Dec 2015.
Morgenthau, H. J. (1978). *Politics among nations: The struggle for power and peace* (5th rev ed.). New York: Knopf/Aufl.
Morton, A. D. (2005). The age of absolutism: Capitalism, the modern states-system and international relations. *Review of International Studies, 31*(03), 495–517. doi:10.1017/S0260210505006601.
Neal, L., & Williamson, J. G. (2014). *The Cambridge history of capitalism*. Cambridge: Cambridge University Press.
Pinker, S. (2002). *The blank slate: The modern denial of human nature*. New York: Viking.
Pinker, S. (2011). *The better angels of our nature: Why violence has declined*. New York: Viking.
Porpora, D. (2016). Some reservations about flourishing. In M. S. Archer (Ed.), *Morphogenesis and the good life*. Dordrecht: Springer.
Ricks, T. E. (2006). *Fiasco: The American military adventure in Iraq*. New York/London: Penguin Press.
Rosen, James. 2011. Why George W. Bush is the Arab Spring's forgotten man. *McClatchy*. http://www.mcclatchydc.com/news/nation-world/world/article24718339.html. Accessed 19 Dec 2015.
Rosenberg, Justin. 2015. International relations in the prison of political science: Is there a way out? In *E.H. Carr Annual Lecture*. Aberystwyth.
Security Global. 2016. http://www.globalsecurity.org/military/world/war/. Accessed 5 May 2016.
Shafer-Landau, R. (2003). *Moral realism: A defence*. Oxford: Clarendon Press.
Soper, K. (2001). Realism, humanism and the politics of nature. *Theoria: A Journal of Social and Political Theory, 98*(December), 55–71.
Speer, J. P. (1968). Hans Morgenthau and the world state. *World Politics, 20*(2), 207–227. doi:10.2307/2009796.
Spruyt, H. (2002). The origins, development, and possible decline of the modern state. *Annual Review of Political Science, 5*(1), 127–149. doi:10.1146/annurev.polisci.5.101501.145837.
Wendt, A. (2003). Why a world state is inevitable. *European Journal of International Relations, 9*(4), 491–542. doi:10.1177/135406610394001.
Wight, C. (2001). The continuity of change, or a change in continuity? *International Studies Review, 3*(1), 81–89. doi:10.1111/1521-9488.00226.
Wight, C. (2004). Theorizing the mechanisms of conceptual and semiotic space. *Philosophy of the Social Sciences, 34*(2), 283–299.
Wight, C. (2013). Morphogenesis, continuity and change in the international political system. In M. S. Archer (Ed.), *Social morphogenesis* (pp. 85–104). Dordrecht: Springer.
Wight, C. (2015). Mechanisms and models: Some examples from international relations. In M. S. Archer (Ed.), *Generative mechanisms transforming the social order*. London: Springer.
Young, J. (2007). *The vertigo of late modernit*. Los Angeles/London: Sage.
Žižek, S. (1999). *The ticklish subject: The absent centre of political ontology*. London: Verso.
Žižek, S. (2012). Trouble in paradise: From the end of history to the end of capitalism. *London Review of Books, 35*(14), 11–12.

Chapter 13
Creating Common Good: The Global Sustainable Information Society as the Good Society

Wolfgang Hofkirchner

The Commons

At a first glance, it might seem surprising that among sociology and other social sciences as well as philosophy there has been growing attention to issues of eudaimonia, the good life, flourishing, happiness, conviviality, the good society, and other cognate terms, since humanity lives under circumstances that not only put the thriving of individuals and society at stake but even threaten their survival. Surviving is possible without thriving but thriving is not possible without surviving. Why then focus on thriving instead on surviving? On closer scrutiny, however, the answer becomes clear: survival is at stake for the same reason for which eudaimonia, good life, flourishing, happiness, conviviality, and the good society are at stake. It is for that very reason the prolongation of civilised human life on our planet is threatened.

The title is from an exhibition that took place in Vienna 17 November 2015–10 January 2016 in co-operation with Vienna Art Week 2015. See https://www.kunsthauswien.com/en/exhibitions/archive/67-2015/337-creating-common-good.

W. Hofkirchner (✉)
Institute of Design and Technology Assessment, Vienna University of Technology, Argentinierstraße 8, 1040 Vienna, Austria

Bertalanffy Center for the Study of Systems Science, Paulanergasse 13/5, 1040 Vienna, Austria
e-mail: wolfgang.hofkirchner@bcsss.org

M.S. Archer (ed.), *Morphogenesis and Human Flourishing*, Social Morphogenesis,
DOI 10.1007/978-3-319-49469-2_13

The Commons Revisited

Thanks to the frequently praised advent of the so-called information society as well as to the criticism it provoked, new social movements and intellectuals discovered social information (knowledge, data) as another common good that any individual or collective actor should have the right to share and impart in order to be able to thrive. By promoting that notion they paved the way for recalibrating the Marxist idea of communism that should have been brought about by the working classes who were excluded from the disposal of the means of production in the so-called material sphere of society, which made those classes fight for thriving: nowadays multitudes are excluded from a so-called immaterial good too that is needed for thriving, which makes them long for "commonism" or "commonalism".[1] Common(al)ism is a generalisation of Marx's idea of communism – a generalisation that extends from material products via presumed natural givens, which far from being natural need more and more reproductive work by the economies and health care systems, to information including fields such as education or the arts. This summarises all phenomena mentioned under the term of the "commons".[2]

In that context, eudaimonia and related terms require redefinition, in order to rule out egoistic connotations of "flourishing" and introduce a higher goal into the meaning of flourishing as Doug Porpora called for (see Chap. 3). It might be advisable to establish a connexion between agency and structure, individual and society, such that one can speak of the free flourishing of each as depending on the free flourishing of all, whereby "each" indicates the level of individual agents and "all" a higher, structural level or – as Pierpaolo Donati and Margaret Archer call it (Donati and Archer 2015) – the level of the "relational subject". Thus, no term of those that are used for qualifying life should signify either level without spelling out its relationship to the other level.

Accordingly, eudaimonia here refers to a certain quality of the dialectic of agency and structure or individual and society respectively. In systems terms, it depicts a state of a social system in which (1) the structure of the social system is made up of social relations that facilitate the flourishing of the actors in the system and (2) these flourishing actors contribute to the emergence of suitable social relations. This is a self-propelling cycle: the structure provides ever better conditions for the interaction of the actors to flourish and those actors who do flourish produce an ever better structure.

[1] "Commonism" was a word that was used by Woodie Guthrie with reference to the Bible – Briley R. (2006), Woody Sez: The People's Daily World and Indigenous Radicalism, *California History* 84 (1), 35; quoted after Linebaugh (2014, 139). "Commonalism" is used by Rudi Laermans (2011a, b, 2012).

[2] Actually, it was a lecture by Slavoj Zizek given in the first decade of our millennium in Vienna that made me aware of that idea.

If the social system in question is a society, such a state of affairs might characterise the "good society". The acceleration of the mutual conditioning of happy individuals and the good society makes the good society the ideal instance of a morphogenic society. Happier individuals conduct a better life together such that they bring about the formation of relations that improve the promotion of the formation of happier individuals. This positive cycle is a concretisation of the cycle of generic social morphogenesis described in Hofkirchner (2014) in volume II of our book series. That generic social morphogenesis is, in turn, a concretisation of deep morphogenesis characteristic of any evolutionary, self-organising system, including natural systems too:

> Any system shows a dialectic of integration and differentiation. Agents that differ from each other bring about the formation of a structure that integrates; this structure catches up with the differentiation at hand and, at the same time, conditions a new differentiation of the agents which brings about a new integration: ever more differentiated agents bring about the formation of an ever more integrated structure that conditions the formation of ever more differentiated agents. There is divergence and convergence in one. That is the line along which evolution can make progress. [...] After the festschrift for Ludwig von Bertalanffy, it may be called unity through diversity. (Hofkirchner 2014, 128)

Deep morphogenesis is the ground for generic social morphogenesis in social systems. Unity through diversity – integration through differentiation – "appears in social systems as dialectic of 'socialisation' and 'individualisation'" (128). "Socialisation" or 'sociality'

> describes the increase in the "socialness", "commonness", "communitarity", which is a property of the societal relations in accordance with which human life is organised. (129)

"Individualisation" describes the increase in the "individuation", "individuality", which is a property of the actors that they themselves want to bring into being for their own sake. Socialisation is the process in which ever more differentiating individuals bring about the formation of ever more integrating relations, whereas individualisation is the process in which ever more integrating relations allow for the formation of ever more differentiating individuals

How can the socialisation-individualisation cycle be characterized in a more detailed manner? How can the integrating relations be defined and detected? How can those conditions necessary for the flourishing of happy individuals in a good society be further determined? In short, what are these social relations about?

The answer is: the social relations are about commoning,[3] about (the) common(−good)s, the commons, the *commune bonum*, which are values that are added, in material or immaterial respects.

[3]That term is used in Linebaugh, P. (Linebaugh 2014) and on https://blog.commons.at/commons/was-ist-commoning/, meaning, approximately, taking care of something together.

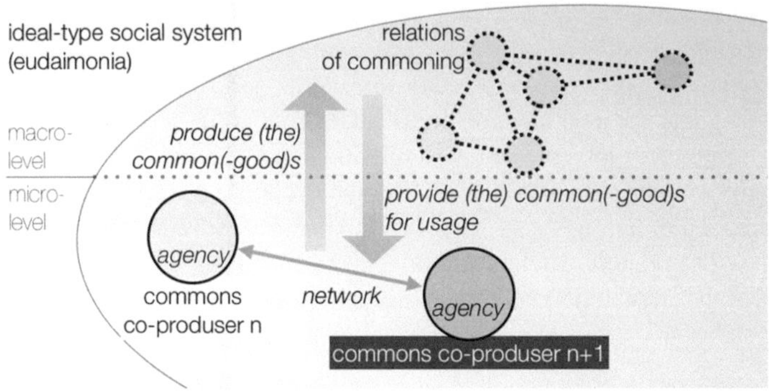

Fig. 13.1 Ideal-type, eudaimonic social system

According to evolutionary systems thinking,

> The rationale of every system is synergy. Because agents when producing a system produce synergetic effects, that is, effects they could not produce when in isolation, systems have a strong incentive to proliferate (Corning 2003). In social systems synergism takes on the form of some social good. Actors contribute together to the good and are common beneficiaries of that good – the good is a common good, it is a commons. (Hofkirchner 2014, 121)

So, since any (self-organised) system is a system by virtue of the synergy it supplies through its organisational relations, any social system is a social system by virtue of the common good it supplies through its organisational relations. The common good is the social manifestation of synergy. Social actors play a major part in adding to those values and themselves share the added values in turn. They are producing and using the commons in common, they are commons' co-produsers.[4] By commonly producing the commons they produce relations of commoning that provide the commons for common usage (see Fig. 13.1).

> Through their action, interaction, and co-action they bring about the formation of societal relations that condition the generation and utilisation of commons in an integrated way, which allows the individuals to differentiate: the more individuals are "individualised", the better they produce the common good; the better the common good is "socialised", the more individuals can become individuated. (Hofkirchner 2014, 129)

[4]It is not a coincidence that the term "produser" and "produsage" came up with modern ICTs that made the users of social network sites the producers of the content of the latter – hence "produsers" (Bruns 2006). This is taken here as a metaphor for any social system production and usage on a generic level.

The Morals of the Commons

It is worth noting that, according to Pierpaolo Donati (Chap. 7), the organising principle of relations of commoning is not the "*do ut des*" principle. It is rather a principle of conviviality[5] or, as Doug Porpora (Chap. 3) might put it, a principle of unconditional love. The ideal of the humane organisation of production and provision of the commons would be: "from each according to their ability, to each according to their need".

According to emergentist systemism, the origin of morality is historically connected to the change in co-operation that led to social systems creating commons (see Hofkirchner 2016). Michael Tomasello who in 2014 had published his theoretical generalisations of empirical findings of experiments with great apes and children on the genesis of human thinking, published in 2016 his generalisations regarding the genesis of morality. He hypothesises two evolutionary steps: a first step from our animal ancestors that like today's chimpanzees formed relationships with kin and other conspecifics in which they favoured "others over themselves" (2016, 3) but were "often, perhaps most often, acting out of self-interest" (159), to early humans who "extended their sense of sympathy beyond kin and friends to collaborative partners" with whom they "developed a common-ground understanding of the ideal way that each role had to be played for joint success", and with whom they developed "original socially shared normative standards" that were impartial and recognised "that self and other were of equivalent status and importance in the collaborative enterprise" (4). From this a natural, second-person plural morality developed in which the "me" was subordinated to "we" in a joint commitment and a normatively constituted "ought" emerged (5); and a second step from those early humans to *Homo sapiens sapiens* with "a kind of scaled-up version of early humans' second-person morality", "a kind of *cultural and group-minded, 'objective' morality*" (6).

> They have become cooperatively rational in that they factor into their decision making (1) that helping partners and compatriots whenever possible is the right thing to do, (2) that others are equally as real and deserving as themselves (and this same recognition may be expected in return), and (3) that a 'we' created by a social commitment makes legitimate decisions for the self and valued others, which creates legitimate obligations among persons with moral identities in moral communities. (160)

With the advent of culture, that is, of separate and distinct cultural groups, the interdependence that caused co-operation reigned "not just at the level of the collaborating dyad, and not just in the domain of foraging, but at the level of the entire cultural group, and in all domains of life" (85).

[5]Ivan Illich was the first to coin that term in a rather scientific context when he published his philosophy of technology book "Tools for Conviviality" (Illich 1973). In recent years, that term gained new attention when intellectuals in France opened the discussion on a political manifesto for the redesign of agency and structure in the social systems of our time (http://convivialism.org). Conviviality can be traced back to the Spanish connotation of sitting together in peace and enjoying drinking and eating together.

Tomasello's ideas can easily be integrated with emergentist systemism and – particularly his idea that human culture comes with a sense of equality[6] – forming the stepping stone for the following elaboration on moral values. The background assumption is that culture underwent a historical differentiation into other domains of society such that we have a logical hierarchy of sublevels on the top of which is culture, followed by politics, economy, ecology, and technology at the bottom. The order results from the fact that every sublevel is a concretisation of the preceding upper level: culture is the level where rules are defined; politics is the level where regulations (specific rules) are decided; economy is the level where resource regimes (specific regulations) are deposed; ecology is the level where the natural infrastructure, the eco-structure (specific resource regimes), is designed; and technology is the level where the technical infrastructure, the techno-structure (specific natural infrastructure), is designed.

That order follows a gradient. The domains at the lower levels are progressively material, the higher ones progressively less material (see Andrea Maccarini in Chap. 5).

Also the lower levels are those that exhibit a faster pace of interaction between the actors and a faster pace of system transformations as compared with the higher levels. So it is no surprise that the techno-structure has the highest rate of innovation and culture the lowest one (when keeping in mind those interrelated habits and values giving ethnic groups an identity that can last for centuries.)

A social systems approach allows a perspective that is factual and normative in one. On the one hand, it is a fact that there are objective functions that need to be carried out in a social system and they are carried out by enactments of the actors' agency. On the other hand, it is a norm when actors are collectively expected to act in a determinate way; it is a value when actors collectively attribute a determinate meaning to an object; it is a moral norm when actors are collectively expected to act in a good way; it is a moral value when actors collectively attribute goodness to an object (see Hofkirchner 2016).

Morality enters the stage because of the commons. That commons are generated and furnished by any social system is an objective fact. That commoning is doing good, is a moral norm for actors. That commons are a good thing, is a moral value for actors. For that reason, any enactment of social agency that contributes to a better fulfilling of the systemic function of yielding the commons is made a moral norm since any actor who is member of that system ought to do so for the sake of the good life, which is, at the same time, for the sake of the perpetuation and improved performance of the system, and any objective systemic property that facilitates the fulfilling of that systemic function is made a moral value since every member of the

[6]Tomasello's working group at the Max Planck Institute for Evolutionary Anthropology in Leipzig gives nice ontogenetic evidence of behaviour that resembles that phylogenetic hypothesis. In an experiment young children are prompted by a device to work together in a subtle way so as to receive an award each. The award is given to them after successfully carrying out the task. Now, if and when the awards are distributed in an uneven way, the child who receives a higher award spontaneously shares the excess part with the other child.

Table 13.1 Systems, facts and actors' values

		systems functions	agency enactments		systemic properties	collective/ individual values	
core social system	culture	self-production	action: self-actualisation	self-expression	social compatibility	justice/ self-worth	equality/ recognition
	politics			self-determination			freedom/ empowerment
	economy			self-subsistence			solidarity, subsidiarity /security
basic eco-social system		self-maintenance	work: self-preservation		ecological compatibility	survivability/ physical well-being	
basic techno-(eco-)social system		self-operation	activity: self-actuation		technological compatibility	thrivability/ performance competence	

community of actors of that system will evaluate it as highly conducive to achieving good life, which is, at the same time, conducive to the functioning of the system. Thus morality is conveyed by the objective functions and properties of the social system. That is, what serves the objective functioning of the social system, appears to the actors as laden with morality.

Any actor plays a role on any of the levels distinguished above. On any level a specific commons is co-produced: on the cultural level it is rules about how to obtain what is seen as the good life; on the political level it is regulations for the conduct of a good life; on the economic level it is resource regimes that allocate the means for a good life; on the ecological level it is the eco-structure, the proper geo- and biospherical conditions of a good life; and on the technological level it is the techno-structure, that supplies instruments for a good life by means of productive forces.

Now let's correlate the facts about the systems perspective with the normativity in the actors' perspective (Table 13.1).

Every commons is co-prodused through individual actors who take part in the systems' dynamics by different types of enactments of their own agency. While actors strive for self-expression, they contribute to the cultural commons; while they strive for self-determination, they contribute to the political commons; and while they strive for self-subsistence, they contribute to the economic commons. Those three enactments can be summarised under the label of actions that are constituted by processes of actualisation of individual selves in the core social system (made up of the levels of culture, politics, and economy). Those individual actions make the social system produce itself (without them the social system would not exist). Both the self-actualisation of the actors and the self-production of the core social system are processes by which each actor as well as the system transcend themselves (both show concomitant drives for change) – typical of the human level of self-organisation.

The ecological level is the first basic level of the core social system, the basic eco-social system. Here the actors act for individual self-preservation. Those enactments constitute work. By work the overall self-maintenance of the social system is served. The technological level is the next basic level, actually, the undermost one, underlying the basic eco-social system. Through actuation of their individual selves the basic techno-(eco-)social system makes the overall social system perform its operations on all its levels.

The property that is required for the self-production of the core social system is called social compatibility. The actors reflect social compatibility as a moral value, namely: justice. The commitment of the collectivity to justice helps each actor achieve self-worth (see Margaret Archer in Chap. 6). Justice itself can be broken down into other moral values that are specific to culture, politics, and economy: as to culture, we know already from Tomasello that it is equality by the collective commitment in which each actor wants to be recognised on an equal footing to be able to express herself; as to politics, the collective moral value is freedom that would grant every actor the power to determine himself by taking part in the common decision-making processes; and as to economy, the collectivity should provide solidarity in conjunction with subsidiarity (Archer and Donati 2008) in order to provide security for everyone's self-subsistence.

The appropriate property of the basic eco-social system that assures the maintenance of the overall social system itself is called ecological compatibility, which is reflected by the actors as the moral value of survivability. Compliance with survivability assures, in turn, their own physical well being when working for preserving themselves. And last but not least, the property needed for the basic techno-(eco-)social system to ensure the capacity of the overall social system to execute its operations is called technological compatibility. The actors look upon technological compatibility as the moral value of thrivability[7] the observance of which increases their individual performative competence to actuate themselves.

Having outlined that, we have arrived at a hierarchy of moral values inherent in systemic properties and moral norms inherent in enactments of the actors that fulfil systems functions. Hierarchy means that the content on the lower level provides a necessary but not sufficient condition for the content on the next higher level. Thrivability does not *per se* determine full-fledged survivability, survivability not full-fledged justice; solidarity with subsidiarity does not entail full-fledged freedom and freedom does not ensure full-fledged equality. The relationships between those level-relative properties, enactments and functions of the system in line with certain values and norms is such that the lower ones form the basis for the emergence of higher ones. Even the highest-level content – normativity grounding equality for individual self-expression and systemic self-production – merely supplies the

[7] I'm hesitant about using the term "productivity" which would be rather appropriate if it had not acquired a certain, narrow, economic meaning and lost another one, in which nature itself is productive, and so are humans by harnessing productive forces. "Thrivability" serves to prevent such an association and links up to the lost meaning.

basis for the emergence of conviviality but not conviviality itself. It provides the preconditions for flourishing but not flourishing itself (see Colin Wight in Chap. 12). However, in hierarchies there are always also shaping influences from the top to the bottom. The sequence of the levels was construed in consideration of that. The higher level has requirements for the level that underlies it. But it will never fully determine the latter and a leap in properties and powers will still remain between them.

Enclosure and Reclaiming of the Commons

In the course of history, a contingent increase in the enclosure of the commons has been hindering their common produsage, thereby bringing about domination and the distortion of conviviality. In other words, by enclosing the commons a group of people originates who dominate the rest of the people. However, today, the enclosure of the commons even threatens civilisation with extinction; it is the ultimate cause of the most serious global challenges: today, not only thriving, but also surviving is at stake. Self-organisation of the good life has become exclusive, commoning relations have become relations of exclusion that deprive increasing numbers of actors of the commons such that actors have been set in competition with each other.

Instead of the self-organisation of rules for the good life, the cultural commons are enclosed. Instead of sharing values in the cultural system that legitimise a good life with respect to equality, there is rather the hegemony of provincialism, nationalism, racism, anti-islamism, fundamentalism among others that exclude groups of certain other cultural actors from the egalitarian setting of rules and denies them the sharing of power over definitions for obtaining the good life.

Instead of the self-organisation of regulations for human flourishing, the political commons are enclosed. Instead of democratisation in the political system that authorises the realization of a good life with respect to freedom, the politics of imposition, such as technocracy, totalitarianism, nepotism and others exclude groups from making regulations and disallows them from sharing power to take free decisions on the conduct of the good life.

Instead of the self-organisation of resources for the good life, the economic commons are enclosed. Instead of sharing wealth in the economic system that allocates the means for a good life with respect to solidarity, wealth dominates as in the financialization of capitalism and the neoliberal destruction of the welfare state, excluding some groups from resources and depriving them from any power to dispose over the means for living a good life.

Instead of the self-organisation of ecologies promoting the good life, the ecological commons are enclosed. Instead of harmony in the eco-social system that supports the good life with proper bio- and geospherical conditions, nature is colonised, which excludes groups from adapting nature and disables them from sharing the power to appropriate nature for survival, which also leads to degradations of nature.

Instead of the self-organisation of the good life by productive forces, the technological commons are enclosed. Instead of fostering the meaningfulness of innovations in the techno-(eco-)social system that are instruments for the good life in terms of productive forces, the domination of the latter by a military-informational complex and transnational corporations excludes groups from shaping technology and disables them from sharing the power of disposition over means for the appropriation of nature for a survivable good life, which even turns productive forces into destructive ones.

Exclusive social relations are antagonistic. Antagonism means logical contradictions, a conflict of mutually exclusive positions, of contrapositions. That is the logic of zero-sum games, which is the case when the active side of the conflict benefits at the cost of the passive side (see Table 5.6 on the ontology of social relations in Hofkirchner 2015, 105).

The moral values of justice (equality, freedom, and solidarity jointly with subsidiarity), of survivability, and of thrivability, and the related moral norms have come under attack. Reclaiming the commons means fighting for those values and norms. Awareness is rising that on every level of society a battle has started for reclaiming the commons.

The Global Sustainable Information Society

Karl Marx focused on the dialectic of productive forces and relations of production. Critical social systems thinking in the age of global challenges needs to extend that focus on a dialectic of, on the one hand, social actors who are more and more concerned about the common fate of humanity in the age of global challenges and, on the other, social relations that, on every level of society, are, in principle, relations of commoning though having been turned more and more into antagonistic relations.

The challenges of today demand mastering by a systems' transformation into a state of society that saves the human world from the danger of decline and makes it survive by making it thrive. That new state needs to adjust the structures that have become obsolete and needs to do justice to the agency that cares for the whole. It needs to make the social systems inclusive through the disclosing of the enclosed commons and, by doing so, can warrant eudaimonia, a good life in a good society, the flourishing of happy individuals in convivial social relations. It needs to accomplish that by letting the increasingly fluctuating activities cascade throughout the societal edifice and change the organisational relations from the technological to the cultural system in a coherent way.[8]

[8]In the sociological literature there seems to be a widespread acceptance of evidence of processes of acceleration except for accelerationists. Both stances, however, would need to focus on the fact that acceleration on the micro-level of a social system (the intensification of interaction of actors) as kind of a quantitative increase does not automatically yield a qualitative change on the macro-level of that very system (new – and desired – social relations), not to speak of such changes in systems

That state of society is the next needful step of social morphogenesis that – at the risk of humanity's devolution – seizes the opportunity of reaching another level of evolution. That state is the state of the Global Sustainable Information Society. It is called Global Sustainable Information Society (GSIS) because its demands are (1) for the first time in the history of Earth, an integration at the level of all humanity; (2) a reorganisation of the social relations within and between the interdependent social systems such that sociogenic dysfunctions with respect to the core social, the eco-social and the techno-(eco-)social systems can be kept below the threshold that would endanger the continuation of social evolution; (3) conscious and conscientious actors who are not only concerned with themselves but even more so with the creation of a new convivial world community. Demand number (1) is globality, demand number (2) sustainability, and demand number (3) informationality. Demand (1) pertains to the spatio-temporal dimension of the transformation to come; demand (2) to the level of organisation; and demand (3) to the state of intelligence.

Globality

The global imperative means that social systems and their actors cannot thrive or survive unless all become nested in a superordinate world system so as to ensure the conditions for further elaboration of societal development. This is grounded in the following insight into the evolution of complex systems: when independent systems have become interdependent, evolution on the same level can become punctuated by the transition to a meta-system that forms a hierarchy; a supra-system can emerge that nests the interdependent systems as co-systems.

The evolution of globality can be conceptualised in the following way (Hofkirchner 2017) (see Fig. 13.2):

- After nomadic life, with human foraging lasting up to the neolithic revolution, after the presumed self-sufficiency of the first agglomerations of human settlements within matrilineal societies (e.g. Eisler 1987; Bornemann 1975; but see also Eller 2000) and after connectivity developed between ancient city-states along historical trade routes (Zimmermann 2014, 2015),
- all those prevailing features of social space have been replaced by strict principles of territoriality manifest in the empires, nation states and regional unions to such a degree that

that rank higher in the hierarchy of nested social systems. What happens on a system's micro-level is just the precondition for the emergence of something new on its macro-level and what happens on one system's level is also precisely the precondition for the emergence of something new on the next higher system's level.

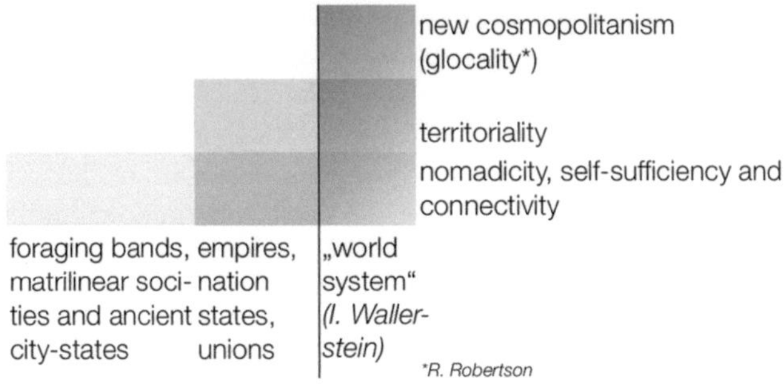

Fig. 13.2 The spatio-temporal dimension of GSIS

- a third step seems possible that negates the exclusive feature of territoriality and resumes 'nomadicity' (Lévy 1997), self-sufficiency and connectivity under novel circumstances. That new feature is a new cosmopolitanism, it is globality that – in the sense of R. Robertson's definition of the term glocalisation (Robertson 1992) – embraces the bottom-up and top-down dynamics in a world system that – though not exactly in the sense in which Immanuel Wallerstein (1988) introduced the term[9] – is a social system of nested social systems that run from the local level up to the global level.

Sustainability

The sustainability imperative means the world system cannot be governed unless actual dysfunctions in the working of social systems are dealt with and possible future ones are prevented, which is substantiated by another insight into evolutionary systems regarding their stability: when the meta-system transition and the re-ontologisation of the new whole system according to the new organising relations has started, the new structure enters into operation that can enable and constrain the interaction of the new co-systems for the sake of a stable development of both the supra-system and the co-systems; unity through diversity can be approached. Stability manifests itself as development from robustness in complex

[9]For Wallerstein the world system had already emerged some 500 years ago. In my view, it was only the interdependence of the social systems comprising different parts of humanity that had reached its utmost extension but was followed then by a phase of intensive growth until the systems' externalities – that the systems tried to get rid of as if any of them were still independent – began to block their own development. In my view, a world system does not deserve the name until the systems in question are gathered under the umbrella of a new transnational governance. In this view, nation states need not to be dissolved when it comes to the world system; they need only to be reworked. Democracy needs to be strengthened from below, in so far as the global level is not hampered.

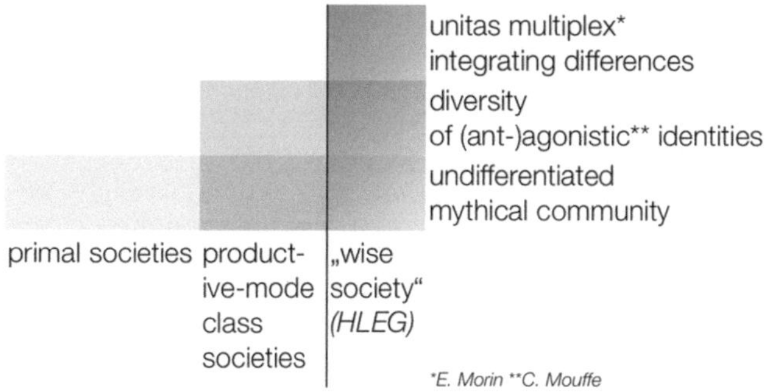

Fig. 13.3 The level of organisation of GSIS

physical systems via resilience (the capacity to bounce-back) in living systems to sustainability in social systems (Hofkirchner 2012).

Again three subsequent levels of organisation can be identified such that two can be reconstructed from history, where the second one is conceived of as a negation of the first and a third can be postulated as the possible negation of the negation (Hofkirchner 2014b, 134–135) (see Fig.13.3):

- primal societies featured the stage of minimally differentiated communities in which mystified top-down projections of a holistic "We" guarded co-operation;
- productive-mode societies that have been producing surplus value came next, with the emergence of heteronomy and class divides, which freed individual competition of "I"-monads against other "I"-monads ("Them") or tactical coalitions of them against others and has brought about an unfolding diversity of antagonistic or agonistic identities. While antagonism signifies contradictions, agonism, a term introduced by Chantal Mouffe (see e.g. Mouffe 2013) but used in a different way here, signifies contrariness, that is, the co-existence of oppositions, the juxtaposition of every difference in its own right (Hofkirchner 2015, 105);
- a possible third step would be the constitution of a "wise society", as put forward by the High-Level Expert Group of the European Commission in 1997, namely an *unitas multiplex* (Morin 1992, 143–144), a universal without totality (Lévy 2001), integrating the differences in synergetic "Me"-"Us"-"Thee" triads – "Me"s and "Thee"s are "I"s and "You"s mediated by all of "Us" and "Us" is the "We" mediated by "Me" and "Thee", from the world system down to the most local system (Hofkirchner 2014, 135) – that foster complementariness, a convergence of mutually supporting propositions, a composition made up of all differences, which is a social relation to be characterised as synergism in contradistinction to antagonism and agonism (Hofkirchner 2015, 105), for it realises the commoning purpose.

Informationality

The informational imperative means: governance cannot be achieved unless sociogenic dysfunctions are reflected upon and a proper information infrastructure underpins these reflections. The evolutionary systems' insight says when the increased complexity of an enclosed system puts the performance or maintenance at risk, the increase in complexity by an enclosing system – already existing or to be installed – can solve the problem; collective intelligence can catch up.

> Intelligence is the capability of self-organising systems to generate that information that contributes in the best way to solving problems that occur to the systems [. . .]. Collective intelligence is emergent from the single intelligences of the co-systems on the level of the suprasystem. Collective intelligence can do better than any single intelligence. In times of crises, systems are prompted to organise themselves onto a higher level to overcome the crises. The better their collective intelligence, that is, the better their problem solving capacity and the better their capability to generate information, the better their handling of the crisis and the order they can reach. This is a reformulation in informational terms of W. Ross Ashby's Law of Requisite Variety. That law states that a system is dynamically stable if the variety (the number of states) of its control mechanism is not less than the variety of that system that is to be controlled. [. . .] that system that is to be controlled can be the system itself or another system. (Hofkirchner 2017, 19)

A three-step logic would give the following sketch in the informational aspect (Hofkirchner 2017) (see Fig. 13.4):

- First, when the transition from our ancestors to *Homo sapiens* started, this was done by the insertion of social factors into the biotic evolution and the reinforcement of their taking effect within the bounds of biotic evolution. An *animal sociale* is formed. As illustrated by Alexei N. Leontyev's (1981, 210–212) hunter beater example in his activity theory and Tomasello's (2014, 36–47) stag hunt example, which stems from game theory and is used in his "shared intentionality" hypothesis to illuminate the co-operative turn in evolution, joint actions, joint goals, and joint attention coevolved together. Dyads with joint intentionality started off social selection by judgements about others and, eventually, when the

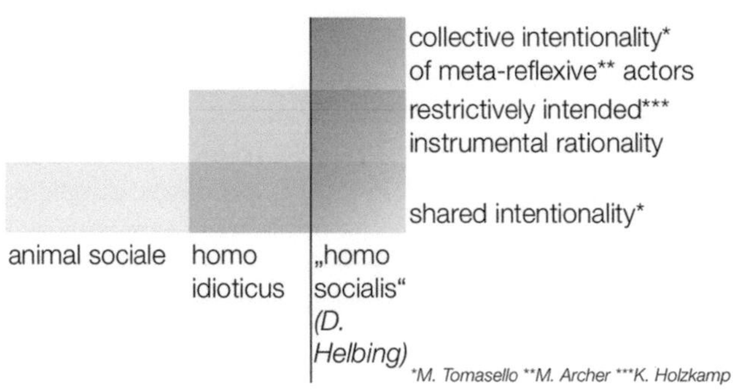

Fig. 13.4 The state of intelligence of GSIS

new factor became so powerful that it took the lead over pre-human evolution and set human evolution going, collective intentionality could be carried out by individuals thinking in conformity with their cultural group (Tomasello 2014, 80–81).
- Second, however, *homo economicus* appeared as a concrete example of generic "*homo idioticus*"[10] who benefitted from "the creation of the private through the enclosure of public or commonly held resources", which "has historically been the primary means by which property has been secured for private use" (Curtis 2013, 12). Instrumental rationality has prevailed since and has used even other persons to further one's personal interests.
- Third, when collective intentionality would be set free from the current restrictions that instrumentalise co-operation for competition against other "Them"-groups, a true "*homo socialis*" (Gintis and Helbing 2015) could enter the stage. New cosmopolitans could enjoy a universalised, extended capability to act through a consciousness and conscience that takes care of the global commons, through a meta-reflexive capability in the sense of Margaret Archer.

According to the Triple-C model referred to in my chapter in volume I of the present series (Hofkirchner 2013, 137), the informational imperative is threefold concerning:

- the actualisation of the cognitive abilities of actors, which allows the reflexive discernment of wisdom to guide acting;
- the actualisation of their communicative abilities, which allows for empathetic understanding of other actors' appeals, thus being an extension and application, of cognition and feeding back to it, and
- the actualisation of their co-operative abilities, which allows them intentionally to share common goals, which is an extension and application of communication and, in turn, feeds back to their communication and – via it – to their cognition.

Cognitive, communicative and co-operative capabilities need to adapt to the challenges of today (Table 13.2).

Cognition in the Age of Global Challenges: Meta-Reflexivity

Cognisability is the ability to reflect, to generalise, and to think in concepts, all of which hang together and enable co-ordination. Reflexivity is for Archer "the regular exercise of the mental ability, shared by all normal people, to consider themselves in relation to their (social) contexts and vice versa" (2007, 4). Reflexivity enables humans to reflect upon themselves as part of a bigger picture, eventually, all the way up to the overarching society itself. The actions of members towards other members of society are mediated by the structure of society, which is a "third" in

[10]My term.

Table 13.2 Required features for GSIS information

	anthropological features		**features required for the Great Bifurcation**
co-operative information	**consensual**	collectively intentional (about the goal, the here and now and the way to the goal)	globally conscientious and conscious: **commonalist**
communicative information	**collaborative**	consilient (help-, truthful, perspectivist)	globally conversational: **all-inclusive**
cognitive information	**co-ordinative**	conceptual (reflexive, able to generalise)	globally concerned: **meta-reflexive**

comparison to their own self (Ego) that is a "first" and another member (Alter) that is a "second" as long as the "first" interacts with the other in a direct way and not via the "third". The reflection of the third is a model for every mode of thinking that is complex thinking. It is a model for grasping the general relationship between elements and system, parts and whole, of which individual and society are merely the model instantiation. It is a model for generalisations and subsuming of the specific under the general. Human cognition is thus concept-dominated rather than sensation-focused, as Robert K. Logan maintained (Logan 2007). A concept is a generalisation of percepts, of sense data, it is a jump to another level that has a new quality. By being reflexive, able to generalise, and conceptual, cognition is empowered to anticipate the co-ordination of tasks, the structure of action.

Now, the Global Sustainable Information Society requires a new feature of cognition: that feature is meta-reflexivity. In order to understand that concept it is worth referring to Margaret Archer who coined the term and Pierpaolo Donati and their example of the performance of an orchestra. The discernment phase that sorts out what matters most to an individual actor (Donati and Archer 2015, 127–142) is a phase in which the actor can refer to the general level of the social order. The finding of an ultimate concern is the precondition for carrying out the deliberation and dedication phases that lead to the collective commitment. Like musicians in an orchestra, individuals constitute "a collectivity that evaluates objectives (discernment), deliberates about realizing its common concerns (deliberation), and commits itself to achieving them (dedication)" (61–62). The point is "about *the orientation of all the musicians to the collective performance*. A collective orientation to a collective 'output' is the core of collective reflexivity". That collective reflexivity emerges from what they call individual meta-reflexivity when practised by each musician. An individual is meta-reflexive if "he reflects *on* the orchestra's performance and about how this performance could be improved were the musicians to relate to each other in a different way", that is, if he seeks "to alter the performance of the whole orchestra" and "to produce a different emergent effect". A meta-reflexive individual is different from an autonomous-reflexive individual – as Archer has named this dominant mode – who is a musician who thinks only about himself and seeks to perfect his own performance disregarding the third; and a meta-reflexive individual is different from a communicative-reflexive individual who simply tries to adapt her performance to the individual performances of the other players, which disregards the third as well. The "group is oriented to the relational goods it produces, to maintaining or improving upon them – and to eradicating any relational evils detected in their collective performance" (61). In the context of global challenges, the orchestra example needs to be generalized to the level of humanity. The solving of global problems needs to have the fate of humanity as its ultimate concern and to be oriented towards the common good for all.

Communication in the Age of Global Challenges: All-inclusiveness

The anthropological feature of communicability is to be collaborative, that is, to be supportive of collaboration by striving for consilience, that is, the bringing together of several perspectives with the objective of bringing about a common perspective on a higher level. This common perspective is convergent on objectivated knowledge, which is achievable through de-anthropomorphisation as Ludwig von Bertalanffy pointed out (e.g. Bertalanffy 2015, 247–248). For that task, communication needs to be helpful and truthful (Tomasello 2014).

The normal functioning of human collective intelligence in communication needs to be topped today by the feature of all-inclusiveness.

> If civilisation today is in urgent need of efficient solutions for global problems, discourse and deliberation must take place as global conversation in order to mobilise any possible effort to create and implement the best ideas. That implies that no actor should be excluded or incapacitated to contribute to the common task of mitigating the challenges. As always with diversity in situations of crises, minority positions might offer potentials to build upon. All humanity needs to be embraced. That's the imperative for communication today. (Hofkirchner 2017, 25)

Co-operation in the Age of Global Challenges: Commonism

The capacity to co-operate is the topmost information ability of actors and social systems as well.

> Co-operative information is anthropologically consensual. Collective intentionality refers to consensus about goals, about the here and now and about the way to reach those goals from the here and now in whole societies that go beyond the kinship groups. It is based on collective action that comes first. And it implies a dynamic at the end of which collective commitment appears, a dynamic that starts with discernment of the ultimate concern of individual actors at the cognitive level, goes on with deliberation and ends up with dedication that translates into collective commitment (Donati and Archer 2015: 127–142, 189). (Hofkirchner 2017, 24)

What is needful nowadays is commonism, the commons-orientation of co-operation that even transcends whole societies. Growing interdependence integrates more and more any commons with the global commons, it becomes part of the global commons and cannot be dealt with without respecting that fact. Therefore global consciousness as well as global conscience needs to develop to do justice to the thriving and surviving of any part of humanity. "Now all commons need to be liberated to save our world. That is the imperative for co-operation today" (Hofkirchner 2017, 24).

Social Morphogenesis Incomplete

It makes sense to characterise social morphogenesis as a process in which the dialectical cycle of the actors' interaction causing the emergence of social relations and of social relations conditioning the emergence of actors' interaction fulfils one loop from an initial state of the social system in question to a significantly different state, that is, the accomplishment of a certain transformation. Such transformations can be intended or not, desired or not. As described above, we are currently in the transformation from an under-complex state of affairs due to dysfunctions in the production and provision of the commons either to a more complex state of governance that we will bring about lest we will perish. Thus we have not yet succeeded in terminating the decisive loop with the advent of the Global Sustainable Information Society that can be furthered by transforming conflicts from antagonisms over agonisms to synergisms as described in volume III of our series (Hofkirchner 2015, 104–111). Having said that, one can judge that the current morphogenic cycle is yet incomplete, though not yet aborted.

The extension and intensification of crises worldwide in the core social systems and the basic eco-social and techno-(eco-)social systems that we are witnessing is evidence of the Great Bifurcation that the evolution of societies has now approached. Those amplified fluctuations are the heralds of a morphogenic society that would match the subsystems and smooth their functioning by reducing the frictions of social information processes if and when activities are implemented that abide by the informational imperatives as outlined above. The Global Sustainable Information Society that would allow a new unity-through-diversity architecture and be the starting point of an ever-more flourishing society with ever-more flourishing actors on an ever-more flourishing planet would then be a kind of such a (concrete utopian) morphogenic society. Deviations from such a wished vision would not denote the completion of a full morphogenic cycle by representing a new social formation.

References

Archer, M. (2007). *Making our way through the world: Human reflexivity and social mobility*. Cambridge: Cambridge University Press.

Archer, M. S., & Donati, P. (Eds.). (2008). *Pursuing the common good: How solidarity and subsidiarity can work together*. Vatican City: Vatican Press.

Bertalanffy, L. V. (2015). *General system theory*. New York: George Braziller.
Bornemann, E. (1975). *Das Patriarchat*. Frankfurt am Main: S. Fischer.
Bruns, A. (2006). Towards produsage: Futures for user-led content production. In: F. Sudweeks, H. Hrachovec, and C. Ess (Eds.), *Proceedings cultural attitudes towards communication and technology 2006*, Tartu, 275–284.
Curtis, N. (2013). *Idiotism: Capitalism and the privatisation of life*. London: Pluto Press.
Donati, P., & Archer, M. S. (2015). *The relational subject*. Cambridge: Cambridge University Press.
Eisler, R. (1987). *The chalice and the blade: Our history, our future*. San Francisco: Harper and Row.
Eller, C. (2000). *The myth of matriarchal prehistory*. Boston: Beacon Press.
European Commission, Directorate-General for Employment, Industrial Relations and Social Affairs (Ed.). (1997). Building the European information society for us all, final policy report of the high-level expert group. Luxembourg: Office for Official Publications of the European Communities.
Gintis, H., & Helbing, D. (2015). Homo socialis: An analytical core for sociological theory. *Review of Behavioral Economics, 2*, 1–59.
Hofkirchner, W. (2012). Sustainability and self-organisation: Sustainability in the perspective of complexity and systems science and ethical considerations. In T. Nishigaki & T. Takenouchi (Eds.), *Information ethics: The future of the humanities*. Nagoya City: V2 Solution Publisher.
Hofkirchner, W. (2013). Self-organisation as the mechanism of development and evolution in social systems. In M. S. Archer (Ed.), *Social morphogenesis* (pp. 125–143). Cham: Springer.
Hofkirchner, W. (2014). On the validity of describing 'morphogenic society' as a system and justifiability of thinking about it as a social formation. In M. S. Archer (Ed.), *Late modernity: Trajectories towards morphogenic society* (pp. 119–141). Cham: Springer.
Hofkirchner, W. (2015). "Mechanisms" at work in information society. In M. S. Archer (Ed.), *Generative mechanisms transforming the social order* (pp. 95–112). Cham: Springer.
Hofkirchner, W. (2016). Ethics from systems: Origin, development and current state of normativity. In M. S. Archer (Ed.), *Morphogenesis and the crisis of normativity* (pp. 239–253). Cham: Springer.
Hofkirchner, W. (2017). Information for a global sustainable information society. In: M. Burgin, and W. Hofkirchner (Eds.), *The future information society. Social and technological problems*, Singapore, World Scientific (in print)
Illich, I. (1973). *Tools for conviviality*. New York: Harper and Row.
Laermans, R. (2011a). The promises of commonalism. In R. De Roo, K. Vanhasebrouck, & L. De Cauter (Eds.), *Art and activism in the age of globalisation* (pp. 240–249). Rotterdam: Nai Publishers.
Laermans, R. (2011b). Artistic collaboration and the promises of commonalism. https://fabricoftrust.files.wordpress.com/2012/05/vortrag_rudi_laermans_tqw3.pdf
Laermans, R. (2012). Teaching theory and the art of not-knowing: Notes on pedagogical commonalism. *Krisis, 1*, 63–73.
Leontyev, A. N. (1981). *Problems of the development of the mind*. Moscow: Progress.
Lévy, P. (1997). *Collective intelligence*. New York etc: Plenium Trade.
Lévy, P. (2001). *Cyberculture*. Minneapolis etc: University of Minnesota Press.
Linebaugh, P. (2014). *Stop, thief! The commons, enclosure, and resistance*. Oakland: PM Press.
Logan, R. (2007). *The extended mind: The emergence of language, the human mind and culture*. Toronto: University of Toronto Press.
Morin, E. (1992). *Method, towards a study of humankind, The Nature of Nature* (Vol. 1). New York etc: Peter Lang.
Mouffe, C. (2013). *Agonistics: Thinking the world politically*. London: Verso.
Robertson, R. (1992). *Globalization*. London: Sage.
Tomasello, M. (2014). *A natural history of human thinking*. Cambridge: Harvard University Press.

Tomasello, M. (2016). *A natural history of human morality*. Cambridge: Harvard University Press.
Wallerstein, I. (1988). *One world, many worlds*. New York: Rienner.
Zimmermann, R. E. (2014). *Η ΝΕΑ ΠΟΛΥ: Neue Stadtbegriffe auf dem Weg in die Heimat*. Berlin: LIT Verlag.
Zimmermann, R. E. (2015). Mesógios - Zur Struktur der Polis-Netzwerke. In R. Faber & A. Lichtenberger (Eds.), *Ein pluriverses Universum: Zivilisationen und Religionen im antiken Mittelmeerraum* (pp. 113–130). Paderborn: Fink.

MIX
Papier aus verantwortungsvollen Quellen
Paper from responsible sources
FSC® C105338

If you have any concerns about our products,
you can contact us on
ProductSafety@springernature.com

In case Publisher is established outside the EU,
the EU authorized representative is:
Springer Nature Customer Service Center GmbH
Europaplatz 3, 69115 Heidelberg, Germany

Printed by Libri Plureos GmbH
in Hamburg, Germany